MY HOUSE IS KILLING ME!

MY HOUSE IS KILLING ME!

A COMPLETE GUIDE TO A HEALTHIER INDOOR ENVIRONMENT

JEFFREY C. MAY AND CONNIE L. MAY

FOREWORD BY JONATHAN M. SAMET, MD
AND ELIZABETH MATSUI, MD, MHS

 JOHNS HOPKINS UNIVERSITY PRESS   BALTIMORE

© 2001, 2020 Jeffrey C. May and Connie L. May
All rights reserved. Published 2020
Printed in Canada on acid-free paper
9 8 7 6 5 4 3 2 1

Johns Hopkins University Press
2715 North Charles Street
Baltimore, Maryland 21218-4363
www.press.jhu.edu

Library of Congress Cataloging-in-Publication Data

Names: May, Jeffrey C., author. | May, Connie L., author.
Title: My house is killing me! : a complete guide to a healthier indoor
environment / Jeffrey C. May and Connie L. May ; foreword by
Jonathan M. Samet, MD and Elizabeth Matsui, MD, MHS.
Description: Second edition. | Baltimore : Johns Hopkins University Press,
2020. | Revised edition of My house is killing me! : the home guide for
families with allergies and asthma / Jeffrey C. May, 2001. | Includes
bibliographical references and index.
Identifiers: LCCN 2019059958 | ISBN 9781421438948 (hardcover) | ISBN
9781421438955 (paperback) | ISBN 9781421438962 (ebook)
Subjects: LCSH: Allergy—Popular works. | Asthma—Popular works. | Indoor
air pollution—Popular works.
Classification: LCC RC585 .M29 2020 | DDC 616.97—dc23
LC record available at https://lccn.loc.gov/2019059958
A catalog record for this book is available from the British Library.

Cover design and interior design by Amanda Weiss

Special discounts are available for bulk purchases of this book. For more information, please contact Special Sales at specialsales@press.jhu.edu.

Johns Hopkins University Press uses environmentally friendly book materials, including recycled text paper that is composed of at least 30 percent post-consumer waste, whenever possible.

CONTENTS

FOREWORD

We write from a shared dual perspective, as clinicians helping to treat patients' perplexing symptoms that are linked to indoor environment issues, and as public health researchers trying to sort out how the many exposures sustained in our homes and other indoor spaces cause health problems and diseases. Circumstances, patients, and populations demand problem solving and finding solutions. What exposures could be causing a person's symptoms? What types of indoor exposures adversely affect population health? For both the patient and the population, finding those exposures is the first step toward ending them.

Evaluating the exposures that we encounter during our lives is complicated. We spend time in many different places across the days, and our senses don't detect all of the exposures or alert us when levels might be dangerous. A person's clinical history of environmental exposures, even if taken with care, is not highly sensitive and reflects only what the person knows about. In our epidemiological studies, trained field teams make observations in homes and elsewhere and may take measurements of chemical pollutants, allergens, and other contaminants according to standardized protocols. With hypothesis-focused research, however, these protocols are not holistic and are not intended to identify all exposures of significance to health.

This gap in understanding indoor environments is where the second edition of *My House Is Killing Me! A Complete Guide to a Healthier Indoor Environment*, by Jeffrey C. May and Connie L. May, proves invaluable. Nearly two decades have passed since the first edition. This second edition broadens the reach and depth of the first, as Jeffrey and Connie have gained more experience and have more wisdom to offer.

Jeffrey and Connie are neither researchers nor clinicians; rather, they are experienced evaluators of indoor environments who know how to find problems that can be damaging to health. The book is organized to cover the full array of problems that can occur, providing both background information and a rich set of case studies. Jeffrey and Connie are storytellers; their stories draw on decades of experience and their own responses to indoor problems. Their stories, which are entertaining while being informative, offer lessons that are hard to draw from lengthy and dry tables of data. They document that problems in indoor environments can seriously damage health and that these problems can be identified and solved.

The tools that the authors use are straightforward, readily available, and buttressed by experience. Jeffrey and Connie know how to take a history of what has happened in a building with water damage, for example, and where to look for problems. Their experience- and insight-guided approach contrasts with the protocol-driven strategies of many commercial firms concerned with remediating indoor air-quality problems. For addressing the complaints of many patients, a report from Jeffrey and Connie might be more helpful than pages of data from a consultant firm.

The book is structured logically, beginning with coverage of the agents that cause problems and then moving to what goes wrong in different rooms and with heating and cooling systems. The four closing chapters address a potpourri of topics: renovation and new construction, environmental hazards, testing and remediation, and cleaning. With this structure, *My House Is Killing Me!* could be read in its entirety, used as a reference, or consulted for a specific problem. The style is nontechnical, and readers will enjoy its many stories and anecdotes. For researchers, this book offers a wealth of experience that could be foundational to planning future studies.

Use this book when you next face a challenging indoor environmental problem—there are many, and they are all too common. As always, if you believe that health problems may be caused by your home, speak with your doctor, who can help with the process of pinpointing the cause.

Jonathan M. Samet, MD
Elizabeth Matsui, MD, MHS

APPRECIATION

Because I learned something every time I completed an indoor air quality investigation, all the people who asked for our help deserve my appreciation. There are, however, some people to whom I'd like to give special thanks. Jack Spengler and Jack McCarthy, as well as Thad Godish in his book *Indoor Air Quality Pollution Control*,[1] provided me with my first glimpse into the world of indoor air quality. John Knowles worked with me to produce the scanning electron micrograph images from my samples. Henri Fennell gave me invaluable information about the installation of spray polyurethane foam insulation. Thanks to Mark Cramer for his comments on air conditioning in hot and humid climates. I am also grateful to the many physicians and other medical professionals who referred patients to me for indoor environmental surveys.

Jeffrey C. May

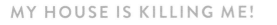

MY HOUSE IS KILLING ME!

INTRODUCTION

We wrote this book not only for people who sneeze, cough, or wheeze in indoor spaces but also for anyone who wants a healthier indoor environment by reducing potential exposures to indoor contaminants, allergens, and irritants. In this second edition we explain why problems related to indoor air quality (IAQ) may occur and include stories of our many experiences helping people improve the quality of their indoor air. We make practical suggestions for eliminating IAQ problems throughout the chapters as well as in the recommendations at the end of each chapter.

This edition includes recent developments in the IAQ field and new stories and photographs from my investigations. We organized parts I and V by topics; the discussions in parts II and III focus on specific areas of a home. Part IV covers mechanical (heating, cooling, ventilating) equipment. We designed the book so that you can read it from start to finish, dip in and out according to certain topics or areas in your home, or use the index to look for certain content. There are also updates in the glossary and resource guide. Unless otherwise indicated, all the photographs and photomicrographs are my work. (We are coauthors of this second edition, but Jeff is the building investigator, so when we write "I" or "my," it means Jeff or Jeff's.)

While we focus on residential buildings, the discussions in the book are also relevant for smaller spaces, including home offices and work spaces carved out of former residential buildings. But much of the information in parts I, IV, and V could apply to other building types. We do not include discussions of catastrophic events such as fires, hurricanes, and floods. These are worthy subjects, but in this book we are concentrating on everyday conditions that could affect human health. I am a building inspector/investigator who specializes in IAQ and am not a remediator, so I don't cover remediation practices in this book. I do, however, offer some guidance to help you be a better "shopper" when it comes to hiring a remediation company. I don't write remediation protocol, but many remediation companies use my reports to plan their work. An IAQ inspection report should be specific enough to be used for this purpose.

I have traveled all over the country and have inspected buildings in California as well as in Virginia, South Carolina, and Florida. These locations have more temperate climates than in New England, where I do most of my inspections. Still, buildings across the United States have similar sources of IAQ problems, such as mechanical equipment and new furnishings, which are common regardless of the climate (for example, air conditioning is used in most climates). And conditions of elevated relative humidity that lead to microbial growth can develop regardless of whether people live in a four-season climate as I do or in a more temperate climate such as Florida. Much of the advice in this book is therefore relevant, regardless of where you live. That said, we do include some discussions that focus on more temperate climates than New England's climate.

Although we make comments about fungi and insects in this book, I am neither a mycologist nor an entomologist. The comments are based largely on the observations I made in my thirty years of investigating IAQ problems. Through microscopy, I have identified particle pollutants in the over 40,000 air and dust (surface) samples that I collected. In so doing, I have gained an intimate understanding of the many potential sources of IAQ problems. Still, I apologize in advance for any academic transgressions in the book (for example, I use the genus and common name of an organism when I don't know the species).

I am not a doctor and will not be giving medical advice. I would never tell people to postpone seeking medical advice or disregard such advice in favor of environmental measures. If you are experiencing symptoms that you suspect may be caused by an indoor environment, talk to your physician. Many of our clients were referred to us by physicians who suspected that environmental conditions were exacerbating or in some cases even causing their patients' symptoms. Sometimes, my work helps a doctor's diagnosis (in one case, a patient had tested negative to certain molds, but the person's blood serum tested positive to the type of mold that I found in the dust samples I gathered from the person's furnace). My experiences have led me to a firm belief that by better controlling the indoor environmental conditions where we live and work, we can minimize the symptoms we or those we know or love may be experiencing because of IAQ problems. I also believe that we can avoid exposures to indoor contaminants that could lead to sensitization and ill health.

If you find this book to be helpful, consider reading the other three books on IAQ that we wrote that discuss additional topics and cover other types of indoor spaces. These three books have also been published by Johns Hopkins University Press. *The Mold Survival Guide*:

For Your Home and for Your Health expands our discussion of mold and will help you identify mold growth or conditions that could lead to indoor mold growth. Part III of that book offers guidance on mold removal, including from personal goods. *Jeff May's Healthy Home Tips* summarizes much of the advice in our books on IAQ but in a workbook style, so you can keep track of the steps you've taken to clean up your indoor environment. *My Office Is Killing Me! The Sick Building Survival Guide* covers conditions that can lead to poor IAQ in larger work spaces as well as in schools. The book also reviews other conditions such as temperature and humidity that can have a negative impact on the physical comfort of building occupants.

We welcome feedback from our readers, so if you have questions or would like to share your success stories as you improve your IAQ, please contact us through our website: www.mayindoorair.com. Finally, we wish you good luck in working to improve your indoor environmental conditions.

PART I.

THE STAGE OF OUR LIVES

SEEING THE INVISIBLE

We accept that when stung by a bee, some people will experience only a small swelling at the site while others may die within minutes. We think it normal that some of us taste food differently, which may be why olives and spinach are loved by some and hated by others. Some people think that cilantro is delicious, while others insist it tastes like soap. Scientists have found that people who think cilantro tastes like soap lack a specific sensor for the aromatic flavor. A chemical called phenylthiocarbamide can be used to test a person's genetically determined sense of taste. For the test, you touch your tongue to a narrow strip containing a minute amount of this chemical. Some people immediately grimace at the bitter taste, while others find the paper tasteless.

We know that we are introducing substances into our bodies every time we eat a meal. Few people recognize, however, that we inhale fragments of the spaces around us with every breath. In a way, the delicate surfaces of our lungs are in contact with our environments just as our skin is. Why, then, do some of us tend to be suspicious or even disbelieving when people with whom we live or work seem to be reacting to some unseen substances in indoor air? Perhaps if we could see these substances the way we can see smoke, we would all be more understanding.

PARTICLES

In just about any room where people are gathered, the air will contain suspended particles that we do not see. These particles include shed

Shine a flashlight into a dark room at night, and you can see airborne dust called "motes." Most of that dust consists of microscopic skin scales, which are normally not visible unless they reflect bright light. Every year, human beings shed approximately one-half to three-quarters of a pound of skin in the form of microscopic skin scales.

C. Weschler, "The Skinny on How Shed Skin Reduces Indoor Air Pollution," *Environmental Science and Technology* 12, no. 8 (2011): 923. doi:10.1021/es60144a011.

skin scales and pet dander particles (people who own pets carry pet dander particles on their clothing). Each person in the room will inhale these particles with every breath. Fortunately, most such particles are benign, and the human respiratory system (including the nose, trachea, and lungs) is designed to capture them and then in some cases to remove or destroy them. We discuss indoor airborne particles in more detail in chapter 2.

CHEMICALS

Air also contains invisible chemicals, some of which we can smell, such as gasoline fumes, ammonia, fragrances, and cooking odors. Some of these chemicals we cannot sense, though, because they are in concentrations below our "odor threshold" (the lowest concentration that our sense of smell can detect). A female *Cecropia* moth secretes a sex pheromone (a chemical substance secreted by an organism that influences behavior) that a male moth can detect miles downwind, yet we cannot sense this chemical. Ants use alarm pheromones to muster their fellow soldiers. We see the troops battling on the pavement, but we don't sense their urgent, airborne messages.

KEEPING AIR CLEAN

To keep fish happy and healthy in an aquarium, water must be aerated, cleaned by a filtering system, and circulated. No one would expect fish to survive in a closed jar of green, cloudy water. If we could see the particles and chemicals in the air in our indoor spaces, the indoor air might look as murky as stagnant water looks in an aquarium. Many new buildings, including homes, are similar to aquariums in the sense that they are tightly constructed environments in which mechanical equipment is supposed to help keep the indoor air healthy and clean. Unfortunately, either by design or because of poor maintenance practices, such equipment can sometimes be the cause of rather than the solution for indoor air quality (IAQ) problems.

FLUIDS FLOW

Air is similar to water in that it is a fluid, and fluids flow. You know that air flows when you are outside and feel breeze on your face or hear the leaves rustling in the wind. Air also flows indoors. Several forces affect the flow of indoor air. Hot air is less dense than cool air, and less dense substances float on top of denser substances, which is why hot air rises and cool air sinks. (The same is true of water, which

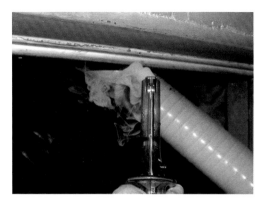

FIGURE 1.1A. Smoke from a Wizard Stick is used to illustrate convective airflows through a window between a heated basement and an adjoining cold and moldy crawl space. The warm air at the basement ceiling flows into the cooler crawl space at the top of the window. The cooler air flows out of the crawl space window and sinks down the foundation wall. In this way, mold spores from the crawl space air are introduced into the basement air.

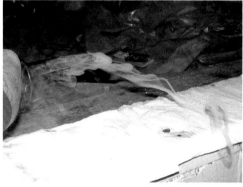

FIGURE 1.1B. Smoke flowing into a basement from a crawl space.

is why water in a pond may feel cooler at your legs than up near your neck.) When the heat inside a building is running, warm air rises up in the building and exits at the top level. Then air from the lower levels, including the basement, flows upward to create a convective cycle of airflow (figs. 1.1A and 1.1B).

Pressure differences also affect the flow of air, because air flows from higher pressure to lower pressure. For example, the operation of a blower in a heating or cooling system in a basement can lower the air pressure. Then exterior air flows into the basement through leaky windows and cracks in the foundation floor or walls. As a result, soil gases (including radon gas) can be drawn into the basement. At the same time the basement is depressurized, the upstairs of the house may be pressurized by the heating or cooling system. When the heat is running, moist indoor air can be forced up into an attic, causing moisture to condense, which can lead to mold growth on the roof sheathing.

In hot and humid climates in which buildings are primarily cooled, an air conditioning system can sometimes reduce a building's air pressure, and warm and humid outdoor air will infiltrate exterior walls (walls facing the exterior). Water will then condense on cooler surfaces in the wall cavities, causing mold problems.

Wind can also affect airflows within a building. When the wind is blowing against an exterior wall, air can flow through cracks into the wall cavity, pressurizing the cavity. Then any odors or mold spores in

Air from a basement or crawl space flows upward to habitable rooms above, so occupants are inhaling air from below-grade (below-ground) spaces, whether they enter the spaces or not.

Some motels constructed in hot, humid climates have acquired the reputation of "mildew motels." In such buildings, the drywall is covered with vinyl wallpaper, which is impervious to moisture. When humid exterior air migrates into exterior wall cavities, the moisture becomes trapped behind the vinyl wallpaper, and mold (mildew) grows on the drywall paper.

the cavity can flow into the room through cracks and openings such as electrical outlets.

We once lived in a leaky Victorian home. The lower third of the walls in my home office was covered with wainscoting that had gaps an eighth of an inch wide between a few of the individual strips of wood. When the wind blew against that side of the house, I experienced asthma symptoms in my office (I am allergic to some types of mold). I took a sample of the air that was flowing through a gap in the wainscoting covering an exterior wall. The sample contained numerous mold spores, confirming that there was mold growth in the wall cavity. The mold growth may have been ancient, but it still caused me to have allergy symptoms. As a temporary solution, I taped over the gaps in the wainscoting along that exterior wall; after that, I stopped coughing in the room.

In newer homes with airtight windows and doors, wind does not affect the air pressure within wall cavities as much. But just turning on a dryer or kitchen exhaust fan can depressurize a tight house, possibly resulting in backdrafting of combustion products from heating equipment.

BUILDING CHARACTERISTICS

Building characteristics can affect IAQ. We once compared 600 "sick" homes (with sick house syndrome, or SHS) in which people were experiencing health symptoms due to poor IAQ with 300 "control" homes that I had inspected as part of real estate purchases. We found that:

- Of SHS homes, 41 percent had forced hot-air heat, compared to 29 percent of homes in the control group.

- Of SHS homes, 37 percent had central air conditioning, compared to 19 percent of the control group.

- Elevated levels of airborne mold spores were found in 81 percent of SHS homes.

- In a subset of 47 SHS homes in which exposed fiberglass insulation in basements and/or crawl spaces was sampled, 74 percent of the insulation batts tested contained significant mold growth. In addition, 31 percent contained mold-eating mites in the sampled dust. (Dust contains biodegradable material that is food for microbes, and fiberglass insulation captures biodegradable dust.)

- In another subset of 37 SHS homes in which the dust on baseboard heating convectors located close to concrete floors was sampled, 37 percent contained significant mold growth in the dust.

Forced hot-air heat and a finished, carpeted basement were more likely to be present in SHS homes than in homes in the control group. Significantly, SHS homes were almost twice as likely to have central air conditioning. If you live in a home with any of these characteristics, you may want to read this book with particular care.

THE SCIENTIFIC METHOD

In the scientific method, a researcher forms a hypothesis and designs experiments to test the hypothesis. If the hypothesis is that an IAQ problem exists only when the contaminants can be measured, are of a certain type, and reach a certain level or concentration, then the researcher goes about trying to prove or disprove the existence of the problem by measuring the concentration of a finite number of known contaminants. If this hypothesis is not supported by the air or dust sampling (and it usually isn't), then it is assumed that there is no IAQ problem present, regardless of what people in the building may be experiencing.

If I receive a report of a strange building odor or allergy or asthma symptoms in a building, I assume there is an indoor environmental issue that should be researched, whether one person or many people are sensing a problem. My task is then to follow the clues that a visual inspection and air and dust sampling provide so that I can find the source or sources of the problem. Only then can appropriate solutions be identified.

I often say to my clients, "Identify the source of the IAQ problem before spending a lot of money on a solution that may not be effective."

In the air samples that I take, I usually find bioaerosol, or particles suspended in the air that are originally from living organisms. For non-bioaerosol particles such as asbestos (an inorganic material), exposure would not result in immediate symptoms. Still, exposures to toxic or carcinogenic inorganic materials pose a health risk and must be investigated.

DISBELIEVERS

I once inspected a house in which the wife's asthma worsened whenever she was in the basement. Her husband, on the other hand, didn't think there was an IAQ problem in the house. I like clients to accompany me when I inspect a property so I can explain why certain conditions cause me concern. The woman didn't want to go into the basement, so her husband accompanied me when I went down into the space. We disturbed moldy floor dust as we walked around the basement. He turned to me and said, "See? There's no problem down here," but I noticed that mucus was dripping from his nose down to his chin. He didn't think he had any allergies, but I could see that he was probably sensitized to the mold spores in the basement dust.

We've often found that only one or two members of a household or work community are sensitized (affected by indoor chemicals, allergens, and other irritants) to substances in indoor air, while other people in the space are not sensitized. Then the sufferers can be treated with impatience or even disbelief. Sensitivity to indoor environmental conditions is more common than many people may think. The American Academy of Allergy, Asthma & Immunology (AAAAI) reports that 10 to 30 percent of the world's population has allergic rhinitis.[1] The Centers for Disease Control and Prevention (CDC) reports that 8.4 percent of children and 7.7 percent of adults have asthma.[2] A survey of over 1,000 adult Americans conducted in 2016 found that 25.9 percent had chemical sensitivities and 12.8 percent had multiple chemical sensitivities (MCS).[3]

You may not be sympathetic toward the suffering of others who are experiencing symptoms in an indoor environment. But such symptoms can afflict any of us at any time, particularly since nowadays people can spend up to 90 percent of their time in buildings, even when they exercise. Building occupants can thus be exposed on a daily basis to contaminated indoor air, and their health may suffer as a consequence.

Cleaning up indoor environments is therefore important for all of us.

SOME RECOMMENDATIONS

- If you are experiencing health symptoms in an indoor space and feel better when away from the space, consider wearing a NIOSH N95 two-strap mask (available at most hardware and building supply stores). If you feel better while wearing the mask, you will know that some particles in the air are causing your symptoms.

- If someone in your home or place of work is suffering health symptoms, support any efforts to find a relationship between indoor environmental conditions and their symptoms.

CAST OF SMALL CHARACTERS—
READ THIS CHAPTER IF YOU DARE!

2.

Let us begin by introducing the cast of small characters, both visible and microscopic, that live beneath our feet and under our noses. Members of this cast—organisms such as dust mites, mold, and yeast—and the creatures that feed on them can cause coughing, itchy eyes, and breathing difficulties. Controlling the growth of such organisms is often the key to eliminating indoor allergy symptoms and air quality problems.

DUST

House dust is its own universe, providing nutrition and shelter for an entire community of microscopic life. I can gather a lot of information about how someone lives by looking at the contents of house dust, which consists mostly of human skin scales. The presence of other particles in dust depends on the inhabitants. If you have a bird, dog, or cat, pet skin scales (dander) join the mix. If you own a down quilt or down pillows, I'll find feather fibers from the bedding in my samples. I always find clothing fibers (lint), and if a house has carpets, I find carpet fibers. In or near a bathroom, either talcum-powder particles or cornstarch granules may be present in the air, depending on the type of body powder used. In a den where people munch snacks while watching TV, I find microscopic crumbs from cookies and potato chips in the dust from the sofa cushions. I find more soil particles and plant debris in the rooms where people first enter from the outside. If I'm sampling in the spring, I sometimes find pollen particles and other plant materials scattered throughout the house but mostly in carpeting under the windows. If I find pollen in a carpet in the winter, I suspect that the residents don't vacuum adequately.

Small particles of dust measuring approximately 1 micron (0.00004 inch) in diameter tend to remain suspended in still air for hours (particles smaller than 1 micron are permanently suspended in air). Larger spherical particles above 50 microns (0.002 inch) in diameter generally settle out of still air within seconds and form layers of visible dust on tables, shelves, and other surfaces. Thin, flat particles (like skin scales) have more air resistance and stay aloft longer. Regardless of the shape of settled particles, when we walk on carpets or move any stationary object, the settled dust particles are agitated and become airborne again (re-aerosolized).

PARTICULATE MATTER

Professionals refer to particles suspended in air as PM, for particulate matter, and they divide PM into two broad ranges of sizes: PM_{10} (all particles less than 10 microns in diameter) and $PM_{2.5}$ (all particles less than 2.5 microns in diameter). The particles in the PM_{10} group that are larger than 2.5 microns are referred to as the "coarse fraction" of PM, and particles smaller than 2.5 microns are referred to as the "fine fraction" of PM. There is even a category of ultrafine (UF) particles: those that are less than 0.1 micron in diameter. Photocopiers can be a major source of UF particles indoors. The health effects of inhaling these emissions are being studied.

The inhalation of PM_{10} particles poses a health risk because such particles can get deep into the lung, and smaller $PM_{2.5}$ particles may even move from the alveoli in the lungs directly into the bloodstream. The US Environmental Protection Agency (EPA) lists some of the health effects such exposures may cause, including increased asthma symptoms and premature death for people with heart or lung disease.[1] A paper published in the *Journal of Medical Toxicology* states that "PM exposure causes a small but significant increase in human morbidity and mortality."[2]

Most studies of the effects of PM focus on the presence of small particles in outdoor air. But in modern life, people spend up to 90 percent of their time inside buildings. Since all the air in a building ultimately must come from the outdoors, and since many fine and all ultrafine particles from outdoors are permanently suspended in the air, these particles will be found in the indoor air. What can people do to reduce exposures to PM indoors? Reducing dust levels indoors is a good start; using HEPA (high-efficiency particulate arrestance) air purifiers is another. We discuss other steps people can take throughout this book.

I use an Allergenco air sampler and Burkard samplers to collect airborne particles. An Allergenco sampler has a blower that pulls in air through a narrow slit at a precise rate. The airstream then hits a flat glass slide and is forced to take a sharp turn. The particles in the air have so much momentum that they cannot make that turn. They continue to travel in a straight path until they hit the slide and stick on its thin layer of grease. The Allergenco can be programmed to take multiple samples on a single slide, so I can compare them to see how the numbers and types of particles change over time as the activity in the space changes. A Burkard sampler is a similar device that also collects dust particles on a greased microscope slide, but it can take only one sample at a time on each slide. Regardless of which type of sampler I use, I add biological stain to the adhered particles, put a cover glass on the slide, and look at the sample with a microscope.

Most IAQ professionals use disposable, plastic cassettes to collect dust. Each cassette is attached to a pump that draws air in through the cassette. Particles in the air are deposited on a sticky glass surface that is then analyzed through microscopy. The difference between what most IAQ professionals do and what I do is that they send the cassettes to labs for analysis, whereas I analyze my own dust samples.

In a clean home with hardwood floors and leather furniture, I do not see many particles in my samples, even with a reasonable amount of room activity. In a home with wall-to-wall carpeting and upholstered furniture, however, my air samples are sometimes so thickly layered with particles that it's difficult to distinguish among them.

Let's examine the sources of some of these particles.

DUST MITES

Dust is home to dust mites, whose body parts as well as fecal pellets are considered some of the most common causes of allergy and asthma symptoms in the world. Dust mites are microarthropods, or invertebrates generally smaller than 2 millimeters in size. Dust mites are about 0.01 inch (0.25 millimeter) long and are usually invisible to the naked eye, though you could see a mite crawling on a black background. When I collect samples in houses infested with dust mites, I am likely to find microscopic mite legs and mite fecal pellets in the air after dust on surfaces has been disturbed. In a mite-infested environment, over 100,000 mite fecal pellets may be found in a gram of dust, and these pellets can become re-aerosolized and be inhaled. Mite fecal pellets, whatever the species, may contain allergenic materials such as mite digestive enzymes or mold spores.

It takes about a month for a dust mite egg to hatch and the mite to mature to an adult. An adult female mite may live another month. Once inseminated, a female mite is called a gravid female and can produce up to 200 fertilized eggs. Mites lay their eggs in skin-laden house dust and eat protein, including shed skin scales. Since we shed so many skin scales, the food for mites is essentially in infinite supply.

Our sloughed-off skin scales are small enough to slip through the weave of pillowcases, sheets, and mattress pads, and the scales gather inside our pillows and mattresses. You could beat a bed pillow for half an hour, and there would still be enough food left for thousands of mites. I've found dust mite infestations in heavy, padded coats as well as in armchairs, couches, and cushioned office chairs upon which people sit for extended periods of time. You might be wondering how dust mites travel from one home to another. If you sit on a mite-infested cushion in another person's house, a gravid female mite could attach to your clothing. Then the female mite could drop onto a surface in your home and lay her fertilized eggs. This is why I always avoid sitting on cushioned furniture in clients' and even friends' and relatives' homes!

CLIMATE FOR DUST MITES

Dust mites take the moisture they need directly from the air, where moisture is present in the vapor form. Relative humidity (RH) is a measure of how much water vapor is in the air as compared with the maximum amount of moisture the air can contain at a given temperature, or how close air is to being saturated. Air at 80 percent RH can still contain more moisture. Air at 100 percent RH looks just the same but can hold no more water vapor. RH is an important concept to understand in the battle against IAQ problems, because microscopic life—including mites—flourishes at higher RH.

When we are in bed, moisture from our bodies raises the RH in the mattress and pillows. When we breathe into our pillows, mites (if present) congregate to imbibe the moisture. Warm quilts or thick, soft mattress pads soak up our body moisture and thus may be teeming with mites. Those of us who sweat a great deal or sleep under piles of blankets or in overheated bedrooms risk greater infestations. In RH above 70 percent, mites can grow in dust without added moisture from our bodies. As the RH rises, dust mites increase their rate of reproduction, intake of skin scales, and defecation. If we keep the RH in our homes no higher than 50 percent, we will help reduce the chances of air quality problems due to dust mites, mold, and other organisms.

Mite infestations are not as common as some people think. Mites are very fragile, and they dry out and die in dry conditions. When the RH is low (below 70 percent), mites congregate in clusters to conserve their moisture. In New England where I live, only about a third of the beds I sample are infested with mites. Dust mites colonize thicker material where moisture levels tend to remain more constant. Thinner materials dry out faster and thus do not provide the best living and breeding conditions for mites.

DUST MITE ENCASINGS

One easy solution to the threat of exposure to dust mite allergens from mattresses, pillows, quilts, and box springs is the installation of mite encasings. On a new mattress or pillow, an encasing can prevent a mite infestation. In an already mite-infested mattress or pillow, the encasing must also prevent mite allergens from exiting. Some encasings can even prevent the moisture critical to mite survival from entering the mattress or pillow.

Dust mite encasings have gone through four iterations. The first generation was made out of thin vinyl plastic. These encasings were effective barriers but were not popular because they were crinkly and felt sweaty. The second generation was made of nonwoven material, but a mite could crawl through the gaps between the fibers. The third generation consisted of woven polyester or cotton with thin, solid polyurethane lining at the interior. The lining prevented mite allergens and mites from exiting or entering the mattress. The encasings also prevented moisture from our bodies from readily entering the mattress.

But consumers wanted a softer product without the polyurethane lining, so the most current and fourth generation of encasings, woven cotton or polyester with more than 400 threads to an inch, lack the lining. Manufacturers rightly claim that dust mites cannot enter the mattress owing to the small spaces between the fibers. Manufacturers also claim that dust mite allergens within an infested mattress cannot exit this kind of dust mite encasing.

I have found this last claim by manufacturers to be inaccurate, because while most dust mite allergens are on particles too large to pass through this generation of encasings, some dust mite allergens can still pass through the spaces between the threads. In one home I inspected, a mother had installed a fourth-generation dust mite encasing on her son's dust mite–infested mattress. Her son was allergic to dust mites, and even with the new encasing on his mattress he continued to suffer allergy symptoms when in bed.

Another problem with this last generation of dust mite encasings is that they are permeable to body moisture. In an older mattress with a

When the relative humidity (RH) is 100 percent, water vapor will condense onto any surface that is below the temperature of the air around it. Imagine you are sitting outside in Florida on a 75°F day, and the RH of the air around you is 100 percent. If you are holding a drink at 76°F, moisture will not condense on the glass. If you lower the temperature of the liquid below 75°F with an ice cube, you will see condensation on the glass. The temperature of air that is at 100 percent RH is called the dew point.

preexisting dust mite infestation, there are enough skin scales present to feed the mites for years. When the sleeper's body moisture enters the mattress, the dust mites can live happily on, producing allergens as if no dust mite encasing were present. For mattresses already in use, I always recommend the third generation of dust mite encasings with polyurethane liners. On a mattress that has never been slept on, however, the tightly woven cotton or polyester dust mite encasing without a polyurethane liner is fine. People sit on other people's beds, so if you or anyone in your family has dust mite allergies, it's important to put dust mite encasings on all mattresses and bed pillows in your home, as well as on box springs if present.

THE VARIETY OF MITES

Dust mites such as *Dermatophagoides pteronyssinus* and *Dermatophagoides farinae* are only two of over a dozen common species of mites found in houses. Another kind of mite, *Cheyletus eruditus*, preys on dust mites. In the samples I take of dust, I have found many other varieties of mites, including mold-eating mites such as *Tyrophagus putrescentiae*. When mold-eating mites are present, building occupants are exposed to allergens from the mites as well as from the mold spores. I occasionally accept samples by mail from people wondering what their dust contains. One fellow was concerned about some fine brown dust that he had repeatedly wiped away from the countertop at the edge of his stainless-steel kitchen sink. The tape sample that he sent me contained thousands of mite droppings, some mite eggs, and Acari (storage) mites that were no doubt eating the bits of food trapped between the sink lip and the laminate counter top (figs. 2.1 and 2.2).

Tyroglyphus farina (also known as a storage mite) lives in stored grains. Another species of storage mite, *Glycyphagus domesticus*, is called grocer's itch mite because it thrives on flour and wheat. In one case I read about allergy to storage mites, a child had a severe asthmatic reaction in a pizzeria after the raw dough coated with dry flour was flattened and flung spinning into the air. When the flour became airborne, mite allergens were dispersed. I know someone with a severe mite allergy who occasionally falls into a stupor and sleeps for several hours after eating a sandwich. Although there is no apparent pattern to these incidents, I suspect they occur when storage mite–contaminated flour is consumed.

A negative reaction to one type of dust mite allergy testing does not rule out allergy to other mite species, and unfortunately allergy testing is not available for many common species of mites.

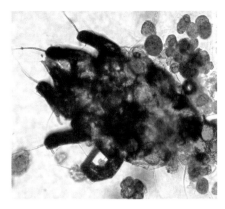

FIGURE 2.1. A storage mite and its fecal pellets were in the dust exiting from beneath the rim of a stainless steel kitchen sink set into a laminate countertop. Storage mites were thriving on sink moisture and food bits trapped under the sink rim (200× light micrograph).

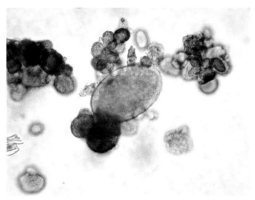

FIGURE 2.2. This micrograph shows more storage mite fecal pellets and a 300-micron storage mite egg at the center (200× light micrograph).

FROM MITES TO MOLD AND MUSHROOMS

Mold needs the same conditions for growth as mites need: moisture and nutrients. In basements where the RH is over 70 percent, the foundation walls and floors are often blackened by mold colonies that are home to mold-eating mites. In one home, an entire wall in a basement room was covered by what appeared to be black mold. When I looked at a sample of the dark dust, I found that it consisted of mold spores, nearly all of them clumped within fecal pellets from microarthropods (including mites). If such fecal pellets get wet and stay damp for a few hours, viable mold spores within may germinate.

Molds are fungi (singular fungus). There are two major divisions of fungi: macrofungi and microfungi.

MACROFUNGI

Macrofungi grow in very damp conditions, digest wood, and can cause wood decay. The spore-forming structures of macrofungi are large and visible and are called mushrooms or toadstools. One man called me because there was a musty odor in one of the rooms in his condominium. The room had an exterior wall, and there was a flat roof above the room. Whenever I investigate a property, I routinely look at the exterior for any visible signs of water problems that might negatively affect the exterior or interior. I found a mushroom growing out of the siding of this building. The man had never noticed the mushroom and thought that it might have appeared suddenly.

Mushrooms often appear overnight, but most of the fungal mass is invisibly spread out in the soil or substrate. When conditions are right, the nutrients for the mushroom structure gather below the surface and it bursts through. In this case there was a roof leak, and water had been entering the sheathing behind the siding. The fungal mass had spread out throughout the sheathing, and the mushroom appeared at a gap between two clapboards. There must have been extensive wood decay behind the clapboards, but the siding was made out of cedar, which is resistant to wood decay.

Macrofungi can rot wood in buildings, but unless someone works in a mushroom-growing facility, macrofungal spores rarely cause health symptoms indoors. Exposure to microfungal spores, however, can cause allergy symptoms, and microfungi are commonly found in damp, indoor environments. This is why I focus on microfungi in this discussion.

MICROFUNGI

The spore-forming structures of microfungi are microscopic, and with few exceptions, microfungi don't cause wood decay because they cannot digest the structural components of wood. Microfungi consume organic materials such as wood sugars, leaves, food bits, fruit, paper, cotton, soap, oil, paint, and surface dust. Many people believe that microfungi cannot grow in fiberglass insulation or on metal or concrete, but this isn't the case. Microfungi can grow on or in the dust on any surface, including the dust captured in fiberglass insulation. And many microfungal species can flourish at high RH conditions in the absence of any liquid water. Familiar forms of microfungi include the molds often seen on bathroom ceilings and foundation walls.

Microfungi are typically referred to as mold or mildew, though to a biologist, mildew refers to a mold that grows on a living plant. For the sake of discussions in this book, we will be referring to microfungi as mold.

MOLD REPRODUCTION AND GROWTH

Microfungi produce microscopic spores in great numbers. Some spores form in clumps that are stuck together. Others form in long, fragile chains that are easily dispersed into the air if the mold is disturbed. If adequate moisture is present when a spore lands on a suitable food source, it uses nutrients stored within it to start growing, just the way a plant seed does. The spore sends out a small extension called a hypha (or "hyphae" if plural), similar to the root from a germinating seed. This is the beginning of a microfungal colony.

Mammals digest food within their own bodies. Microfungi secrete enzymes from the growing tips of the hyphae to digest food sources outside the organism. The resulting nutrients diffuse into the organism through the cell wall at the hyphal tip. The hypha elongates, splits, lengthens, and eventually creates a complex network of hyphae called a mycelium. Often the mycelium is white and furry, but as many mold colonies mature, the hyphae may acquire the color of the colonies' spores (black, yellow, brown, or green). Within days, a single spore can produce a mature colony containing millions of spores.

One genus of mold, *Penicillium*, comprises hundreds of known species; some produce the antibiotic penicillin, others turn milk curd into cheese, and still others create the blue-green growth found on long-forgotten oranges at the back of a refrigerator drawer. Another genus of mold, *Aspergillus*, is commonly found indoors, especially in damp basements; exposure to *Aspergillus* spores through inhalation is the cause of many allergy and respiratory symptoms.

People who are sensitized to mold spores will react allergically if they inhale airborne spores. They may cough, sneeze, experience eye irritation, or wheeze. But mold can bother people who do not have mold allergy. The content of every mold spore is different, but the cell walls are similar. It is now believed that components of the cell wall (called glucans) of all mold spores can inflame lung tissue.[3] Mold can also produce musty odors that some people find irritating.

One family asked me to help them determine the source of a strong musty odor in their home. The odor originated in the old basement carpet, and they removed it. The smell went away, and they installed new nylon carpeting that was supposed to be non-allergenic. Two months later, they went on a two-week summer vacation, leaving the central air conditioning on. They again noticed the musty odor when they returned. I found that the condensate pump for the central air conditioning had broken, allowing water to leak out of the basement mechanical closet and into the new carpeting.

I cut out a small piece of the carpet and took it to a scanning electron microscopist (see "Scanning electron micrograph" in the glossary). I had expected to find mold growing at the bottom of the fibers in the backing where the dust ultimately accumulates. The microscopist and I spent an hour examining the fingernail-sized sample, and much to our surprise, we found mold at the top of the nylon fiber loops rather than at the bottom. Since the carpet

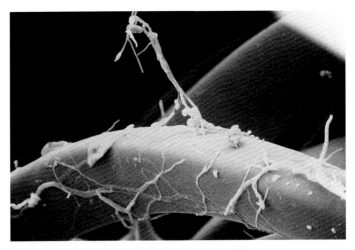

FIGURE 2.3. This scanning electron micrograph (SEM) shows a fiber from a two-month-old nylon carpet with mold hyphae creeping like a vine along the surface. Most of the hyphae are wrapped around the thicker carpet fiber, but a hypha projects upward. Other hyphae not visible in the micrograph had spread from one nylon fiber to the next. The invisible mold growth gave the nearly new carpet its musty odor (450× SEM).

was new, the dust that had settled from the air onto the nylon fibers had not yet fallen down to the backing, and the germinating spores had sent out hyphae where the food source was.

The microscopist and I could see the hyphae growing like ivy on a telephone pole, clinging to carpet fibers and lengthening as they grew toward and consumed the dust particles. That the carpeting material was nylon (and sold as nonallergenic) did not deter mold growth within it, for as is often the case with synthetic carpeting, the mold was consuming the dust rather than the carpet fibers. The family eliminated the problem by replacing the condensate pump and the contaminated section of carpet near the mechanical closet (fig. 2.3).

MYCOTOXINS

Under certain conditions, some mold species produce mycotoxins (toxic substances produced by fungi). Scientists do not yet know for certain what functions mycotoxins may serve for the organisms, but the more closely investigators look at different species of molds, the more often they find mycotoxins. *Aspergillus flavus*, a common mold that grows on nuts and grains and can be found in homes, can produce aflatoxin B_1 (a kind of mycotoxin), one of several chemicals that are among the most carcinogenic compounds known. The black mold *Stachybotrys chartarum*, commonly found on chronically damp drywall, can also produce a series of mycotoxins called tricothecenes that are poisonous. (*Stachybotrys chartarum* is commonly referred to as "toxic black mold." *Cladosporium* mold is also black, and people often mistake this mold for *Stachybotrys* mold.)

In the 1930s, Russian horses started dying in large numbers. Symptoms included inflammation of the skin and respiratory tract and hemorrhaging. Death sometimes occurred within twenty-four hours of the time symptoms first appeared. The horses' feed was found to be contaminated with *Stachybotrys chartarum*. In the mid-1990s, based on evidence from cases at Cleveland's Rainbow Babies and Children's Hospital, Dr. Dorr Dearborn associated *Stachybotrys* with pulmonary hemosiderosis (bleeding in the lungs). Though some disputed his conclusions, Dr. Dearborn believed that several infant deaths were caused by this mold. In the same decade, a house in Texas became so contaminated by *Stachybotrys* that the family had to abandon the property and bulldoze the house. The husband experienced memory loss, and the child became asthmatic. The man who was investigating the case threw up for hours after spending thirty minutes in the contaminated building.

BACTERIA

So far we've discussed relatively well-known sources of allergens such as mites and mold. Bacteria, which we know cause respiratory and other infections, can also lead to allergy-type reactions. Actinomycetes, organisms that produce small spores and grow the way mold grows, are actually filamentous bacteria. Actinomycetes are present in soil and produce its characteristic earthy odor. Chronic inhalation of actinomycete spores can lead to the pulmonary disease "farmer's lung," a serious respiratory illness that is a type of hypersensitivity pneumonitis (HP).

YEAST

The yeast we add to dough to make bread rise is another fungus, and some types of yeast can cause allergy.

MATE ALLERGY OR SELF-ALLERGY?

More than once I've heard people say their allergies started after their partners moved in. Papers in the medical literature point to a possible scientific reason: several common fungi called dermatophytes can cause medical conditions such as dermatitis and dandruff.

These fungi can exist in two forms. In a petri dish culture they grow the way mold grows, in colonies with hyphae, but on human skin they revert to cells. Individual yeast cells reproduce by simply dividing into parent and daughter cells. These yeast cells are the size of mold spores and thus can be inhaled. Fortunately, unlike mold spores, dermatophytes cells do not easily become airborne because they adhere to the oily surface of the skin scales they grow on. Recently, two proteins that are allergens have been identified on the surface of yeast cells. One study found that almost 10 percent of hairdressers in Finland reacted with allergic symptoms to the yeasts that cause dandruff and dermatitis.[4]

I learned about inhalant yeast allergy when a client asked me to investigate his apartment, where he had been experiencing severe asthma symptoms. He was desperate because after he spent time at home, his breathing became so labored that he could barely walk to his car or go out to shop for food. He felt better whenever he was away for more than two days.

I was pretty sure I would find mold and mites, but I was surprised. The man was a fastidious housekeeper; there was little dust anywhere, and I could find no source of excess moisture. Yet the dust samples I collected from his bedding and favorite TV chair were full of skin scales covered with yeast. Walking on the carpet also produced large numbers of individual, respirable yeast cells. Although I had no trouble breathing in the apartment, the man was convinced his home was contaminated. I can only assume that the yeast was subsisting on the skin scales shed by his body. In this case the man may well have been allergic to something that his own body was "feeding."

One woman called me because her three-year-old son was experiencing rashes and severe respiratory symptoms that she thought might have been caused by some condition in her home. I took many air and surface samples in the home but was most concerned about the sample from the hide rug in the boy's bedroom. The rug had been purchased shortly before her son's birth and had been present in his bedroom ever since. The sample from the rug contained hundreds of yeast cells. As soon as I examined the sample, I called the woman and told her to immediately remove the rug from the room. During our conversation she recalled that when she first received the rug, it had a musty smell. The next day she called the company that had sold her the rug, and they offered her a refund.

The bad news is that it is difficult to test for a particular yeast allergy because the allergens are not stable and thus can't be easily stored in solution and kept in the doctor's refrigerator for testing. The good news is that their instability makes them easier to destroy.

I suspect that thoroughly treating all the furniture and carpeting with steam vapor from a steam vapor machine would destroy most of the unstable allergens. Pure steam is water vapor alone, without liquid water. Many allergens are denatured at the temperature of pure steam. We discuss some uses of steam vapor in chapter 24.

SOME RECOMMENDATIONS

- If you have dust or mite allergy, put dust mite encasings on any mattresses, bed pillows, and box springs. I recommend the type of encasings with polyurethane liners. If the mattresses and pillows have never been used, however, the tightly woven encasings should be sufficient.

- Never remove a dust mite encasing from a mattress or box spring, because doing so could release mite allergens. If you want to wash an encasing now and then, install two encasings and never remove the inner encasing.

- To kill dust mites and denature some allergens, you can put thick blankets and quilts in a dryer every few weeks on medium heat for approximately ten minutes.

3.

"TROJAN HORSE" ALLERGENS

Many allergens are associated with discrete particles that can be seen using a microscope. For example, pollen grains and mold spores are relatively easy to distinguish visually. But the actual allergens associated with these particles are chemicals on the surface or at the interior of the particle. Any particular particle such as a pollen grain or mold spore can be associated with a dozen or more individual chemical allergens. Many of these chemical allergens are water-soluble proteins and can coat or be absorbed by particles that are not in and of themselves allergenic.

It is therefore my hypothesis that particles such as rust and soot that are not allergenic themselves can still act as "Trojan Horse" allergens, because they are in our midst but investigators looking for particulate allergens do not see them as threats.

These Trojan Horse allergens can also be called "surrogate allergens," because in a way they are substitutes for allergen sources such as pollen grains and mold spores. The idea of surrogate allergens is not as strange as it may sound. Let's start with an example of a surrogate allergen that is well accepted: the powder that used to be applied to latex gloves.

LATEX GLOVES AND DONNING POWDER

The latex rubber used in gloves is uncured and is therefore somewhat tacky. To prevent the rubber surfaces from sticking together, donning powder was added to the gloves during manufacturing. This powder

Ancient Greece had been engaged in a ten-year battle trying to take over the independent, walled city of Troy. According to legend, the Greek soldiers pretended to give up the battle for Troy after leaving behind a huge wooden horse as an offering to the goddess Athena. The Trojans dragged the horse into the walled city, not realizing that the Greeks had hidden fighters inside the hollow horse. At night, the Greek soldiers returned and were able to enter Troy after the hidden fighters exited the horse and opened the city gates.

consisted of cornstarch, which is made up of microscopic granules containing starch. These granules were in intimate contact with the surface of the rubber and the allergens that naturally occur in the latex rubber (and that come from a plant). Then the granules became coated with the allergens from the latex rubber, thus becoming surrogate allergens.

Exposure to these starch granules was a risk for those who were allergic to latex rubber proteins or who became allergic over time through exposure to the latex gloves or the donning powder. Allergy to latex rubber was first described in 1927; however, it was not until the 1980s that people recognized that allergic rashes were caused by contact with proteins in the latex rubber. Inhalation of these granules could cause an anaphylactic reaction (an extreme, potentially life-threatening reaction to an allergen) in someone highly allergic to latex. In 1984, a case of anaphylaxis was associated with a reaction to latex gloves. The first death due to anaphylactic shock associated with a latex glove occurred in 1991.[1] Since the problematic allergic sensitivity was more closely associated with medical personnel, latex gloves are no longer in wide use in medical facilities in the United States.

I consider the latex allergen on a cornstarch particle as a surrogate allergen because the starch granule is acting as a surrogate for the latex rubber allergen. The possibility of other such surrogate allergens has been investigated by Heidi Ormstad, a researcher in Norway (although she refers to surrogate allergens in her journal articles as "adjuvant allergens"). She used a sophisticated technique called "immunogold labeling" to show that aerosolized microscopic soot particles can carry cat, dog, and birch allergens on their surfaces.[2]

Now let's move to more surrogate allergens that are not well recognized.

KITTY LITTER BOXES

Many cat owners use corn-based kitty litter. Cats urinate on the litter, which then may dry out between the cat's visits to the litter box. When the cat stirs up the litter, some cornstarch granules with dried urine on them can be aerosolized. I have taken air samples in homes in which corn-based kitty litter was in use and have sometimes found large numbers of cornstarch granules in the air throughout the houses, no matter where the litter boxes were located. Cats have allergens in their saliva, their sebaceous (skin) gland secretions, and in their urine. I believe that the cornstarch granules become coated with these allergens and could thus serve as surrogates for cat allergens.

Any type of kitty litter can be a source of aerosolized allergens. Sometimes families with cat allergy cannot part with their cat. One way to reduce emissions from a kitty litter box is to have the box enclosed in a larger housing with an opening at the side for the cat to enter and an opening at the top for a duct. The duct could be attached to either an exhaust fan venting to the exterior or to a HEPA-filtered air purifier. The operation of the fan could be controlled by a motion detector and timer, so that as soon as the cat entered the litter box, the fan would turn on and stay on for a set amount of time, say, ten minutes. This arrangement is much like installing a laboratory hood over a kitty litter box.

DOG AND CAT SKIN SCALES

When speaking about cat allergens, doctors and others often refer to cat dander. Cat and dog dander particles consist of skin scales that the animals shed (skin scales that human beings shed could also be called human dander particles). Whether they are shed or not, dog, cat, and human skin scales consist of a protein called keratin. This protein by itself is not allergenic; if it were, everyone might suffer from "human allergies," because skin scales are the most common suspended particles in indoor air. If keratin is not allergenic, then why can cat or dog dander particles be allergenic? The animals' skin glands have secretions that contain allergens, and those secretions can coat animals' skin scales.

The cat allergen on keratin particles is soluble in water. There are some manufacturers who make vacuum cleaners that use water instead of a vacuum bag to trap dust. Cat allergens in the air of a home where a cat resided were measured before and after vacuuming using a water-based vacuum.[3] The concentration of cat allergens in the air was higher after cleaning with the vacuum than before the cleaning began, presumably because cat allergens dissolved in the water and were re-aerosolized by the vacuum's exhaust. The allergens were even present on smaller particles in the air after the vacuuming stopped. (The researchers found that filtering the exhaust could prevent the re-aerosolization of cat allergens.)

BIRDS

Allergy to birds is much less common than is allergy to cats and dogs; nonetheless, bird dander particles also consist of keratin, which can carry allergens from excretions from a bird's skin.

In addition to shedding dander particles, birds also release large numbers of small (1 to 3 microns in size) particles of keratin called

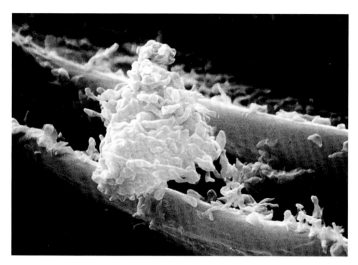

FIGURE 3.1. In this scanning electron micrograph (SEM), a dander particle spans two strut-like structures from a cockatiel's wing feather. Note the bean-shaped bloom particles littering the feather surfaces and piled up in a cluster on the dander. In every home where cockatiels live, the air is filled with these 1- to 3-micron-sized bloom particles that settle out of the air to form a fine white powder on room surfaces. The bloom particles help to keep a bird's feathers dry; the particles are coated with bird allergens and are thus surrogate allergens (4,000× SEM).

"bloom," which help to repel water from a bird's feathers. In homes with several pet birds, a fine white powder consisting of bird-bloom particles can be found settled on surfaces and can even be intermingled with regular house dust. These bloom particles are coated with bird allergen, and because they are so small, they can be inhaled deep into the lung, delivering allergens even into the alveoli (allergic alveolitis is also known as pigeon breeder's lung) (fig. 3.1).

One of my clients owned two cockatiels that he sometimes allowed to fly free around his carpeted office. He became breathless one day after some mild exercise, and his physician determined that he had hypersensitivity pneumonitis (HP), a serious respiratory illness. I took a Burkard air sample in his office and a second sample close to one of his birds while it flapped its wings. I found that both samples contained numerous bird dander and bird-bloom particles. He gave the birds away and cleaned the surfaces in his house, and his health improved dramatically.

I have taken what I call "pat" samples from hundreds of feather-filled quilts and pillows. (In a pat sample, I gently pat a surface with a spatula and then collect the aerosol that is emitted from the surface.) In about one-third of these samples, the aerosol contained bird-bloom particles. (This suggests to me that the feathers had not been adequately cleaned prior to being used as fill for the quilts and pillows.)

There are some serious health conditions that can be associated with exposure to bird allergens, including pigeon breeder's lung and bird fancier's lung, both of which are forms of hypersensitivity pneumonitis, a serious respiratory disease.

Physicians have now identified a rare respiratory condition known as "duvet lung." Duvet lung is a form of hypersensitivity pneumonitis caused by exposure to bird bloom from feather (down) quilts.

N. Inas et al., "A Clinical Study of Hypersensitivity Pneumonitis Presumably Caused by Feather Duvets," *Annals of Asthma, Allergy and Immunology* 96, no. 1 (January 2006): 98–104.

The potential allergenicity of feathers is one reason why many allergists recommend that their patients avoid feather-filled bedding.

I received a call from a fellow who had been diagnosed with HP. Since HP is an illness caused by environmental exposures, his physician advised him to schedule an environmental investigation of his home. In the course of our initial phone discussion I asked if he had any feather quilts. He mentioned that his daughter had given him an expensive feather quilt for Christmas and that in February he started to experience respiratory symptoms. Within a year he was having severe shortness of breath and chronic coughing: symptoms of HP.

Since I was familiar with situations in which feather-filled goods caused health symptoms, I recommended that the fellow send me the quilt before he made an appointment for me to investigate the home. The quilt arrived by mail in a surprisingly small box, as it had been vacuum packed. I am allergic to bird bloom and thus was a bit fearful about being exposed to the quilt's emissions, so I decided to open the box outdoors. I cut open the tape at the box flaps and made a small slit in the plastic bag containing the compressed quilt. As soon as air entered the slit, the quilt grew out of the box like some kind of threatening, boneless alien in a sci-fi horror movie. I never did remove the quilt from the box but rather took a "pat" sample of the bulge sticking out of the box. The sample contained the highest concentration of bird-bloom particles I have ever seen in a sample from a feather-filled object. (I quickly stuffed the quilt bulge back into the box, taped it shut, and mailed the box back to the owner!)

Apparently the feathers in this high-end quilt were emitting large numbers of bird-bloom particles. When HP is caused by exposure to bird bloom, the illness is seen primarily in individuals keeping live birds as pets, yet in this case the man's HP had presumably been caused by exposure to the quilt. The man reported to me that his health improved dramatically after he removed the quilt from his bed.

CARPETS AND RUGS

The assertion that wool can cause allergy symptoms has for years created quite a debate among allergists, some of whom maintain that it is the lanolin in the wool that causes allergies. Other allergists contend that the irritation caused by wool is not really an allergic response.

Wool consists of hair from sheep. Keratin in hair—whether from a human being, a dog, a cat, a bird, or a sheep—actually contains two different structural forms. The outer "skin" layer of the hair fiber is called the cuticle, which consists of keratin in what is known as beta-

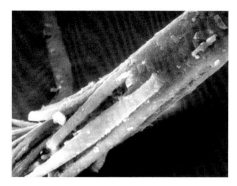

FIGURE 3.2. Wool hair with the cortex exposed. The intact cuticle is at the upper right, with some respirable fragments of cuticle on the surface. At the bottom left, the cuticle has disintegrated and is missing; the individual cortex fibers (a ropelike structure within the hair) are visible. This is the sheep hair equivalent of a human split end (1,000× SEM).

pleated sheet form because the molecules are aligned in thin, curved layers. The cuticle at the exterior of a hair is wrapped around the cortex, a second form of keratin called alpha helix. This form of keratin consists of strands of protein in the form of fibers. The individual cortex fibers can have sharp points at the ends. If you have a split end, the cuticle has peeled away from a portion of the hair, allowing the cortex fibers to stick out (fig. 3.2).

The structures of the cuticle and cortex allow hair to be flexible. The plates that make up the cuticle of the hair are not strongly attached to each other, allowing the hairs to bend similar to the way that a snake's skin scales allow it to coil. There are also microscopic air gaps between the cuticle layers and between the individual, ropelike fibers of the cortex. All these microscopic gaps in the structural proteins make the hairs somewhat porous. In fact, when placed in warm water, a hair absorbs enough moisture to increase in diameter by more than 10 percent.

As noted, keratin is not known to be allergenic, but the porosity of hair may account for its potential allergenicity. Imagine that the wool from your rug or sweater came from a sweaty sheep that had slept on moldy hay. The allergens from the sweat glands and the moldy hay could have infused into the gaps in the cuticle and cortex in much the same way that hair dye fills hair and changes its color. If the wool fibers are washed enough, perhaps most of the sheep's body odor, other potentially odorous compounds, and allergens will be rinsed out. I believe that one of the reasons that damp wool has a particular odor is because when the wool is damp, some of the odor molecules from sheep sweat that are trapped between the cuticle and cortex are released.

I have taken hundreds of samples from wool rugs. I observed respirable fragments of wool cuticle particles and somewhat larger fragments of wool cortex particles in about half of these samples. For some unknown reason the wool fibers had become brittle and were breaking up. If there are any allergens remaining trapped in the gaps of the wool hairs, I believe that the keratin fragments of wool cuticle and wool cortex particles may serve as surrogate allergens. Such particles can be aerosolized when people walk across a degrading wool rug's surface. In a few buildings that I inspected in which occupants were experiencing coughing and eye irritation, I found high concentrations of wool cuticle particles in the indoor air. I therefore believe that, even in the absence of allergens on the keratin particles, large numbers of these aerosolized particles can be irritants. So, in the end, I guess that both sides of the argument are correct: wool cortex and wool cuticle particles can be both irritating and allergenic.

What about carpets and rugs that are not made from wool? Even the most thorough cleaning and washing cannot remove all the biodegradable dust captured in carpet fibers. If rugs or carpets are washed and do not dry out quickly enough, the moisture and dust provide conditions conducive to microbial growth. We discuss this issue in greater detail in chapter 24.

MECHANICAL SYSTEMS AND EQUIPMENT

Many reservoirs in the components of mechanical systems are fabricated from galvanized iron (iron that is coated with a thin layer of zinc). The zinc protects the iron from rusting for a while, but eventually the zinc corrodes, and then the iron can rust. Rust particles can become coated with by-products of microbial growth in the reservoirs. When the particles are aerosolized, they can expose building occupants to allergens.

I once investigated an air quality problem in a computer facility inside a high-rise building. The room in question was a server room filled from floor to ceiling with humming computer servers. Dry air is conducive to electrostatic sparks, which would have been a risk to the numerous sensitive electronic components, so a humidifier in the room kept the relative humidity (RH) rather high. When I entered the room, I coughed a bit owing to the allergenicity of the air. I took an air sample in the space, and there were almost no particles in the sample. This made sense, since there was virtually no human activity in the space and few surfaces upon which dust could settle. The only particles in the sample were micron-sized (and thus respirable) rust particles from the humidifier, which must have had microbial growth in the water in a rusted tray, making the rust particles surrogate allergens.

I often find dried-up rusty scum in the condensate pans for air conditioning systems in both large and small buildings including homes. The scum in these pans forms during the cooling season, when the galvanized iron pans are full of water that condenses from the air conditioning coils. If there is dust in a pan (which there almost always is), microbial growth ensues in the wet dust (this is why air from some air conditioning systems or units emits a musty or bacterial odor when first turned on). The rust particles in the pan become coated with allergens, and when the particles are aerosolized, they become surrogate allergens. The puddles of slime and rust dry out in the winter because there is no longer any moisture condensing on the cooling coil. But rust particles covered with allergens from the microbial growth in condensate pans can be aerosolized when the heat is running. Since many ducted, mechanical systems provide heat in the winter as well as cooling in the summer, building occupants can be exposed to surrogate allergens year-round.

In my opinion, just about any liquid reservoir in mechanical systems and equipment that contains microbial growth can produce surrogate allergens. We discuss mechanical systems in part IV.

POLLEN GRAINS

In Australia, emergency room visits for asthma increase sharply after some thunderstorms.[4] One theory holds that the cause for this phenomenon is a sudden increase in the amount of pollen allergens in the air. Pollen grains often contain many small granules of starch. These granules are surrounded by pollen allergens consisting of proteins. When exposed to rain, some pollen grains burst, and then allergen-coated starch granules are released into the air, making the starch granules surrogate allergens (fig. 3.3).

Pollen grains are relatively large, often greater than 60 microns (60 millionths of a meter) in size, and are therefore trapped in the nose, where they release allergens and cause sneezing. The starch granules in the pollen grains are much smaller, however, about 5 microns in size, and are small enough to carry pollen allergens deep into the lung, causing a more significant exposure. This may explain the increase in emergency room admissions for asthma during thunderstorms.

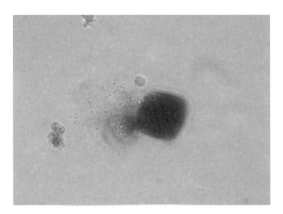

FIGURE 3.3. The pollen grain in this micrograph is stained pink with acid fuchsin (which colors protein pink). The lactic acid medium for the stain caused the pollen to burst open and release starch granules that are coated with allergenic protein. If the starch granules had been released into the air, they would have become surrogate allergens owing to the protein residue coating the granules (450× light micrograph).

SO WHAT?

In nearly all air quality investigations of buildings where occupants are suffering health symptoms, most laboratory technicians examining the air and dust samples taken in these environments only identify discrete allergens. Unfortunately, surrogate allergens cannot be identified by microscopy because they do not have the familiar shapes (such as the shapes of pollen grains, pet dander particles, mold spores, and bacteria) that microscopists typically look for. When no indoor allergens are identified, most IAQ investigators conclude that any symptoms that the building occupants are experiencing are not caused by indoor conditions. At that point some people may suspect that the building occupants experiencing symptoms are suffering from "psychological problems."

Then the responsibility for the "fix" is shifted from the building or management personnel to the sufferers themselves. Luckily, a growing number of physicians are recognizing the relationship between indoor environmental conditions and health symptoms. IAQ professionals and laboratory technicians should also understand how surrogate allergens can negatively affect the health of building occupants.

SOME RECOMMENDATIONS

- If you or anyone in your household has allergies, asthma, or other environmental sensitivities, avoid using feather-filled goods, including bedding.

- If you are allergic to wool or find wearing wool clothing irritating, consider avoiding having wool rugs or carpets in your home.

- Treatment with steam vapor will not prevent the emission of wool cuticle and cortex particles from a rug or carpet with deteriorating wool fibers.

- If you are concerned about potential exposure to cat allergens, build an exhaust hood for your kitty litter box.

4.

CREEPY CRAWLERS (APOLOGIES FOR THE TITLE!)

It was not until the 1960s that the medical community had sufficient evidence to accept the theory that dust mites cause allergy. Now physicians recognize that fecal material and body parts from other arthropods and microarthropods may also cause allergy and asthma symptoms; cockroaches are a well-known example.

In addition to mold growth and dust mites, I have found many creatures such as silverfish, booklice, and carpet beetles (dermestids) in some of my clients' carpeting. All of these creatures, including carpet beetles, produce allergenic fecal matter. It is my theory that a so-called house dust allergy could largely be a diagnosis of allergy to arthropod and microarthropod fecal matter in dust.

CARPET BEETLES

Except for entomologists and pest control operators (PCOs), few people have ever seen or heard of a carpet beetle, yet they are common in indoor environments. Two common types of carpet beetles are the black carpet beetle (*Attagenus megatoma*) and the varied carpet beetle (*Athrenus verbasci*). The adults of both species are about 3 millimeters (0.12 inch) long, but the former is black and the latter is multicolored (with white, yellow, and brown scales). Carpet beetles lay their eggs in larger dead animals and insects; a dead moth is a favorite place. The eggs hatch and produce young that molt (shed the outer layer) into hairy larvae that feed on anything that contains protein, including fur and dead animals and insects. Like other larvae, they have voracious appetites and do nothing but eat, defecate, and molt.

Many valuable collections of butterflies and other insects have been turned to frass by these creatures. Carpet beetle larvae are also the scourge of museums with mounted specimens because they love hair. They don't care where the hair comes from; it can be from a mighty stuffed lion, from the wool fibers in an Oriental rug, from your body, or from the body of a beloved pet. In dust samples from carpeting and beds, I have seen hairs that larvae have gnawed to points resembling roughly sharpened pencils. You can see in the fecal pellets of these creatures the chewed bits of whatever they have been feeding on.

Although these fecal pellets are far too large to become airborne (about 140 microns, or 0.0055 inch in size), I was curious to know if they could be broken apart. I crushed a pellet and accidentally breathed in the dust. My throat swelled, and I immediately had trouble breathing. After that experience, I read about research by doctors from Spain who document allergy to carpet beetles.[1] In *Urban Entomology*, Walter Ebeling also describes cases of allergy to dermestids, possibly due to the beetles' hairs and body parts.[2]

I was afforded the wonderful opportunity of observing my first carpet beetles because of a recommendation from Harvard's entomologist Gary Alpert. He suggested that I find a dead moth, place it in a container, and watch. Sure enough, a carpet beetle larva emerged (actually, I didn't realize until two mature carpet beetles appeared that for weeks I had been observing twins!). I was able to obtain moth wing feathers with bites as well as pristine larval fecal pellets from this little slide box (figs. 4.1 and 4.2).

Carpet beetle frass may even be useful to crime investigators. I received an email from a forensic chemist who had been searching the Internet for information on carpet beetles when she found our website. She wondered if it would be possible to determine whether the chewed-up hair in carpet beetle frass contained hair dye. She was circumspect about why she needed this information, but I can only assume that the police were attempting to identify a decomposed body by looking at the hair fragments in the frass.

"LITTERATURE"

The dust that has settled on books seems to bother many people with allergies. There is nothing special about the dust on books except that

If you move a piece of furniture, you may find the carcass of a moth or bee on the floor surrounded by a circular thin layer of brown dust 2.5 centimeters (1 inch) or so in diameter. This dust could be the frass (fecal pellets) of a carpet beetle larva that has fed on the dead insect.

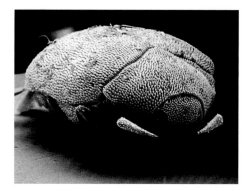

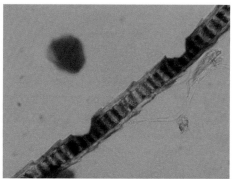

FIGURE 4.1. This scanning electron micrograph (SEM) shows one of the adult carpet beetles that emerged from a dead moth that I collected. At some point after the moth died, an adult carpet beetle laid its eggs in the moth. After I collected the moth, two larvae hatched from the eggs and proceeded to chew up the moth. Looking at the remaining moth parts with a microscope, I learned how to identify the bites of carpet beetle larvae (40× SEM).

FIGURE 4.2. The cat hair in this micrograph came from the carpet dust in a home that at one time had a carpet beetle infestation. The round particle at the upper left is a skin scale stained pink with acid fuchsin. The long cat hair is partially stained pink and contains two missing chunks, bites taken by a carpet beetle larva. Adult carpet beetles do not cause the damage associated with these microarthropods (400× light micrograph).

it often sits there longer than the dust on other surfaces. Once the book is disturbed, the particles become airborne.

We may think of the words inside as intellectual nourishment, but the particles that settle on the exposed top edge of a book provide real sustenance for a wide variety of microarthropod and arthropod life. When I look at book dust, I may find booklice, settled pollen grains, mold spores, spider silk, mites or their body parts, or microarthropod fecal material. In book dust that has nurtured microarthropods, I find chewed pollen grains or even fecal pellets consisting entirely of partially digested pollen. What starts out as benign settled dust on top of a book becomes over time a conglomerate of allergenic "bug poop." So don't be surprised if you sneeze in the library stacks. Books that have been stored in musty spaces can contain allergenic dust, so it's best to avoid buying used books that smell musty, even if you are a teacher and want to augment your classroom's library.

BOOKLICE

Booklice, also called psocids, are about 1.5 millimeters (0.06 inch) long and are sometimes found feeding on the dust on books that are stored in damp basements. Psocids aren't really lice, but they resemble them. I met my first booklouse while I was reading at my desk and saw a small, buff-colored bug scurrying across the page. I trapped the unknown creature on a piece of sticky tape and placed the tape on a glass slide to view under my microscope. While I was observing the microarthropod, it ejected a small dark pellet about 9 microns (0.0035 inch) in diameter from the end of its abdomen.

Suddenly, I had the unique opportunity to observe an uncontaminated fecal pellet from a known source. I managed to get the pellet to adhere to a tiny drop of water suspended at the end of a pin and to transfer the drop to a microscope slide. I crushed the pellet, added acid fuchsin stain, and observed that it contained skin scales and a mold spore. I thus discovered that these microarthropods forage in the dust for mold spores and skin scales the way mites do.

Unlike mite fecal pellets, which are known allergens, the entire booklouse fecal pellet is too large to become readily airborne. But I did see respirable crystals (possibly coated with allergens) drifting away from the surface of the pellet before I crushed it. There has been a study of allergy to booklice,[3] but this is territory for further allergy research.

BOOKLICE IN PILLOWS

I received a desperate call from a young couple with a baby. The parents woke up one night surrounded by hundreds of bugs. They assumed that the infestation was in their bedroom, so they moved to the guest bedroom, only to wake up the following night to again find hundreds of bugs. When I visited the home, they were spending the night in sleeping bags in the living room. They carried their expensive organic pillows with them when they moved from their bedroom to the guest room and then to the living room. I cut into one of the pillows, and it was crawling with booklice that were eating the moldy millet grain filling in the pillows. The couple threw out the pillows, and the seller refunded their money (fig. 4.3).

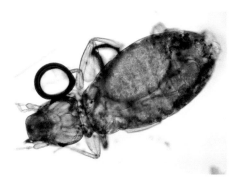

FIGURE 4.3. This one-millimeter female booklouse (also called a psocid) emerged from a grain-filled pillow along with hundreds of its kin, terrifying a young couple at night. There is a large oval egg in the psocid's abdomen (the colorless circle above the psocid's head is an air bubble). Psocids are annoying pests, but they do not bite (80× light micrograph).

WOOL MOTHS

Wool carpeting and clothing can attract wool moths, and moth fecal material and body parts may cause allergic symptoms in some people. I had my own problem with wool moths. My brother and sister-in-law gave us an imported woven-wool wall hanging containing muted shades of red, gold, and brown that matched our decor. One day Connie noticed that one of the tassels had fallen off the bottom. She took a closer look at the fabric and noticed that all the tassels were frayed; in some spots the yarn had been reduced to the thickness of a thread. She looked at the back of the fabric, and to her horror she saw hundreds of quivering moths and writhing larvae embedded in the material.

The hanging was directly above a radiator. I put on a NIOSH N95 two-strap, fine-particle face mask, threw the hanging away, and then vacuumed up and saved the dust on the floor below and behind the radiator. With a light microscope, I could see that the dust consisted of nearly pure larval frass. The fecal pellets had different colors, the same muted tones as the hanging. At very high magnification (30,000 power) with an electron microscope (see "Scanning electron micrograph" in the glossary), I could see that the surface of each pellet consisted of nearly spherical crystals called spherules (possibly containing guanine, a chemical insects excrete), all bound together by some unknown coating. Later, I tapped a box containing some of the frass and took a Burkard sample of the air above it. I found some of the approximately 1-micron (0.00004-inch) spherules in the air, and I surmised that my tapping had dislodged them from the surface of the fecal pellets. Although the intact pellets were too large to become airborne, the spherules were not, and these may have contained surface allergens (fig. 4.4).

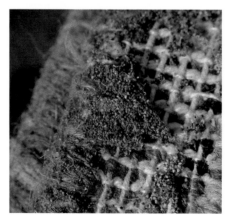

FIGURE 4.4. This photograph shows the backside of a deteriorated wool Oriental rug that Connie and I discarded after discovering a wool moth infestation. The grid (warp and weft) onto which the wool fibers were attached is covered with the droppings of the wool moth larvae that fed on the fibers. If you look carefully, you can see that each small dropping has the color of a fiber from the rug.

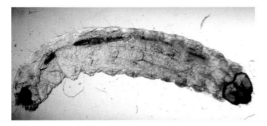

FIGURE 4.5. This wool moth larva is about three-eighths of an inch long and came from our infested wool rug. The head is at the right, and the anus is at the left. Near the upper edge of the larva is the narrow digestive tube that stretches from the head to the anus. Within the tube are several straight amber sections of a wool fiber that were gnawed off one at a time. The partially digested fiber sections accumulate in a fecal pellet in the anus and retain their original color (light micrograph).

Wool moth larvae have a simple way of destroying your wool fibers. I discovered this after I accidentally created a transparent larva by placing it in lactic acid to prepare to view it under a microscope. After a few days, the normally white larva became completely transparent. I could see into its digestive tube, which started at the mouth and ended about three-eighths of an inch away at the anus. The digestive tube contained several evenly spaced bits of wool fiber that the larva had gnawed off and ingested. The barely digested fibers flowed to the end of the tube, where they accumulated in a fecal pellet the colors of the individual fibers being eaten (fig. 4.5).

SPIDERS

Although some people regard spiders in their homes as beneficial, most people know how poisonous a black widow or brown recluse spider can be. Some people have had severe reactions to the bites of less threatening spiders. I also believe spiders are a source of fecal allergens. If you look under a spider web, you will find clusters of white dots that resemble paint spatters about 1 to 2 millimeters (0.04 to 0.08 inch) in diameter, some containing a dark bull's-eye. These clusters are the spider's fecal material. The dots consist of microscopic crystals about 1 micron (0.00004 inch) in size that can become airborne if disturbed by our footsteps. I think that though the crystals consist of almost pure guanine, each is stuck to its neighbors by an allergenic coating that could contain digested spider proteins.

To obtain spider droppings for a scanning electron micrograph, I set up a blind in the corner of my office where I had noticed a small web with a spider in the middle. I placed the bottom half of an empty petri dish directly beneath the spider. It must have seen its own reflection in the shiny surface, because it jumped down and attacked the petri dish. I was thrilled that I had such an aggressive subject, since the spider would be energetic in capturing prey and would thus yield my much sought-after fecal material. I even placed a small night-light on the floor near the web to lure prey to the spot. Unfortunately, Connie swooped away the entire apparatus to make way for her vacuuming before I could gather any results.

Undaunted, I repeated the experiment in the winter, but this time I hid the petri dish in a closet and left it beneath a spider web for a month. When I collected the dish, I found it contained not only spider droppings but also four dried-up booklice the spider had preyed on. This experiment provided not only fecal material but also insight into house ecology, since I was reminded of the unseen battles that take place in the hidden corners of our homes every day. The experiment also reinforced my belief that spider droppings may be allergenic, because I started to cough and wheeze as soon as the electron microscopist disturbed the material.

The presence of many spiders in your home means that too much moisture is present. Spiders prey only on living bugs, so they get their liquids from what they eat, and mites are on their menu. In turn, mites as well as booklice and many other small household pests absorb moisture directly from the humidity in the air, and high relative humidity can lead to mold growth. So much for the theory that spiders are a healthy sign!

COCKROACHES

Cockroaches are particularly prevalent in cities and are one of the pests recognized as causing asthma symptoms. A National Library of Medicine–NIH report stated that "cockroach sensitization is a specific and major contributor to asthma morbidity for individuals who are exposed to high levels of cockroach allergens."[4]

Once while I was living in a dormitory, I walked over to a large paper train schedule taped to the wall near our common kitchen. As I pointed to the departure time, I touched the paper. A cockroach dropped to the floor and scurried off. Horrified but curious, I lifted the edge of the schedule and peeked behind it. I had accidentally discovered a roach harborage or shelter where there were hundreds of motionless insects, packed nearly pest to pest. Cockroaches spend the daylight hours in their harborage, attracted to each other and to the location by aggregation pheromones in the abundant feces they leave there.

A cockroach harborage is usually near a supply of food and moisture, most commonly in kitchens and bathrooms. Cockroaches prefer narrow spaces and are often found in the dead space between a kitchen cabinet and the wall or in crevices associated with shelves holding food. Harborages are also common under appliances such as stoves or refrigerators or in appliance insulation. In larger infestations the roaches can even be found inside televisions and dressers. Cockroaches tend to move about at the floor-wall joint rather than in the middle of a room, so the best way to determine the extent of an infestation is to set out sticky traps along likely travel routes. By doing this methodically, you might even find the harborage.

Cockroaches are nocturnal and forage at night. They will eat just about anything, including garbage. The best way to minimize the likelihood of a cockroach infestation is to store all foods in closed containers (don't leave pet food out overnight). Cockroach allergens may be found in food where roaches have foraged; if you eat the food, you ingest the allergens. When kitchen or pantry dust containing cockroach droppings and body parts is disturbed, these allergens can become airborne and be inhaled (though scientists have found that much of roach allergen aerosol is on particles larger than 10 microns [0.0004 inch], so these allergens remain airborne only briefly).

An adult of one of the more common species of cockroaches, *Blattella germanica* or the German cockroach, grows to about 12.7 millimeters (half an inch). These creatures are hardy and can live up to 20 days without food or water. This means that roaches can move into your home on furniture that has been purchased from a yard sale or stored in a moving truck. After German cockroaches mate, the female produces an egg case containing about 30 eggs. She carries the case, which resembles a brown purse about 8 by 3 millimeters (0.3 by 0.1 inch) in size, until the eggs are ready to hatch (in about a month). The nymphs that hatch are still immature, are about 3 millimeters (0.12 inch) long, and look gray to black. Over about 60 days, they will molt six or seven times before becoming adults. An individual roach may live 200 days, and a single female can produce up to 300 offspring. Within a year under warm and moist conditions, a few roaches can theoretically grow into a colony of millions.

One of my clients told me that friends of his with a significant cockroach infestation discovered in the middle of the winter that the roaches were nesting in the gasket of their dishwasher. They decided the simplest way to kill the pests was to freeze them. They disconnected the dishwasher and put it outside, which eliminated the problem in the appliance. They continued to have roaches in the kitchen,

It is believed that cockroaches can spread certain illnesses. For example, if the cockroaches eat food contaminated with *Salmonella*, the bacteria that cause food poisoning, viable *Salmonella* can be found in the roach feces. Should this fecal material end up in food eaten by humans, the roach feces may transmit the *Salmonella* and cause food poisoning.

however, so they applied their special treatment to the entire house. They drained the plumbing, turned off the heat, and left the house vacant. By freezing the pests, they were able to get rid of their roaches without using pesticides. If you live in a warm climate, though, shipping your home to Alaska is probably not an option. A borate-based pesticide (based on boric acid) would be a relatively safe choice, since these pesticides contain no solvents and do not evaporate. Many people with chemical sensitivities are highly sensitized to pesticides. The blankets that moving companies use may be sprayed with pesticide to kill roaches that might otherwise be hitchhiking with furnishings from one home to another. If you are sensitive to pesticides and are planning to hire a moving company, be sure that your possessions are wrapped in new, pesticide-free blankets.

We had a client who lived in a very rural area. Her son was diagnosed with cockroach allergy even though his mother had never seen a cockroach in her life and certainly not in her home. The family's home, however, had an infestation of Asian ladybugs. It turns out that there is cross-reactivity between the ladybug allergens and cockroach allergens.[5]

BED BUGS

Bed bugs have plagued human beings for centuries, but through the use of pesticides these bugs had been eliminated as a major indoor pest by the twentieth century. Then, starting in about the 1990s, bed bug infestations reemerged in most countries. Some people hypothesized that the reappearance of the bugs was because the pesticide dichlorodiphenyltrichloroethane, or DDT, was no longer being used. By the beginning of the twenty-first century, most health departments in urban areas had experienced large increases in the number of calls regarding bed bugs. Newspapers published stories of travelers who acquired infestations in their homes after staying in hotels. There were even some jury awards of thousands of dollars to hotel guests who claimed that their bed bug infestations originated from overnight hotel stays.

Sometimes feeding in large numbers, bed bugs typically snack on their sleeping hosts at night. The sites where bed bugs have bitten can become inflamed and itch, particularly if one is allergic to the proteins in the pest's saliva. I have never seen a major bed bug infestation (and hope never to do so!), but on a few occasions people called us because they were concerned about bites they acquired in bed at night. Apart from the itching and irritation caused by bed bugs bites and the psychological horror of having a bed bug infestation, my concern about bed bugs is exposure to allergens from bed bug detritus: the body parts and droppings they leave in the environment.

Bed bugs (like roaches) create concealed harborage sites where they congregate during their inactive daytime periods. Common harborage sites include the edge seams of mattresses and box spring covers, undersides of labels and buttons on mattresses, and cracks and crevices in box springs. In some infestations, harborage sites can be found within a few feet of the host's bed behind pictures hanging on the wall or even in electrical outlet boxes or the hollow legs of metal chairs. If the harborage sites can be located, the site must be thoroughly HEPA vacuumed (along with the rest of the mattress, box spring, and room surfaces) using a vacuum with a bag; the vacuum cleaner bag should then be sealed and placed outdoors.

I use a CPAP (continuous positive airway pressure) machine to assist my breathing at night. I brought my CPAP along when I had to spend one night in a hospital. The nurse would not allow me to use the device until it was inspected by a respiratory therapist. I could not imagine why this was necessary since I use the CPAP every night without a problem, so I asked the purpose of the inspection. I was told that the respiratory therapist had to make sure that there were no bed bugs or roaches in the device that could infest the hospital! The therapist looked the CPAP over and said it was clean, thankfully.

Whenever Connie and I stay in a hotel, before we move our possessions into a room, we always peel back the bedding from both bottom corners of the bed to expose the mattress. Any blood or other small stains on the mattress could suggest that a bed bug infestation may be present. We have found such stains only once, at a fairly expensive hotel where I was attending a conference. Needless to say we demanded and received another room (at a discount)!

There are many useful products available online to minimize the likelihood of a bed bug infestation. These products include bed and box spring encasings, water traps for bed legs (assuming a harborage isn't in the bed itself), and sticky traps with sex attractants.

ANTS

I have never heard that people have allergic reactions to ants unless bitten. If you do have an ant infestation, I don't recommend liquid or spray pesticides, because chronic exposure to these products can make people chemically sensitive, particularly if these products are incorrectly applied. If you must use pesticide, choose ant baits or a borate pesticide.

Sticky paper traps can give you an idea of the kinds of insects that are in your kitchen (if you really want to know!).

We once had a red ant problem in our kitchen that I discovered when I opened a cabinet that rested on the floor. I was reaching for a cereal box when I noticed that the walls, shelves, and packages were crawling with small red ants. There was a gap between two floorboards that ran under the cabinet. The ants were moving in two well-organized lines inside the crack: one line in, one line out. Ants in the "out" line were carrying bits of my breakfast away to the nest. They disappeared under the baseboard at the outside wall.

When I went into the basement, I could see the marching battalions traveling horizontally in the same two lines in opposite directions along the sill toward the framing beneath the kitchen door. The ant line turned upward directly beneath the threshold. When I went upstairs and outside the kitchen, I could see the army crawling up and down the trim board under the threshold and along a joist beneath the exterior deck. At the end of the joist they marched along a vertical deck support post that went into the soil. The ants were exiting and entering from the bottom of a piece of flagstone resting on the soil next to the post. I lifted the flagstone, and there were my cornflakes. (Often the best solution is patience. Follow the ants as they carry the food home, and then destroy the nest.)

CARPENTER ANTS

Sometimes air quality problems are caused not by the pests themselves but by the damp conditions that attract them. Carpenter ants carve out their nests in wet wood because, like most insects, they thrive in humid environments. When you see evidence of a carpenter ant infestation, you may also find moist wood or another environment that is not only attractive to the ants but also conducive to the growth of mold.

One homeowner called me because she was plagued by big black carpenter ants in her kitchen. She joked that when she baked cookies for her children, she had to set aside extra ones as decoys for the ants. The ants moved in soon after completion of their kitchen addition, an octagonal space containing built-in benches around a table. The roof had a very low slope, the gutters were narrow, and the building lacked an overhang. Water that overflowed the gutters ran directly down the siding rather than away from it. I lifted the hinged seat in the new kitchen addition and measured the moisture content of the drywall with a Tramex meter. The reading suggested excessive moisture, the most likely source of which was rain running down the outside wall.

I recommended that they remove some of the drywall from inside the seats to see if there was decay. I later received a hysterical phone call. At the bottom of each stud bay they opened was a seething, checkered mass of black ants and white ant eggs. Their contractor removed the bottom few inches of drywall from all sides of the addition, and in each bay he found a carpenter ant nest. Though the scene was hideous, there was no damage to the wood. The ants had not needed to chew their way into or through the wood because there were plenty of small gaps and spaces for them to enter the stud bays, and the bays themselves were roomy enough for the nests. The fiberglass insulation kept the temperature constant, and the leaks kept the humidity at Floridian levels.

THE MOIST ATTIC

Because most attics are isolated and are generally open to the environment in one way or another, bees, ants, silverfish, and even cockroaches can nest either in the insulation or on the framing. One homeowner asked me to figure out why there was so much moisture in her attic. I opened the pull-down stairway and ascended. There were insulation batts between the floor joists, and there was no flooring. The batts were installed upside down, with the vapor barrier facing the attic. I poked my finger through the aluminum foil barrier and was able to squeeze water out of the tuft of fiberglass insulation that I removed from the hole.

Moisture was rising up from several sources in the rooms below: an unvented dryer, several room humidifiers, and normal everyday activities such as showering, cooking, and even breathing. I noticed many holes in the vapor barrier. The attic did not have adequate ventilation to the exterior, so I suspected that, in the winter, moisture was condensing on the roof sheathing, dripping from the nails, pooling on top of the vapor barrier, and leaking through rips into the insulation.

I was surprised at how much moisture I found, even though I understood why it was there. But what lay ahead was like a scene from a horror movie. As I walked carefully on top of the framing through the tropical attic to the opposite gable end, my attention was drawn to an oval damp spot on the brick chimney where moisture was condensing on the masonry that must have been below the dew point of the humid attic air. I saw a textured black circle several feet in diameter on top of the vapor barrier near the chimney. As I neared the area I realized that the circle consisted of thousands of carpenter ants, basking motionless in the warm, moist attic atmosphere. I was so unsettled that I tiptoed away, afraid that the vibrations of my steps would raise the hordes and send them scurrying in my direction.

STINGING INSECTS

BEES

In one home I inspected, I asked why many of the living room windows were taped shut. The homeowner told me that he was trying to keep bees out of his home. I thought that the bees were more likely entering through the fireplace, since I had seen what resembled a busy airport of bees flying in and out at the top of his chimney. He asked if I thought that a fire in the fireplace would "smoke them out." I recommended instead that he call a PCO who specialized in beehive removal.

Weeks later, he told me that the PCO had wanted too much money to remove the hive and kill the bees, so the man decided instead to smoke the bees out. The heat from the fire that he lit in his fireplace melted the wax in the hive, and half of the hive fell from the top of the chimney down into the fireplace. Dozens of bees flew into the house, and the man was stung seven times before he escaped. Luckily, he wasn't allergic to bee stings, but now his chimney was lined with wax and honey in addition to creosote, so the chimney had to be cleaned.

In the living room of another house I inspected, I noticed a slight bubbling in the paint above a sliding door. I crossed the room to have a better look. I accidentally touched the paint when I pointed to the spot. A large section of the wall caved in, leaving a big hole. The chunk that fell out consisted solely of paint that was thinner than a piece of paper. There had been a beehive in the wall, and in expanding their hive the insects had removed all the plaster and paper from the drywall. Outside the sliding door was an obvious hole where bees had entered and exited. Luckily for me, the hive by that time was inactive.

This wasn't the case in another home. A woman noticed a stain on the wall of her family room. She rubbed her finger over it and discovered that the sticky film was honey. She looked carefully over the wall and saw small drops of honey everywhere. She called a PCO who found an active beehive within the wall cavities. He killed the bees and removed more than 50 pounds of honey from the hive! In this case, a small hole to the interior of the home might have been deadly. (If you wish to avoid killing bees, you might consider calling a beekeeper to remove a hive.)

YELLOW JACKETS

We have our own tale to tell about stinging insects. Connie and I used to live in a house with a mudroom at the rear entrance. One day she noticed that yellow jackets were flying in and out of a hole above the back door. Connie is afraid of bees, wasps, and yellow jackets, so she asked me to call a PCO. Unfortunately, we lived in a college town, and it was September, when schools open for the academic year. Every PCO I called was busy for a few days, removing bees from college dorms. One PCO said he'd come to the house in three days. In the meantime, yellow jackets found their way to our bedroom by flying upward through wall cavities. I didn't mind because I knew that the insects would be quiescent at night, but Connie was terrified.

She slept on the living room couch for one night and then called me the following afternoon.

"Where are you?" I asked.

"I've moved into a hotel," she replied, "and will come back when the beehive is gone."

I called the PCO to relay our situation, and he agreed to come over the following afternoon to rescue us.

PESTICIDES

Wherever possible, I prefer to see physical means used rather than pesticides to kill microarthropods and arthropods. The simplest way to do this is by using steam from a steam vapor machine (such machines are discussed in chap. 24). When the nozzle tool is placed less than an inch from a surface, the temperature of the steam (water vapor) will kill most microarthropods and arthropods, including mites as well as bed bugs. In addition to the edge seams, every surface of the entire bed must be thoroughly heated with the steam vapor using a wide tool. For more widespread major infestations, an entire home or building may be heated (called thermal treatment) to about 120°F with air blasted from gas heaters.

If you suspect that a small clothing item or book may contain bed bugs, and you are absolutely certain that there is no metal or foil (including metalized thread) present, you can place the dry item in a microwave for about 10 seconds to kill any microarthropods and arthropods that may be present.

Some people use pesticides to get rid of ants and bees. My own mother-in-law used to spray pesticides liberally when she saw ants on kitchen shelves and bees around windows. Another woman with an ant invasion in her kitchen drilled holes and sprayed volatile pesticide (a liquid that evaporates) into every stud bay in the kitchen. She became chemically sensitive and could not tolerate even perfume. The woman is convinced that her sensitivity began shortly after her exposure to the pesticide.

Most people get upset when they see ants running around their kitchen or bees flying up against their windows. Often the first thought is to run out and buy a can of spray pesticide. I encourage you to resist this impulse. I don't recommend using pesticides indoors, because these chemicals can have toxic effects on the hunter as well as the hunted. It's much better to use ant baits (which keep the chemical fairly well contained), a rolled-up newspaper, or a sticky insect strip. You can also try to capture a bee in a paper cup and release it outside. After all, the bee wants to get out of your home, right? That's why it's buzzing up against a window.

SOME RECOMMENDATIONS

- The tops of books should be vacuumed periodically with a HEPA vacuum (a vacuum with high-efficiency particulate arrestance filtration).

- If you are particularly sensitive to mold or arthropod or micro-arthropod fecal pellets, store your books in closed cases.

- Be careful about accepting or buying books that may have been stored in damp spaces.

- Limit the use of pesticides indoors.

- Don't over-humidify your home.

- Check the hotel mattress for evidence of bed bug activity before moving your possessions into the room.

THE THREE Ps—
PETS, PESTS, AND PEOPLE

PETS

Before I became allergic to pets, I loved them. I grew up with a dog and even had a cat in my apartment while in graduate school. There are millions of dogs and cats in the United States, and I understand the enormous amount of love and companionship that pets add to the lives of families. For those of you who are pet lovers, please excuse my focusing on the negative aspect of pet ownership, but I am trying to help those who suffer from pet allergies.

Pets are soft and cuddly, but their fur acts like a "living dust mop" that can pick up allergenic dust from the surroundings. Dogs and cats like to hide under furniture, and they can pick up and spread the moldy dust that I often find on the bottoms of older couches and easy chairs. Many people keep their kitty litter boxes in moldy basements, and cats can spread spores from basement mold to the upstairs.

Some people who own beloved pets continue to keep the animals around even though the owners' eyes swell and their noses run. I had one client who was so attached to her dog that she built a heated shed in her backyard for the pet. She walked the dog and allowed herself to pet the animal every day, but she quickly washed her hands afterward to avoid having an allergic reaction. It's virtually impossible for someone who is highly allergic to a pet to share a home with the animal without experiencing some difficulty. Many people are willing to endure allergy symptoms, though, as a consequence of living with their beloved pets. Sniffling is one thing; asthma is another. And if not cared for properly, dogs and cats can cause unpleasant odors.

One client in her seventies called me because, after a life completely free of allergies, she suddenly developed asthma. She had two enormous puppies that were not house-trained and often "made mistakes" on her white wall-to-wall carpeting. As a result, she had to wash the carpeting frequently. There were biodegradable materials, including skin scales and dog waste, trapped in the carpet fibers. When moisture was introduced, the carpet became a haven for mold and bacteria. When I sampled air in the room, I found that about 30 percent of the particles were related to biological growth in the carpet. When I described the situation to my client, her response was, "I will never get rid of my poochies!"

Another person contacted me because he noticed a disturbing odor in the finished basement of a house he was thinking of purchasing. He and his family really liked the property, but they were considering walking away from it if they could not determine the cause of the odor. I parked in front of the house and noticed two dogs frolicking in the fenced front yard. The real estate broker who met me at the site said that he thought the odor was emanating from the automatic fragrance emitters that were spraying perfume into the basement at regular intervals. I asked the broker to turn these emitters off.

The house was sixty years old, and the basement contained a billiards room with mahogany-paneled walls and an oak parquet floor. A carton of a dozen aerosol air fresheners was on a shelf above the built-in bar. When I shined a bright flashlight beam along the floor, I could see that the oak strips were warped and swollen. The room reeked of animal urine. Numerous nail holes with oval black stains in the wood floor suggested that the floor had once been carpeted.

I checked the wood floor with a moisture meter, which measures resistance to the flow of electric current. The readings were off the scale. It was a wretchedly humid day, but the high meter readings were due not to moisture in the wood but to salts from animal urine. Outside, I explained to my client that the only way to get rid of the odor completely was to remove the antique flooring. It was a shame because the wood was exquisite.

Another family had their new house completely cleaned before they moved in because their son was so allergic to dogs that he experienced anaphylaxis from exposure to dog allergen. The prior occupants had a dog, so the family hired me to advise them on what to do to make the home habitable for their son. I told them that they might never be able to remove all the dog allergens from the house, but I advised them to eliminate all the carpeting, replace the furnace and all

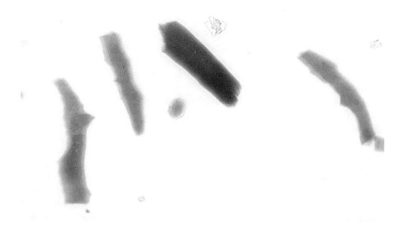

FIGURE 5.1. The four long, irregularly shaped "rectangles" are poodle dander particles. The smaller, oval particle near the center is either a *Penicillium* or an *Aspergillus* mold spore, referred to as a Pen/Asp spore (since spores from these two different genera cannot be readily distinguished by microscopy). All of the biological particles took up the pink acid fuchsin stain. The small, colorless particles are inorganic particles, which do not take up stain (500× light micrograph).

the ductwork, and eliminate all dust from electric boxes, light fixtures, walls, and ceilings. The only things they saved were the expensive curtains the wife wanted to keep. She stored the curtains in tightly sealed plastic bags, hoping that later she could have them cleaned to remove whatever dog allergens might be present. The family moved into the home, and for months their son experienced no allergy symptoms. One day his mother opened the bag with the curtains to show them to a friend. She didn't even remove the curtains from the bag, but nonetheless some dog allergens were released into the air. Her son went into anaphylactic shock and had to be rushed to a hospital (fig. 5.1).

DOG BEDS

I've taken dust samples from deeply cushioned dog beds, many of which contained some mold spores and evidence of mite infestation. Such beds may be cozy for dogs, but they are also hard to clean. As dogs drool and shed their skin scales (dander), they create conditions conducive to microbial growth. Dogs carry mite and mold allergens on their bodies. If a dog picks up a gravid female mite from the dog bed, mite infestations can spread to other furniture in your home, including your own bed. In some cases, dogs can even develop allergic reactions such as skin irritation and asthma. These are the reasons why I recommend that blankets be used as dog beds, and that the blankets be washed on a regular basis.

CATS

One boy who slept with his cat every night woke up each morning with a rash on his face. The parents identified the source of the irritation when they realized that the cat spent much of the day sleeping in the exposed fiberglass ceiling insulation in their basement. Fiberglass fibers often have sharp ends similar to broken glass. When the boy slept with his face next to his cuddly pet, his skin was irritated by the insulation fibers stuck to the animal's fur.

OTHER MAMMAL PETS

Some people have pet gerbils and guinea pigs that they keep in cages. Many of these animals shed dander or fur, and if their cages are not kept sparkling clean, microbial growth can occur in the sawdust or other bedding at the bottom of the cage (urine and spilled water supply the moisture needed for microbial growth). Children like to play with animals like this, so they may remove the animals from their cages, exposing themselves to pet allergens.

I investigated one home in which the owners had two pet ferrets before they had any children. They kept the ferret cages in a carpeted room on the first floor, but the ferrets were allowed out of their cages to wander throughout the home. The couple kept small triangular litter boxes in every corner of the home because the ferrets could not be house-trained. They called me after they had their first child because the infant was developing asthma. The couple had converted the ferrets' old room into the infant's bedroom, and they hadn't replaced the carpet. The woman told me that she loved the animals and couldn't bear the thought of parting with them, so the couple wanted to be sure that the ferrets weren't the cause of their child's health symptoms.

I was looking around the finished basement and was startled when large lumps within the couch started moving around. The woman said that the ferrets liked to spend the day inside the couch. She somehow extracted them and I asked to take a photograph of her and her beloved pets. She held each ferret on an outstretched bare arm. When she put the animals down, she had welts on the skin of each arm where the ferrets had lain. Apparently, she and her infant were allergic to the ferrets. I recommended that she replace the carpeting in the infant's bedroom and try to find another loving home for the ferrets.

FISH

One day I received a call from a retired professor. Although he had never had any allergies before, now he was wheezing and sniffling and could no longer enjoy his new leisure life. Occasionally, his symptoms even appeared at his favorite seafood restaurant. Once when he was sitting there with friends, his nose ran so much that he had to apologize and leave before the meal was finished. He had even been told to see a psychiatrist because his nose started to run whenever he entered two specific areas of his home.

There were tropical fish tanks in both his home and the restaurant. The tank in his den at home had a black plastic cover with a hinged access panel so he could feed the fish. I lifted the cover and saw a layer of fine brown "dust" adhering to the underside. I took a sticky-tape sample of the dust and looked at it under my microscope. Dust mites were there, wriggling and stuck to the tape, but the brown dust consisted entirely of damp mite fecal pellets that were being digested by bacteria. When the man threw fish food flakes into the tank, some of the flakes stuck to the underside of the opened cover. It's not surprising that I found this microcosm, since fish food is as appealing to dust mites as skin scales are. (Dust mite colonies in laboratories are fed high-protein fish flakes.)

I didn't find many whole dust mite fecal pellets in the air in the room, but I did find fragments of pellets as well as clumps of bacteria and small bits of partially digested skin scales. The irony is that sometimes the only pets that people with asthma can have are fish, and in this case (and perhaps in others) the fish tank was a source of allergens. The man cleaned the fish tank and its lid as well as the surfaces in the room, and his nose stopped dripping when he was at home.

Fish tanks are also the source of other problems that can lead to IAQ issues. Sometimes a filter placed on the outside of the tank leaks onto shelves, the wall, and the floors. One unfortunate youngster was enthusiastic about feeding his fish, and he often spilled fish food onto the floor near the tank. Water from the leaking exterior filter dripped onto the fish flakes, and mold soon proliferated in the carpet. Another tank's leaking filter led to mold growth on the M, N, and O volumes of an encyclopedia on a shelf below the aquarium. Filtration and aeration systems placed inside a fish tank bubble through the water, and algae and other bioaerosols are dispersed into the room when the bubbles break at the water's surface.

Children who have pet allergies are sometimes allowed to have fish tanks in their bedrooms. Not a great idea.

PESTS

MICE

Significant mouse infestations can cause unpleasant odors, one of the most familiar of which is that of a dead mouse. This odor smells like rotten meat and usually dissipates within a few weeks after the mouse has died, most likely in a wall cavity out of view.

One couple looking for a new home fell in love with a house that had a spacious, unfinished basement that was insulated with exposed fiberglass. The woman noticed on their first visit to the property that there was a litter box in the basement for the owners' two cats. Although the woman was highly allergic to cats, the couple decided to buy the house anyway. Before they moved in, they asked me for advice on how they could renovate the basement in a way that would remove allergens, because they hoped to carve two home offices out of the space.

There was evidence of moisture in the basement, so I was concerned about cat dander particles as well as mold that may have accumulated in the fiberglass insulation. I recommended that they have all the insulation removed, the joists and subfloor HEPA vacuumed, and all accessible wood structures spray-painted before moving in or constructing any finished basement rooms.

They both called me to report on the progress being made after the work had begun. As the insulation was being removed, so many mouse droppings fell down that the concrete floor beneath was barely visible. When people walked across the floor, their feet crunched mouse skeletons that were swaddled in fiberglass. The cats that lived in that house must have been pretty lazy! And I was worried about cat dander particles.

There is another odor associated with a mouse infestation. Mice communicate through their urine, so they leave a trail of it wherever they go. The alpha mouse has a particular pheromone in his urine, and a female mouse indicates when she is in estrus with a pheromone in her urine. Mouse urine contains mouse urinary proteins (MUPs), the purpose of which is to help the pheromones persist in the urine trails. Some of these MUPs are allergens. As mice skitter along their urine trails, they wet the dust under their paws anew with more urine, and they aerosolize some of the dust with their movements (figs. 5.2 and 5.3).

Mice typically follow the same paths throughout a building and therefore leave well-defined trails of purplish-stained urine. These trails can be found on electric cables, PVC pipes, the vertical corners of foundation concrete, the tops of foundation walls, and on foundation walls under joists and beams where the structural members block the rodents' passage on top of the foundation, forcing them to run around and under the wood. It's amazing how mice seem to be able to move horizontally and vertically up a smooth foundation wall! Mouse urine trails on the tops of foundation walls and other horizontal surfaces can also be littered with mouse droppings.

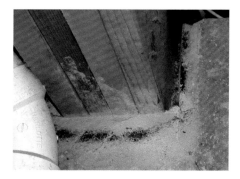

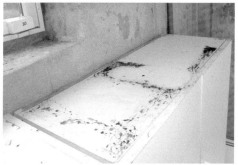

FIGURE 5.2. This photograph, taken in a basement, shows a rust-colored mouse urine trail on foundation concrete. Mice are adept climbers; they can scale a vertical concrete surface. Mice typically run along the top of a foundation wall, but in this case they encountered the sizable wooden main beam and were forced to travel under it in order to continue their trip along the foundation top.

FIGURE 5.3. These mouse urine trails were left by mice racing around the top of a shelf where there had been stored items. The obstacles, probably cans and boxes, are no longer present. The mouse urine trails probably represent dozens of trips made by more than one mouse.

On three occasions I was curious about what might be in the dust in mouse urine trails, so I took tape samples from the trails. In all cases, there was *Aspergillus* mold growth or other types of mold growth in the dust. It makes sense that dust that is intermittently dampened will become moldy. The result is that in addition to smelling the odor of mouse urine trails, people are also being exposed to allergenic mold spores.

I recently investigated a home with two odor problems. A prior owner had a dog that was not well cared for and therefore damaged furnishings and surfaces. The home's new owners thought that the dog was the cause of the odor and eliminated carpet and even subflooring stained with dog urine. After this work was completed, another odor remained that was caused by a mouse infestation. There were extensive mouse urine trails as well as mouse droppings on top of ceiling tiles and behind walls in the finished basement. The new owners ended up tearing out the entire finished basement, finding a shocking number of mouse carcasses and droppings. The mice had been entering the house from the exterior through an opening around piping for the air conditioning compressor. They probably had been attracted by the dog food that the previous owner had kept stored in the basement. The opening was sealed as part of the basement remediation work (fig. 5.4).

In another home with a massive mouse infestation I found the rodent entry point: a golf-ball-sized hole in the foundation. The hole was not readily visible from the front of the house because the

A study of indoor asthma symptoms correlated an increased presence of mouse allergens with exacerbated asthma symptoms.

E. Matsui, "Management of Rodent Exposure and Allergy in the Pediatric Population," *Current Allergy and Asthma Reports* 136, no. 10 (December 2013): 681–686; Johns Hopkins Medicine, "High Levels of Airborne Mouse Allergen in Inner-City Homes Could Trigger Asthma Attacks," press release, February 10, 2005, https://www.hopkinsmedicine.org/Press_releases/2005/02_10a_05.html.

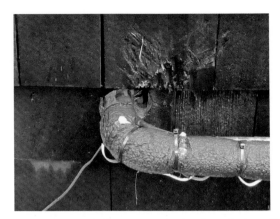

FIGURE 5.4. A mouse entry hole appears in shingles alongside air conditioning lines at the rear exterior of a home that had an enormous mouse problem. An insulated hose from an air conditioning compressor entered the exterior shingled wall, and there was a round hole alongside the piping. The round hole was likely partially chewed out by mice to expand the opening. The scratch marks in the shingle above the hole are probably from a frustrated animal, possibly a dog or a big cat that tried to chase the mice before they entered the hole.

opening was beneath the front entry stairs. The occupants sealed the entry hole and trapped as many mice as they could that remained in the house. To get rid of the odor caused by the infestation, they removed all the basement ceiling tiles, which were covered with mouse droppings on the top side. The owners asked me to return to the site to find out why the mouse odor remained despite all their efforts to get rid of it. They had removed the drywall from a ceiling soffit. When I looked into this soffit with a mirror and flashlight, I could see that a plank running from the front of the basement to the rear was deeply stained with mouse urine. The couple removed the board, and the odor problem was solved.

I have heard many folks and even PCOs (pest control operators) lament that mouse infestations are inevitable, especially in wooded areas. Nonsense! The only reason that mice find their way into buildings is because people are not careful enough about sealing up rodent entryways. If you look carefully around your home (don't forget to check the soffit and ridge vents), eliminate any pest openings, and trap the rodents within, you should be able to end a mouse infestation.

SHREWS

It's annoying to have an indoor mouse invasion, but shrews are a whole step up in the "annoying pest" category!

In the last few years we have received many phone calls from occupants who were desperate to find out the sources of powerful, unpleasant odors in their homes. The odors were caused by shrews in nearly every case. We have had more than 60 cases where shrew infestations made the indoor air quality intolerable in homes, schools, and offices. Sometimes the odor smells skunk-like and chemical, and other times the odor is intensely musty.

Shrews have odiferous body musk; they smell so unpleasant that they have few natural predators. Shrews also defecate in thick piles that become wet with their urine, leading to mold growth that is responsible for the musty odor associated with these animals. Shrews are often mistaken for mice because they, too, are small and gray but they have longer snouts. Shrews are primarily meat eaters; their prey includes mice, larger soil larvae, and slugs. Shews can be vicious; some species have toxic venom to paralyze their prey.

Before my first shrew case, I had never even heard of these animals or even the word (except for in Shakespeare's famous play, *The Taming of the Shrew*). In that first case, we sent some droppings to a state agricultural lab, which confirmed that the droppings were from shrews. I have found shrew infestations in wall cavities even on the second floor. In one case a young couple expecting their first child moved out of their master bedroom for fear that their unborn child would be affected by the stench in the room. In another case a family sealed off a beautiful study in their home with plastic sheeting to prevent the odor from permeating their entire house. I even found a substantial shrew infestation in fiberglass insulation above the drop ceilings in two classrooms in a daycare facility. The school had stopped using the classrooms because the odor was so strong.

Why have shrews begun to inhabit buildings? My theory is that when people started putting garbage out in plastic bags rather than metal pails, the outdoor food supply for rodents increased dramatically. This led to an explosion in the mouse population. Since shrews eat mice, an increase in the shrew population followed. Shrews in the outdoor environment nest in the ground and in stone walls (you may notice a strong skunk-like chemical odor from shrew musk when you walk by a stone wall). Shrews may also choose to nest near or even in your home and defecate inside or just outside the building.

One of the characteristics of shrew odors is that they can be intermittent, depending on wind direction. If shrews are nesting under the landing of a home or just outside of the foundation, people may notice a powerful odor outside or even inside the home when the wind blows toward the nest and forces the odor into the house. If the shrews are nesting in an exterior wall cavity (a wall that faces the exterior), the wall cavity will be pressurized when wind blows against that side of the building. Then air will flow from the cavity through outlets and other gaps into the room, carrying the odors of the shrews and their droppings. A day later, if the wind direction switches, there may be little or no odor at all.

Interestingly, there is little awareness among PCOs about the problem of shrew infestation. Perhaps it's because most people mistakenly think the odor is caused by mold, and therefore they do not contact a pest control company for help. I have given presentations at two PCO conferences, and when I asked how many of them had ever encountered a shrew problem, not one of the more than 100 listeners' hands was raised.

Because shrews are primarily meat eaters, they can be trapped using a standard mouse snap trap, but the trap should be baited with beef jerky rather than cheese. If you place a trap outdoors, put a box over the trap (to keep larger animals out) and a rock on top of the box to hold it in place. Cut two small "mouse holes" in the box to allow the shrew to enter. Make certain that the trap is secure to a base so that it will not flip when tripped. Shrews are present in pairs, so if you catch one you will probably catch another, so don't give up.

PEOPLE

Spiritualists believe that people are surrounded by an aura or energy field. Some believers say they can see the colors in peoples' auras. Being a pragmatist (as well as a scientist), I see the human aura in a different light.

I agree that every individual has an aura consisting of body odors (bad breath, underarm odor, etc.) and fragrances from the cleaning and personal care products that people use. Everyone also has what I call a "dust aura." Each of us is surrounded by a cloud of dust particles that emanate from our hair, our skin, and our clothing. These particles consist of our own skin scales as well as particles such as dust mite droppings, mold spores, and pet dander particles that we pick up on our bodies and in our clothing and hair as we go about our daily business. Dog and cat allergens have been found in classrooms in which no pets have ever been present[1] because children and teachers carry allergens from their pets into school with them. Other children and adults may react to such pet allergens.

I have many allergies, including dog, cat, dust mite, and mold. Connie and I were staying in a hotel for a conference at which I was giving a presentation. I put on my jacket and tie and entered the hallway to get on the elevator. A young woman was rushing down the hallway with her wheeled suitcase to catch the elevator. I started coughing as she walked by me. At first I thought my reaction might have been due to an allergy to the dust on my jacket, so I rushed back into the room to use my inhaler and change jackets. Connie pointed out that I had worn the same jacket the prior evening and had not experienced any problem. It was then that I realized that it must have been the young woman's dust aura to which I had reacted. Despite the cleanliness of her appearance, some allergens were being emitted from her clothing. I waited for a few moments for the hallway dust to settle and then entered the hallway and had no problem breathing. But I made sure to take a different elevator down to the lobby.

FRAGRANCES

I once saw a client of mine being interviewed on a television show about people who are bothered by scented products. One day while she was crossing the street to go to her physician's office, a car stopped in front of her. The window was open, and the driver was drenched with aftershave. She was wheezing by the time she reached the doctor's office.

There seems to be a growing awareness that scents can be irritating to some people. Even so, many cleaning and body products contain fragrances.

The office of one of Connie's doctors posts a sign asking patients not to wear any scented products when they enter the space. I applaud such efforts to reduce the use of fragrances. I am sensitive to fragrances myself. I sometimes cannot walk down the laundry detergent aisle in a supermarket without wheezing, and I also cough and wheeze around scented candles and fragrance emitters. Fragrances are chemicals, after all, and their use adds to the chemical load in indoor as well as outdoor air.

SMOKE GETS IN OUR LUNGS

When health is an issue, it sometimes takes decades for the scientific community to recognize a danger. Lead was a common ingredient in gasoline, paint, and food cans until the second half of the twentieth century, when its use in such products was banned. Asbestos has been recognized as a carcinogen, but that discovery came too late for pipe fitters and shipbuilders who were exposed to asbestos dust from insulation.

The public recognition that smoking causes lung cancer and heart disease is relatively recent (in the mid-1960s, the US Surgeon General started issuing warnings about the dangers of tobacco smoking).[2] People still smoke, though, and even exposure to secondhand smoke is a serious health concern. Cigarette smoke contains hundreds of known toxins, including formaldehyde, carbon monoxide, and hydrogen cyanide. One of the cruelest things to do to a child with asthma is to smoke in the child's home. Even a person without asthma might be sensitive to cigarette smoke. If you, anyone you love, or anyone in your household is sensitive to cigarette smoke or has asthma, it is essential that no one smokes there. In addition, avoid going into any bars or restaurants that allow smoking.

I worry about secondhand exposure to marijuana smoke. Research is being undertaken on this subject,[3] but it makes sense that exposure to any kind of smoke, including smoke produced by burning substances that contain chemicals injurious to human health, poses a threat. I am also concerned about exposure to the aerosol produced by vaping. In addition to nicotine, this aerosol contains numerous chemicals that could be harmful to the person who is vaping and potentially unhealthy to others nearby.[4,5,6] The Surgeon General's 2018 advisory on e-cigarettes states: "In addition to nicotine, the aerosol that users inhale and exhale from e-cigarettes can potentially expose both themselves and bystanders to other harmful substances, including heavy metals, volatile organic compounds, and ultrafine particles that can be inhaled deeply into the lungs."[7] This caution is warranted. On one of its websites, the Centers for Disease Control and Prevention reports that "As of October 1, 2019, 1,080 lung injury cases associated with e-cigarette, or vaping, products have been reported to the CDC from 48 states and 1 U.S. territory. Eighteen deaths have been confirmed in 15 states."[8]

People sometimes call me because they are bothered by smoke in their apartments. Sometimes the odor comes from a smoker several floors below and is carried by hidden air currents within the building's structure. We discuss the issue of smoke and odor infiltration in apartments in chapter 14, on multi-unit buildings.

SOME RECOMMENDATIONS

FRAGRANCES

- If someone who lives in your home or spends a great deal of time there has allergies or asthma, avoid using perfumed products.

PESTS

- If you find mouse urine trails inside your home, use a HEPA vacuum to remove the dust, and then disinfect the surface with either a dilute bleach solution (one part bleach to sixteen parts water) or with any suitable cleaning product (see chap. 24 for cautions about using bleach). When doing this work, wear a NIOSH N95 two-strap mask (available at building supply stores) and operate a fan on exhaust to vent air from the work area.

- Be sure you have an airtight inner door at the foot of your bulkhead stairs.

- Any openings between an attached garage and the house that could allow rodent entry should be sealed.

- Add gaskets or sweeps to your garage doors as needed to make them tightly fitting.

- Look carefully around the exterior of your home for any gaps or openings (including around pipes and cables) that could be rodent pathways and seal them as needed with metal mesh and foam, masonry, or wood as appropriate.

- Use mousetraps bated with beef jerky to catch shrews.

- Trim plantings around a building to leave an 18-inch to 2-foot free space, so you can keep an eye out for rodent activity (as well as moisture problems).

PETS

- Use old blankets for dog beds. Wash the blankets on a regular basis.

- Keep pet food in an airtight container, preferably not in a location where pests can find pet food bits that may fall on the floor.

- Keep the area around your pet food dish clean.

- Keep dogs, cats, hamsters, and other pets as well as fish tanks out of bedrooms.

- If anyone in your household is experiencing allergic reactions to your pet dog or cat, try to find a new loving home for the animal.

- If you or anyone in your household has pet allergies, be careful about accepting furniture, rugs, or curtains from people who may own pets.

- People who own pets should not lie on the bed of anyone who has pet allergies.

- If your child has pet allergies or is allergic to mites, ask that rabbits, mice, gerbils, guinea pigs, and other animals as well as fish tanks not be allowed in his or her classroom or even in the school library.

SMOKING

- There should be absolutely no smoking (including cigarettes, marijuana, vaping, etc.) in the home of a person with asthma. Children should also be protected from such exposures.

6.

THE SET

In the first five chapters we introduced a cast of characters both microscopic and visible that inhabit the "stages" of our homes. Now we will look at the "set" on which these creatures act out their roles, including our rugs and furniture. Whether the drama that unfolds is a tragedy or comedy depends on the conditions within our homes.

CARPETING AND AREA RUGS

Many carpets and rugs are fine, but some are fiber jungles alive with mites, carpet beetles, mold, or pet dander particles. Even new carpeting and rugs can be contaminated if they have been stored in damp or dirty spaces. If you moved into a new home that already had carpeting or you acquired used or even antique rugs, you may not know whether people who used such carpeting or rugs had dogs or cats, or whether the carpeting or rugs were already infested with mold or mites before you added them to your décor (figs. 6.1 and 6.2).

UNWANTED GUESTS

I have taken many samples of the air above Oriental rugs after patting them to disturb the dust. One woman had trouble breathing in the office corner of her living room. The dust from the rug contained significant amounts of *Aspergillus* mold. She had bought the rug from an antique dealer and had no idea who had owned it or under what conditions the rug had been stored. In a family with allergies or asthma, previously owned rugs must be chosen with great care and professionally cleaned before use.

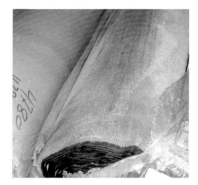

FIGURE 6.1. These two rolls of carpet were in a hotel storage area, where they were about to be cut up and installed in hotel guest rooms. I noticed the stain at the edge and top of the roll (with torn plastic) at the right. The top of the roll looked as if it had been stored on a floor that got wet.

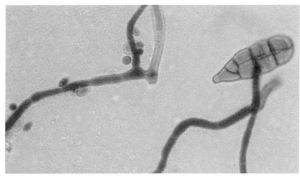

FIGURE 6.2. This micrograph shows mold spores and hyphae. Curious to see if there was any mold growth in the roll of hotel carpet that appeared to have gotten wet, I pressed some sticky tape onto the discolored area of the carpet backing to remove a dust sample, cut off a section of the tape, stained it with acid fuchsin, and looked at the piece of tape with a microscope. There was already mold growth on the carpet backing; the micrograph depicts pink-stained hyphae and a large brown *Alternaria* spore. There are some smaller pink-stained spores alongside the hyphae. I hope that I never stay in a hotel room containing this section of carpet (500× light micrograph)!

Carpeting and rugs can become contaminated if vacuumed infrequently or washed by amateurs. Just as pillows and mattresses emit allergens when compressed, carpet fibers can emit thousands of airborne allergens with every step. And once present in the dust, some allergens can cause symptoms for the life of the carpet or rug. Both rugs and wall-to-wall carpets can harbor the same ecosystems, but a contaminated rug can be rolled up (carefully!), removed, and professionally washed. Contaminated wall-to-wall carpeting, on the other hand, is usually left in place far too long.

Moisture and carpets do not make a good combination. I received a call from a management company that was dealing with a complaint from a first-floor tenant. The building was slab-on-grade, meaning there was no basement, and the flooring of the unit was carpeting on concrete. Though the management company had replaced all the carpeting in the bedroom before the tenant moved in two months earlier, the tenant claimed that mold grew on his shoes when he kept them under his bed. I was skeptical, but I took room air samples and bulk samples of the dust under the bed for microscopic analysis. There were spores in the air, which didn't surprise me, but I was amazed to see that there was *Aspergillus* mold growing on the surface of the carpeting beneath the bed.

How did this happen? Many factors were involved. The tenant spent little time in the apartment, and he kept the windows closed so that airflow in and out of the unit was at a minimum. It was a humid

When lead-containing paint was in common usage, many carpets became contaminated with toxic lead dust. Even after numerous passes with a vacuum, all the dust can never be removed from a carpet. Carpets contaminated with lead dust must be replaced.

summer, and the air both inside and outside the apartment was laden with moisture. The carpeting in this apartment was laid directly on the "cool" concrete, which may have created dew-point conditions. The tenant took long hot showers in the morning and did not air out the bathroom afterward to reduce moisture levels. In addition, a downspout was creating puddles outside the building at the edge of the concrete slab. I recommended that the management company install a dehumidifier in the unit, that the downspout be redirected away from the building, that the tenant air out the apartment after he took a shower, and that the wall-to-wall carpet be replaced. Then, so long as the relative humidity near the floor was kept at no more than 50 percent, mold would no longer be an issue.

I once inspected a school building in which the carpets had been washed over the summer. Since school was not in session, the air conditioning was not operating while the building was closed up. The carpets therefore remained damp long enough for microbial growth to ensue. The carpets were so moldy that they all had to be replaced.

Carpets and rugs can be treated with steam vapor from a steam vapor machine (see chap. 24). Wall-to-wall carpeting and area rugs that still smell musty after being treated with steam vapor or that are still causing occupants to have health symptoms should be removed under containment conditions. Wherever environmentally sensitive people live or work, solid flooring rather than carpeting should be installed, because solid flooring is easier to clean and does not capture the same amount of biodegradable dust. (I once calculated that a square foot of carpet has 70 times more surface area than a square foot of hard flooring, so a carpet can capture more dust.)

I am familiar with the argument that carpets help clean indoor air because they capture dust the way a filter captures dust, but this analogy doesn't hold up because we don't walk across a filter. If we did, that activity would aerosolize the dust, which is what happens when people walk across carpeting or area rugs. The aerosolized dust will be allergenic if the carpet or rug contains mold or bacterial growth. I've worked with many clients who replaced the carpeting in the rooms in their new home but left the carpeting on the stairs and in hallways. Often this carpeting has experienced the most foot traffic and can be contaminated with microbial growth.

OTHER CARPETING CONCERNS

Chemicals emitted from new wall-to-wall carpeting can be irritating. In most cases the odor disappears within a few days with no lasting negative effects, but sometimes carpets continue to off-gas for a long time.

Even the US Environmental Protection Agency (EPA) had problems in its own offices with emissions from new carpeting.[1] Thirty thousand square yards of new carpet were installed during a 1987 renovation. Within months, about 60 employees complained of symptoms such as hoarseness and headaches. Many studies were done, some pointing to off-gassing of chemicals from the carpet backing and some claiming that the illnesses were psychogenic (the result of mass hysteria). Ultimately, all the carpeting was replaced with carpeting that had a different kind of backing, and nearly all of the complaints stopped.

One day I received a call from a woman who was experiencing eye irritation and had to revert to glasses after ten years of wearing her contact lenses without difficulty. The irritation started shortly after she and her husband moved into their new home, which had wall-to-wall carpeting on every floor. She insisted her eye problem was somehow related to the house. Her husband, a contractor who had designed and built the house as a gift to her, was deeply offended.

The couple answered my knock together when I came to inspect the house. The woman welcomed me warmly, but her husband was silent and seemed skeptical and hostile. Moments later as I stood in the doorway, my eyes and lips started to burn. I detected the strong, characteristic odor of new carpeting. Perhaps you have noticed this smell in homes or stores. The odor has been attributed to 4-phenylcyclohexene (4-PC), a chemical in carpet backing made with styrene-butadiene plastic (the same chemical that caused the odor in the EPA's headquarters). Both the wife and I were affected by this chemical but the husband was not.

The carpeting in the basement was made with a different backing and had no 4-PC odor. After my visit the husband and wife tried moving their bedroom from the second floor of the gracious twelve-room house into the partially finished basement, and all her symptoms went away. The husband was finally convinced that the upstairs carpeting had caused a problem for his wife.

OFF-GASSING

Carpeting is only one of many materials that can off-gas annoying and even irritating chemicals that cause headaches, hoarseness, and other symptoms in some sensitized individuals. Some vinyl-fiberglass screens, leveling compounds, and adhesives can off-gas for weeks, months, or even years. Heat can intensify the off-gassing. I used to have a booth at the annual Old House Fair in Boston, sponsored by the Boston Preservation Alliance. One year I set up a vinyl-fiberglass screen (from my own storm door) with a hot lamp shining on it to demonstrate off-gassing. A homeowner sniffed the screen and exclaimed, "That's the smell that's been driving me crazy in my house for the past three years!"

One woman called me because she wanted to eliminate a burning odor she had been noticing in her condominium for quite some time. She had just come home from the hospital with her newborn baby and was concerned about the child's health as well as her own. The other unit in the two-family building had recently converted from oil to gas heat. She had already called the gas company and fire department to investigate potential sources of the odor to no avail. The man from the fire department had even implied that she might be unbalanced and hysterical after pregnancy and childbirth.

She told me that the smell was strongest in the dining room and in the late morning. As soon as I arrived, I smelled the acrid odor of heated vinyl-fiberglass insect screens. The screens were installed between the new storm windows and the old, leaky double-hung sash windows. The smell was strongest at the south-facing dining room wall, which started warming in the sun around ten o'clock in the morning. The owner told me that the odor hadn't started until several months after the windows were installed, so at first she had a hard time believing the screens could be causing the odor, even though she immediately recognized the smell when she sniffed the air near the windows. Then she remembered that just before the odor began, her neighbors had cut down two large trees that had been shading the dining room windows. The sun was now hitting that side of the building and the screens with greater intensity, heating the plastic and causing the odor. She replaced the vinyl with aluminum screening and then enjoyed the increased sunlight in her rooms without enduring the smell.

In another case a couple was planning to move into a condominium with a spectacular view. An entire wall of living room windows faced the setting sun. Unfortunately, the unit, which had been renovated three years earlier, was permeated by a peculiar smell that they found upsetting. When I entered the apartment hall, I noted a chemical odor not unlike one I had encountered in other homes but more pungent. The sun's rays were intense in the afternoon, and there was a vinyl-fiberglass scrim (fine-mesh screen) to shade out the bright light. I suspected that the scrim was an odor emitter, so I walked over to the windows and took a sniff. Indeed, the scrim had a peculiar chemical odor similar to the one that had greeted me on entry.

The affable building manager who had already spent hours trying to sort out this problem offered to take away the scrim. He removed screws, anchors, and brackets and managed to eliminate all the offending scrim, at which point I noticed that the vinyl-fiberglass insect screens on the casement windows were also odor emitters. We removed these as well, and I recommended that the woman air out the apartment for several days.

Weeks later, I received a call telling me a different odor was now present. This time the odor appeared to be coming from the carpeting. Since the couple had considered installing wood flooring anyway, they decided to eliminate the carpet. I was called back the day before the new oak floor was scheduled to be installed. With all the carpeting gone, the apartment reeked more strongly than ever with a new chemical odor. Even though the insect screens, scrim, and carpeting were odor sources, it ultimately turned out that the biggest culprit was the polymer-containing leveling compound under the carpeting and pad. The leveling compound had to be removed to solve this newly identified problem.

In another situation a man had a carpeted office space in the basement of his older home. An adjacent section of the basement had a dirt floor. The man developed serious respiratory distress and decided to move out of the property. He built a new house with a beautiful basement office with a private entrance at grade (at ground level). Two years later he called and asked if I had any idea why he became hoarse whenever he spent a long time in his office. I went to his house and found that the air in the basement was irritating. The most likely source seemed to be the vinyl tile floor (he had avoided carpeting this time). But the man still had an unused box of tiles, and they had no odor at all. I therefore suspected the floor adhesive was the culprit. I removed a tile from one of the closets and carried it upstairs, and he and I both took a sniff. That was it! Subsequent air testing revealed high concentrations of many chemicals from the adhesive, even though it had been applied months before. In this case the owner did nothing about the tile floor, which stopped off-gassing in about two years.

The best way to minimize chances of off-gassing like this is to spread a layer of the adhesive on a sample surface outside your home and let it dry for a few days (or weeks, if you have the time) before installing a new floor. If the smell lingers, find another adhesive.

THE SMELLY LIGHT

A retired woman reported feeling ill from some odor whenever she read in front of her fireplace on cloudy days. The fireplace could have been a source of combustion gases from the boiler in the basement, but it was tested repeatedly for carbon monoxide, and no gases were

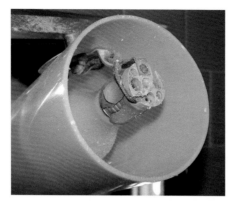

FIGURE 6.3. Lamp with melted plastic base. The nylon plastic insulation around the threaded Edison metal base into which the bulb of this bathroom lamp is screwed is darkened and partially decomposed. When nylon plastic is heated, it may produce a strong chemical odor that smells like rotting, dead fish. An entire portion of the home stunk from this single bit of decomposed plastic.

ever found to be coming into the room. She and everyone involved in the original investigation suspected that the weather might have something to do with the odor. The key, however, was her new reading lamp. On cloudy days she had to turn the lamp on to read her book. The plastic surrounding the threaded metal bulb socket was decomposing when the lamp was on, producing an odor that made her feel sick. The same burning odor appeared in another home after the living room table lamps were rewired (fig. 6.3).

PAINTS AND VARNISHES

Many clients call us because they moved into a new home or because they had their home repainted or their floors redone, and the resulting odors were irritating. Connie and I had the floors redone in a Victorian we used to own, and the finish that had been applied to the floor in one room emitted an odor that was so irritating that I could not go into the room for over a month until the solvents off-gassed. Off-gassing can be accelerated by reducing the boundary layer of air on surfaces (see chap. 23).

FURNITURE

Furniture, too, can be the source of indoor air quality problems.

OFF-GASSING

New furniture made from medium-density fiberboard or particle board can off-gas chemicals such as formaldehyde, which can irritate mucous membranes. The odor will usually dissipate in a matter of weeks or months, but occasionally furniture will continue to off-gas for more than a year. I heard about a woman who purchased a new couch; she began to feel ill shortly after she put the couch in her living room. The sicker she got, the longer she spent resting on her new couch. Doctors determined that she was sensitive to the formaldehyde emitted by the couch. She got rid of the piece and felt better.

When Connie and I purchased our new home, I installed surface-mounted medicine cabinets in the bathroom. The cabinets were made of fiberboard. The odor of the interior of the cabinets was so bothersome that I covered the entire interior back wall with tape made of aluminum foil tape, which prevents emission of all chemicals including formaldehyde. The exterior of the cabinets looks fine, but the interiors have a silver lining.

Furniture finishes can also off-gas. One client was ready to move out of his condominium unless he could determine the source of an unpleasant odor in every room. He had purchased a matching set of furniture with many pieces spread throughout the home. It turned out that the varnish on every piece of furniture was off-gassing a chemical called butyric acid (which smells like vomit), a chemical left over from the manufacturing of the varnish. I recommended that he damp-wipe every surface with a dilute solution of ammonia (a base) to neutralize the odor. If that did not solve the problem, he would have to replace the pieces.

If you have chemical sensitivities or react to formaldehyde, I suggest you buy furniture made from solid wood and be sure it is not coated with varnish containing urea formaldehyde or butyric acid. If your new furniture has a lingering odor that is irritating, you might have to return it.

BIOLOGICAL CONTAMINATION

One woman called me because she noticed a strong odor of mold in the basement of a house that she and her partner were considering buying. They had already had the home inspected, and the inspector had recommended they call me to see if I could help them find the source of the odor.

It was a warm summer day, and all the windows were open when I arrived. Were the owners too warm, or were they trying to air the place out? I wondered. Despite the balmy temperatures I felt quite a chill as the buyer and I walked in past the real estate agents and the owner. A $30,000 commission was in jeopardy, and my nose and microscope might stand in the way of the deal.

It was an older home, and the basement had a stone foundation. In one end was a couch in front of a television set; the sellers' children used this corner as a play area. There was a strong mold odor at this end of the basement. I suspected the couch might be the culprit, so I tapped it and took a Burkard air sample of the dust cloud that rose from the surface. As if to deny that there was any problem, the

Exposed fiberglass and particle board surfaces can be sealed with aluminum foil and foil tape to reduce off-gassing.

real estate agent slumped noisily down onto the couch and relaxed into a comfortable position, commenting that she noticed no odor. When I looked at the air sample with a microscope, I found vast numbers of *Aspergillus* mold spores along with mite fecal pellets.

My clients didn't buy the house, but not because of the odor. We had noticed that the floor sagged at the first-floor entry. Luckily there was a hole around a radiator pipe in the hall, so I inserted my borescope to see if there was any moisture damage. Instead I found substantial structural decay from termites (termites too prefer damp spaces; we discuss termites in chap. 13).

Allergens accompany contaminated furniture. One asthmatic teenager was proud of the couch in her bedroom because it added a sitting area to the room. She spent many of her evening hours lounging on the couch, reading or chatting on the telephone with her friends. The shape of her body was pressed permanently into the cushions. Because her asthma could not be well controlled, her parents allowed nothing in the bedroom except her beloved couch, a dresser, and her bed. The room was Spartan: there were no rugs on the floor, no curtains on the windows, no books on the shelves, and none of the bric-a-brac one would expect to find in a teenager's room. I pounded the couch cushion with my hand and took a brief Burkard air sample to collect the dust particles. I found that the sample contained many *Aspergillus* mold spores. When I talked to the parents, they immediately remembered that the couch had previously been used in a damp basement family room.

In another home, a baby with serious mite and cat allergies was having asthma symptoms. The parents kept the baby's room scrupulously clean; the only furniture was a crib with a mattress covered in plastic and a cushioned chair for the nursing mother. My sample of the chair dust revealed long-forgotten secrets. The parents never realized that the nursing chair (a present from the baby's grandmother) had been stored for years in a damp basement where Granny's cat spent long hours on hot summer days curled up on the chair. In consequence the cushion was contaminated with mold, mites, and cat dander particles. Every time the mother sat down to nurse her infant, a cloud of invisible airborne allergens surrounded the two of them.

Connie inherited a wooden coffee table from her parents. The piece had a cribbage board carved into its surface. It wasn't worth much, but she had fond memories of playing cribbage on it as a child. When she and her siblings grew up and moved away, her parents had stored the table in their barn. We set the table in front of our couch in the family room. I noticed an odor coming from the table the first

Old chairs or sofas that have been stored in barns or basements may have become infested with microarthropods and arthropods such as mites and spiders or even with small mammals such as mice. Antique bureaus may have mold growth, particularly in hard-to-see places like the backs or the bottoms of drawers. Allergens in the dust can get shaken onto clothing when drawers are opened and closed.

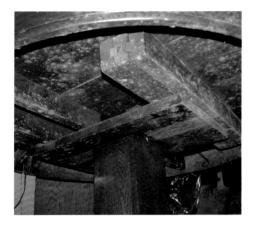

FIGURE 6.4. This round table was stored in a damp basement. The top of the table was clean, but the bottom was covered with white mold colonies. Often, people who buy antiques fail to inspect the backs and bottoms of their purchases. Then their homes may smell musty, much the way that most antique stores smell.

time we played cribbage on it. I turned it over and found the bottom was completely covered with *Penicillium* mold. We went back to using our portable plastic cribbage set (fig. 6.4).

INTERMITTENT OCCUPANCY

Homes with intermittent occupancy can develop mold problems, particularly in properties near large bodies of water. One couple bought a home overlooking the ocean and used it primarily as a vacation home, enjoying the place during the summer as well as on weekends and over the holidays in the winter. The house was closed up for the rest of the year, with the heat turned down low. When they returned to the house now and then from late fall to late spring, they'd fill the indoor air with moisture from showering and cooking. When they left, they closed the house up again and turned down the heat. Moisture would then condense on cool surfaces, leading to mold growth on the backs and bottoms of furniture, including beds. When they retired, they moved into the house full-time and then began to experience allergy and asthma symptoms.

They were worried about the basement, which contained some minor mold growth. But I found *Aspergillus* mold on the backs and bottoms of most of the pieces of solid wooden furniture, as well as in the cushioning in upholstered pieces and in many of their rugs. They could clean the solid pieces but had to replace the cushioned furniture. Some of the rugs could be cleaned, but I encouraged them to replace some that were particularly contaminated.

"HOUSES" OF WORSHIP

I investigated IAQ problems in two 100-year-old churches in which the clergy were experiencing allergy symptoms. There were mold exposure issues in both churches, but one of the most interesting problems had to do with the churches' organs.

The blowers furnished air for the organs. In one church, the blower was located at the bottom of a stairwell full of mold. In the other church, the blower was in a moldy closet, one wall of which was a damp, dusty foundation wall. Curious as to how the air quality might change in the nave after one of these organs was turned on, I asked the minister to play the organ. He had never played that organ before and was excited to do so. Within minutes of his dramatic musical expression, I began to cough and had to put on a fine-particle mask for relief. I wondered how many other churchgoers were bothered by each organ's emissions. The organ system in one of these two churches was cleaned out, and pounds of dust were removed. I recommended that the blowers be cleaned and that they be located in more suitable, mold-free environments.

PLANTS

Believe it or not, Christmas trees can be a source of mold or other allergens. They are cut long before they are sold and may have been stored under damp conditions. Before purchasing a Christmas tree, look it over carefully to be sure it is not moldy. Consider using an artificial tree if you, anyone in your household, or a frequent visitor has mold allergies.

Many people like to keep plants in their houses all year round. In most cases the plants aren't a problem so long as the soil is kept free of moldy leaves and there is a moisture-proof barrier under each pot. But some people are careless; they give their indoor plants so much water that they might as well be using a garden hose. In one home I inspected, a plant had been watered carelessly and moisture had soaked into the living room carpet, creating a large stain. I found several species of mites living on the mold, moisture, and other nutrients in the stain. If a clay pot is sitting directly on carpeting or a rug, mold and mites can flourish in the carpet fibers because the water from the damp soil evaporates through the clay bottom. Some plants should not be welcomed into the homes of allergy sufferers. One particular species, *Ficus benjamina* (weeping fig), has been associated with skin rashes and asthma symptoms.[2] Irritating oils from this popular indoor plant can soak into the dust on the leaves, and the dust can become airborne when the plant is disturbed (the dust then acts as a surrogate allergen). I had a client who experienced skin irritation whenever she even vacuumed near her ficus.

FRAGRANCES STINK

In chapter 5 we discouraged people from using fragranced body products, but there are many fragranced products that should not be used on our "home set," including plug-in scent emitters and scented cleaning and laundry products. When our children were growing up, toy stores even sold "scratch 'n sniff" stickers, and more recently at a birthday party that our grandson attended, fragranced bubble solution was given out to every child as the party favor. I understand that some hotels are even using fragranced paints and sprays, supposedly to enhance the appeal of their lobbies and guest rooms.

One couple I worked with had three children who were experiencing chronic coughing in their impeccably maintained home. The parents had done almost everything they could to reduce allergens, including encasing mattresses and pillows in dust mite covers and installing hardwood floors in most of the rooms. After my first site visit, they had the contaminated ducts and air conditioning equipment cleaned and eliminated most of the remaining carpeting. The children continued to cough. On a subsequent visit I found that their mother was using laundry detergent that contained fabric softener, fragrance, and enzymes. All the clothing and bedding in the house had the overpowering odor of this detergent; in addition, whenever anything was disturbed, bits of microscopic lint containing detergent residues became airborne. (We discuss other problems with some laundry products in chap. 10.)

When I was teaching high school chemistry, I would occasionally pass around a small vial containing a chemical called cinnamaldehyde, the essential oil from cinnamon (and the odor of a popular red pill-shaped hard candy). The oil has a pleasing but pungent odor. I warned students to only carefully sniff the bottle, but one student became so enamored with the scent that she put a little on her skin. She immediately developed a brief rash. Amyl alcohol, a constituent of some liquors and fragrances, can also bother people. One good whiff of the vapors from the pure liquid will make people cough within 20 seconds.

Fragrances are so much a part of our landscape that we are often not even aware of them, but once you begin using fragrance-free products, you will be surprised at how much you notice scents. Our house is now fragrance-free. Whenever I am near anyone who uses a strongly scented shampoo, cologne, aftershave, or even deodorant, I am acutely aware of the scent, and more often than not, it causes me to cough.

We all react with varying degrees and in different ways to our environments. For those who have allergies and asthma or are chemically

The Centers for Disease Control and Prevention (CDC) recognized the potential for fragrances to cause health symptoms and in 2009 issued an "Indoor Environmental Quality Policy" that prohibited the use of fragranced products in spaces owned, rented, or leased by the CDC.

Centers for Disease Control and Prevention, Office of Health and Safety, Office of the Director, *Indoor Environmental Quality Policy*, CDC-SM-2009-01 (Atlanta, GA: June 22, 2009).

sensitive, heavy fragrances can exacerbate breathing difficulties and other physical reactions. I therefore recommend that people who are vulnerable use perfume-free products. In my opinion, everyone should avoid using heavily scented products. Even if you aren't sensitive, someone in your household or who visits your home might be.

SOME RECOMMENDATIONS

CARPETING

- New carpeting should be allowed to off-gas either before installation or before you use the room. If you wonder whether new carpeting is off-gassing, use the paper aluminum foil/paper towel test described in chapter 23.

- Rugs and carpets can be treated with steam vapor from a steam vapor machine.

- Families with allergies or asthma should not have a great deal of carpeting or many area rugs in their homes.

- If contaminated carpeting cannot be removed, cover it with a dust-impervious barrier (such as the adhesive-backed plastic called "carpet protector" that painters use), over which you can place a rug.

FURNITURE

- Use a mirror and a bright flashlight to check for mold growth at the bottoms or backs of pieces of furniture.

- Don't use furniture that has been stored in damp or moldy spaces (though wooden furniture that has gotten moldy can sometimes be disinfected, cleaned of all mold, and varnished or shellacked inside and out to seal in residual dust).

- The surfaces of other hard-surfaced items (plastic, metal, glass) covered with mold can usually just be cleaned.

- Thoroughly clean used furniture, no matter its value, before bringing such pieces into your home.

- Wear gloves and a NIOSH N95 two-strap mask when cleaning moldy furniture. Whenever possible, do this work outdoors. If you must do the work indoors, isolate and ventilate the work space, and HEPA vacuum surfaces in the space afterward to remove allergenic dust (see chap. 24).

- Avoid purchasing (or inheriting) used furniture with cushions.

- Cushioned, upholstered items that are moldy should be discarded or disinfected and re-cushioned and reupholstered.

- If you are sensitive to formaldehyde, avoid furniture made from medium-density fiberboard or particle board.

- Refer to part III of our book *The Mold Survival Guide: For Your Home and for Your Health* (published by Johns Hopkins University Press), which focuses on mold removal, including from personal goods.

ODORS AND FRAGRANCES

- If you notice a chemical smell in a room, try to determine what's new in the room. Sniff window blinds, insect screens, any other plastic items (lamps, television sets, computer monitors), and new carpeting and padding.

- If you are sensitized to fragrances, avoid burning scented candles. Don't wear perfume and cologne or store such substances in your home.

- If someone who lives in your home or spends a great deal of time there has allergies or asthma, avoid using fragranced products.

PLANTS

- Pots should be set on moisture-proof barriers.

- Don't let dead leaves accumulate on the soil.

- Over-humidifying your home may make your plants happy but can also promote biological growth.

- Consider having an artificial Christmas tree.

PART II.
DAILY
LIFE

When we go to bed at night, we lock our front doors, thinking we are keeping ourselves safe from any dangers that lurk outside. But what's inside our houses can also be threatening.

LIVING ROOMS, FAMILY ROOMS, AND DINING AREAS

7.

LIVING ROOMS AND FAMILY ROOMS

BURNING WOOD

A young mother was laying logs in the fireplace. Her infant, who had been asleep on the couch, began to awaken. The mother jumped up to keep the baby from rolling off, and in her haste she stubbed her toe badly against the coffee table. She was in such pain that she rushed to the emergency room, taking the baby with her and entirely forgetting about the open fireplace damper. In the middle of the night her husband was awakened by moaning coming from the bathroom. He found his wife sitting on the toilet, doubled over as if in pain from what he assumed was her recently injured toe.

As soon as the wife was back in bed, she heard a loud thud and looked down to see her husband unconscious on the floor. Luckily she quickly realized that her nausea and her husband's collapse were the result of carbon monoxide (CO) poisoning. She threw open the bedroom window, ran to get the baby, and rushed back to her husband, who had already regained consciousness from the fresh air. Scantily dressed, the family fled into the freezing winter air.

I was asked to investigate why this happened. Warm air rises and cold air sinks. A chimney built in the middle of a house stays warm even when it's cold out because the chimney is surrounded by warm interior walls and warm air from the house rises through the flue, creating a draft.

This chimney, however, was built at an exterior wall and was thus outside of the house. Unless there is a fire in the fireplace, an exterior chimney remains near the temperature of the outside air. In winter the colder air from outside sinks into such a chimney and enters the house. This is called downdrafting. The fire department determined that a defective boiler in the house was producing high levels of CO: a tasteless, odorless, lethal gas (how CO gas forms is discussed later in this chapter). The flue for the fireplace was next to the boiler flue in the same chimney. On that particular night, wind blew CO gas from the boiler flue at the top of the chimney across to the adjacent fireplace flue. The gas was carried down into the house through the open fireplace damper, which had been inadvertently left open. In the middle of the night the mother, father, and baby were within minutes of dying.

I have heard of similar cases occurring when the heating system flue was adjacent to the fireplace flue in an exterior chimney. One older couple experienced intermittent headaches and nausea. They had the town health and fire departments test for CO on numerous occasions, but none was ever detected because the wind had shifted by the time the investigators arrived. One investigator figured out what was happening and recommended that the couple keep their fireplace damper closed unless they were burning wood. That solved the problem. It's a good idea to keep the damper or fireplace doors closed when a fireplace is not in use (but never close a damper when there are warm embers remaining in the fireplace). If you have a heating system with a flue in a chimney that also has a fireplace flue, be sure to maintain the system and have a technician check periodically for CO levels in the combustion gases from the heating system.

Even without downdrafting, fireplaces and woodburning stoves can create smoke in homes. Smoke can be irritating for children or adults who have asthma, so I recommend that they avoid burning wood. Even if you have no allergies, if you are planning to install a woodburning device and you live in a densely populated area, please consider the health of people with asthma who may be downwind.

I have another concern about wood. Some people may be allergic to the mold or insects that grow in firewood. When wood is carried through the house or stored inside, allergens can enter the air or fall onto carpeting. If you can't resist the appeal of a working fireplace, your firewood should be moved and stored carefully.

Wood is composed mostly of cellulose. When cellulose burns, it first thermally decomposes (undergoes a chemical change because of heat), producing water vapor, wood alcohol vapor, and a complex mixture of other chemical vapors. What is left behind in the fireplace is charcoal (which eventually burns) and ash. The alcohol vapor (as well as some other chemical vapors) burns in the flame. Smoke from the wood fire consists of droplets of water vapor and other unburned chemical vapors that have condensed when they hit cool air. But some of these chemicals condense on the cooler chimney flue walls before they meet the outside air and form a tarlike coating called creosote. This coating continues to be exposed to the heat from the fire below, and it is baked into a combustible, charcoal-like glaze. Much the same process happens when we bake an apple pie and the sugary filling oozes out and drips on the bottom of the oven, thermally decomposing into a black glaze (cellulose and sugar both contain glucose).

Creosote has a strong odor, and when downdrafting occurs, the entire house can smell of burned wood. Fireplace and woodstove flues that aren't kept clean fill up with creosote. One family I know had not been careful about having the chimney cleaned each year. One Christmas Day they threw a large bundle of wrapping paper from the presents into the fireplace all at once. The flames crackled, and suddenly a large whoosh! came from the chimney. The creosote lining the flue had caught fire, and flames filled the entire chimney. The house was in danger of burning to the ground, since the flames could have escaped the chimney, which was unlined and full of loose, deteriorated mortar. Even in lined chimneys the extreme heat from a creosote fire can cause a liner to expand, crack, and fail.

The family called the fire department, and the firefighters quickly put out the fire. They also crunched a few of the presents as they walked in and out of the house in their heavy black boots. But better to lose a few presents than the entire house.

Creosote does have some useful applications. For years, a solution of creosote and solvent was applied to wood as a preservative. This is the smell associated with old telephone poles. The odor of creosote can irritate some people, though. A builder I know was renovating his house for his fiancée. To preserve a decayed threshold leading from the living room to the exterior deck, he saturated the wood with an entire gallon of creosote solution. The woman's lungs hurt whenever she entered the house. The builder removed the threshold as well as the concrete near the door and the creosote-soaked soil beneath. He replaced the concrete and threshold, but his fiancée continued to have trouble breathing in the house. Unfortunately, he had put so much creosote into the site that he couldn't remove it all. I recommended the couple install a subslab mitigation system similar to a radon system.

GAS FIREPLACES, CANDLES, AND SOOT

Gas fireplaces offer an easier way to create a romantic ambience than do woodburning fireplaces. Instead of paying for wood, carrying it in, storing it in a corner, vacuuming up chips and sawdust, and cleaning out ashes, all you have to do is flick a switch. But gas fireplaces have drawbacks of their own.

Carbon monoxide is one by-product of a gas flame and is the result of incomplete combustion. In complete combustion, one atom of carbon from fuel combines with two atoms of oxygen from air to produce carbon dioxide (CO_2). In incomplete combustion, the carbon combines with one atom of oxygen, producing CO. Because CO can still combine with oxygen to form carbon dioxide, CO burns in air. (To "burn" in air, a substance must be able to combine chemically with oxygen.)

Soot is another problem caused by gas flames. We expect kerosene and wood fires to create soot, but surprisingly, gas flames can also create soot. When gas burns normally in a stove, the flame is blue because adequate oxygen from the air is premixed with the gas to complete combustion. Combustion is incomplete when the supply of oxygen is inadequate. Then some carbon atoms combine with oxygen to create CO_2, while other carbon atoms combine with oxygen to create CO. Still other carbon atoms do not combine with oxygen at all but combine with each other to produce soot (microscopic particles that become visible when present in large numbers). Soot particles become incandescent and give off the yellow light we associate with firelight. In gas fireplace logs, the gas is not premixed with enough air before it burns, so that the fire will produce the yellow flame people want to see. Soot is the inevitable by-product. (Incandescent carbon particles also produce the yellow flame of burning wood and candles.)

One homeowner had his brother install a gas fireplace in an exterior living room chimney. There was not adequate draft, and CO and soot leaked into the house. Even though the CO level was not high enough to make the people ill, looking at the soot deposits on the wall sickened them. They had to repaint their entire house.

Fireplaces aren't the only source of soot in a living room. Candles also can produce soot, some more than others. Scented jar candles have become popular, but they can bother anyone sensitized to perfumes. Whether scented or not, candles burning in jars flicker more than candles burning freely in the air, because there are turbulent airflows in the jar space around the wick. Incomplete combustion occurs when the flame geometry is disturbed in this way, producing even more soot (fig. 7.1).

Soot deposits are fairly uniform in older homes. In well-insulated newer homes, soot stains on exterior walls and on ceilings near exterior walls can look like stripes at the studs (the wood or metal wall supports to which the drywall is attached) and black dots at nailheads. On an insulated exterior wall, the studs are colder than the bays, and nailheads are even colder than the studs, for they penetrate deeper into the wall and conduct heat toward the outside of the building faster. The room air cools when it comes in contact with the

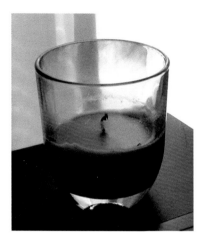

FIGURE 7.1. Soot deposition on the inside wall near the mouth of this jar candle is an indication that the flame is producing soot. Soot particles produced in the flame cannot be seen in the hot air rising from a candle, but soot deposits can be identified on surfaces.

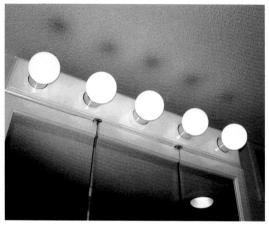

FIGURE 7.2. On the bathroom ceiling above these vanity lights are soot stains. The homeowner burned jar candles in the bathroom. Soot in the air from the candles deposited evenly on most of the surfaces, but warm air rising by convection above the lights caused soot particles in the air to collide and stick more frequently on the ceiling surfaces directly above the warm bulbs.

nailheads and with the plaster or drywall at the studs. This cooler air sinks, and slight air turbulence occurs. Soot deposits increase as more air collides with surfaces, so though soot sticks to the entire exposed surface, there are more soot deposits at the studs and nails. There can also be heavier soot deposits above baseboard heating convectors and light bulbs, again because of increased air flow (warm air rises) (fig. 7.2).

Homeowners I know have repainted rooms more than once to cover soot stains. I heard about one contractor who had been sued by home buyers because the inside walls of some of the houses he had constructed turned black with soot. They blamed the soot on faulty installation of the heating system. As an experiment, the contractor had an engineer burn a candle in a jar for sixty hours in a new home. So much soot was deposited that the entire interior had to be recarpeted and repainted. I know several people who have had to replace all their light-colored carpeting because of soot deposits from jar candles. In some rooms the stains were prominent at the edges where exterior walls met the carpet, probably because the colder air at the exterior wall sank, depositing more soot particles at that carpet edge (fig. 7.3).

I did an experiment in my garage to see what burning a jar candle could do to the air. I burned the jar candle overnight close to a white Styrofoam plate, the lower half of which I covered with aluminum foil (to prevent the exposure of half the plate to garage air). In the morning, I used a particle counter to compare the particle concentration in

Some people think that soot stains are evidence of mold. Soot stains will not disappear when a dilute bleach solution (one part bleach to ten parts water) is applied to them, but mold growth usually does.

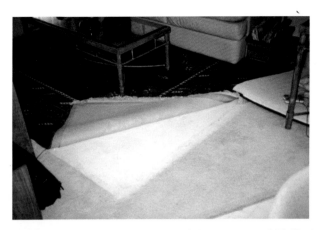

FIGURE 7.3. When a dark rug resting on top of a light carpet was folded back, it became clear that soot had discolored the exposed portion of the carpet. Invisible in air, soot particles from jar candles can deposit on some surprising surfaces. Some people have found plastic containers inside kitchen cabinets and even inside refrigerators blackened by candle soot deposits.

the garage to the particle concentration outdoors. The concentration in the garage was more than 50 times greater than in the outdoor air; to prove that the excess particles were due to candle soot, I removed the foil from the unexposed bottom of the plate. In comparison to the clean bottom, the upper exposed half of the plate had already turned gray from soot deposition. Soot is made visible by its absence, so we tend to notice it when we move out of a house or apartment. When pictures are taken down, you can see the outline of the frame on the wall surface. The pictures protect the wall from the even layer of soot deposited elsewhere, so the area now uncovered looks lighter (fig. 7.4).

Soot is not just a cosmetic concern. People who have allergies or asthma may find that inhaling soot (along with other combustion products) is irritating. One woman we know loved to burn fragranced jar candles, and she burned them in every room. She also suffered from shortness of breath due to asthma. I convinced her to stop burning jar candles during the holiday season, and I gave her a set of battery-operated candles to replace her jar candles. Her asthma symptoms improved markedly. Soot particles can serve as surrogate allergens (see chap. 3), and soot also contains carcinogens (such as benzo[a]pyrene), so long-term exposure should be avoided.

THE SUNKEN LIVING ROOM

I entered a contentious scene when my client, a building manager, warned me to say "nothing to nobody" during the site visit. The disgruntled tenant was complaining of repeated bouts of mold growth

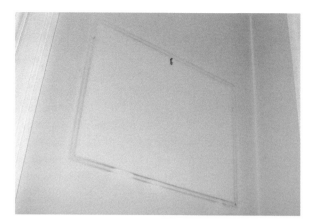

FIGURE 7.4. This photo illustrates the soot pattern that resulted when jar candles were burned in a home. A framed picture was hanging from the hook on the wall, and when the picture was removed, the outline of the frame was left as a black stain. The area behind the picture was not exposed directly to house air and the soot particles that it contained, so it is lighter in color than the walls around the picture.

on the lower six to twelve inches of the living room walls. The condominium owner (the landlord) had replaced the carpeting and had the living room cleaned and repainted. He had even growled to the management company about excessive moisture in the crawl space beneath the adjacent dining room, where dampness from the disconnected dryer vent hose was dripping from the steel beam.

Lint was in the crawl space, and hostility was in the air. The "sunken" living room, constructed slab-on-grade (meaning the concrete pad was poured on soil and no basement was present), had an outside wall with a glass sliding door and was about two feet below the level of the dining room and the rest of the apartment. The living room heat register was inappropriately high on the wall. I determined with an infrared thermometer that the lower two feet of the living room walls were significantly cooler than the wall above. I felt my legs chill below the knees and imagined myself standing in a bowl of stagnant, cold air. The bottom of the living room was in fact like a bowl of liquid, because it contained the denser, cooler air. Once the lower two feet filled with cooler air, the air spilled out over the two-foot-high wall between the living room and the dining room, where it mixed with warmer air. The temperature discontinuity, therefore, was occurring at the level of the adjacent dining room floor.

The moisture content of the air in the sunken living room was fairly uniform throughout, but the relative humidity was higher in the cooler portion of the room; consequently, mold grew on the living room walls. I explained that the tenant must not turn the thermostat down to 60°F every winter day before leaving for work and that

As air cools, its relative humidity (RH) rises; some species of mold can flourish when the RH is over 80 percent.

he should move the furniture away from the cold walls so that warmer room air could heat their surfaces. I also suggested he do all he could to reduce moisture levels in the apartment by taking shorter hot showers and boiling less water on the stove.

I recommended that the landlord install an exhaust fan at the stove that vented to the exterior and a paddle fan in the living room to mix the stratified air and make the room air temperature more uniform. The building manager also needed to repair the disconnected dryer hose in the crawl space to prevent the dining room structure from decaying owing to excess moisture and macrofungal growth in the crawl space (see chap. 2).

RESINOUS CEILINGS AND WALLS

In one case of a mystery odor, a young couple purchased a derelict home and proceeded to renovate it while they were living there. They removed wallpaper, painted walls and trim, and refinished floors, but they were still plagued by an intermittent odor. On cold days this fleeting odor seemed strongest near a particular wall; on other days the odor was strongest at another end of the living room. On some days there was no odor at all.

The odor was reminiscent of marijuana smoke. It occurred to me that all the walls and doors had newer finishes, but the ceilings had never been washed or painted. I borrowed a hair dryer and heated the living room ceiling. Within moments the couple agreed that the odor was suddenly present. Apparently the previous owners had smoked so much marijuana in the living room that the ceiling was coated with resin from the smoke. On days when the steam heat operated, warm air would rise by convection above the living room radiator and heat the ceiling. The warm air would acquire the resin odor, move in an invisible air mass across the ceiling, and, once cooled, sink at an opposite wall. On other days the sun would heat parts of the room and create a different convection pathway for the warmed air, causing the odor to appear elsewhere. The couple cleaned and painted the ceilings, and the odor disappeared.

Tobacco use can cause similar problems. One family moved into a Victorian home with wainscoting in the living room and wood paneling in the family room. There was an omnipresent odor of pipe and cigar smoke in both rooms, yet no one in the family smoked. They had repainted the plaster walls and sanded the floors in the entire house before they moved in, but they had never cleaned the paneling or wainscoting. After they washed these wooden surfaces with a dilute solution of detergent and ammonia, the smell went away.

Exposure to smoke, whether from a fireplace or from tobacco or marijuana products, is bad for our health, and odors may linger.

COUCH POTATO ASTHMA

One couple's teenage son found that his asthma symptoms were worse whenever he was in their family room, where the TV and video games were. As a small child the boy used to lie on the couch and watch Sesame Street. As an elementary school student he played video games from the couch. As a teenager he would stay up late at night, lying on the couch and watching his favorite movies. The cushions were stuffed with down feathers and offered a soft, comfortable retreat.

The couch also offered an extremely high level of dust mite allergens. Whenever the boy moved around on the couch, compressing those cozy down cushions, clouds of sloughed-off skin scales and mite fecal pellets billowed out for him to inhale. He was allergic to mites, and the allergens exacerbated his asthma.

I recommended that the family get rid of the couch and replace it with a leather- or vinyl-covered one, or that they use a futon couch and encase the mattress in a dust mite cover. Families with allergies or asthma should think carefully before purchasing furniture with feather-filled cushions, since these are promising reservoirs for microscopic life and, depending on one's lifestyle, can lead to what I call couch potato asthma.

I believe that a large portion of the increase in asthma can be attributed to our sedentary lifestyle. Years ago, children and parents in this country spent much more time outdoors. Now family time is mostly dedicated to more passive pursuits such as playing video games, surfing the Internet, or watching TV. The longer we spend sitting on cushions or lying on mattresses and couches, the more favorable are the conditions for mite infestations.

GREENHOUSES AND HOT TUBS

Some homeowners add enclosures to their homes for hot tubs, pools, or plants. Such spaces are often near or off living rooms and can contribute more than an exotic flavor to a house. If you are thinking of adding a greenhouse, do all you can to control moisture levels. You will be introducing soil into the indoor spaces of your home, and whatever the soil contains may become airborne when disturbed.

Indoor hot tubs and pools are sources of moisture that can lead to bacteria, mold, and mite colonization, in addition to irritation from the chemicals used to disinfect the water. In one home a hot tub was the source of a powerful bacterial odor. I found the underside of the vinyl cover completely covered with biological growth and mites. In another home with an indoor pool and a powerful mold odor, the pool

Several cases of Legionnaires' disease have occurred after people had heavy indoor exposures to aerosolized dust from potting soil contaminated with *Legionella*.

cover was overgrown with a forest of *Aspergillus* mold, with mites foraging happily within. If you have a hot tub or pool with a cover, be sure both sides of the cover are dust-free and periodically disinfected.

Living rooms and family rooms are important in the private and public life of a household, so these spaces are well trafficked by family members and guests alike. With this level of activity, whatever allergens and irritants are in the room will be stirred up and carried into other parts of the home by airflows. Be sure to keep these rooms as dust-free, dry, and clean as possible.

DINING AREAS

Some people have separate dining rooms, and some people have eat-in kitchens or a combined kitchen, dining area, and family room. Whatever the configuration, since people living in one house often gather together for mealtimes, the environmental conditions in such rooms or areas are worth consideration.

One family installed a kickspace heater in the step down leading to their dining room addition, which was constructed on a crawl space. This was an unusual setup, but their plumber had told them it would be less expensive to have a single blower at the step down leading to the dining room than to install baseboard convectors on the walls of the room. There was no opening in the habitable area for makeup air for the heater, so the blower drew in the air it needed from the basement and the moldy crawl space under the addition. The couple's son experienced asthma symptoms soon after the addition was completed. It turned out he was allergic to mold spores, which of course were being circulated by the heater. (He was so allergic to the air in the moldy basement that he ventured down there only when wearing a face mask.)

I can't tell you how many inherited dining room tables I've looked at that contained mold growth on the underside of the tabletop. Older chairs can also have mold growth on the chair legs or in the chair cushioning, if present. People love older, solid-wood dining room sets, but such pieces have often been stored in musty basements or antique stores. And food spills over the years have provided food for microbes. If you see spots or a white sheen under a dining room table or on dining room chairs, or such pieces smell musty, it's best not to bring them into your home unless the wood surfaces can be cleaned and sealed (see chaps. 6 and 24). (If you or anyone in your family has allergies or asthma, musty upholstery and cushioning should be replaced.)

I never recommend wall-to-wall carpeting or area rugs in a dining area, because spilled food can support microbial growth. If you want to have a rug, however, try to avoid spilling food on it and HEPA vacuum it thoroughly on a regular basis.

SOME RECOMMENDATIONS

DINING AREAS

- Avoid having wall-to-wall carpeting or area rugs in dining areas unless you are willing to HEPA vacuum the carpeting or rug on a regular basis.

FIREPLACES

- Be sure dampers, fireplace doors, or screens are closed when the fireplace is not in use, particularly if you have an exterior chimney.

- Don't ever close a damper when there are still warm embers in the fireplace.

- If the boiler and fireplace flues rise together in the chimney, look into installing a damper that fits onto the top of the fireplace flue.

- If mold affects you or anyone in your household, store firewood outside and be sure the wood stays dry. Try to avoid burning moldy wood.

- HEPA vacuum the area when wood scraps fall to the floor as you carry your wood inside.

- Have chimneys and chimney vent piping cleaned regularly by a professional.

- Do not apply creosote-containing preservatives to surfaces in the interior of your home.

FURNITURE

- If you or anyone in your household has asthma or allergies, use vinyl- or leather-covered furniture rather than upholstered furniture. Avoid down-filled furniture or cushions.

- If you have a sofa bed or futon couch, encase the mattress in a dust mite cover.

- Be careful about introducing older dining room chairs or tables into your home.

HEAT AND HUMIDITY

- To deter mold growth, keep humidity at a comfortable but not too high a level (under 40 percent in winter).

- Keep the living room or family room evenly heated.

INDOOR POOLS AND HOT TUBS

- Periodically disinfect the cover for an indoor hot tub or pool, and keep the cover as dust-free as possible.

SMOKING INDOORS

- Don't smoke or allow others to smoke inside your home.

SOOT STAINS

- Don't burn candles (particularly those in jars) in well-insulated homes.

- Avoid burning tapered candles near airflows (such as near leaky windows or doors), because the airflows will disrupt the flame, leading to incomplete combustion and the production of soot.

ROOMS WITH WATER— THE BATHROOM

8.

A bathroom is usually one of the smallest rooms in the house, but it's a room that experiences a lot of traffic. Wherever water is present, you must pay particular attention to potential sources of indoor air quality problems.

TOILETS

THE HOT SEAT

Using warm water to flush a toilet may sound wasteful, but sometimes it's not a bad idea. In moist climates or on humid days, the toilet tank and connecting pipes are filled with cold water and may be below the dew point, so that moisture from the air condenses on them and drips onto the floor or rug, where odor-causing mold and bacteria can flourish. Mold can also grow in dust on the bottom of the toilet tank (fig. 8.1).

Piping some hot water into the tank can keep the tank above the dew point and prevent condensation. Conversely, too much hot water can create a different problem. On a cold winter day during an inspection of a three-family home, I discovered an illegal basement apartment: one large room functioning as kitchen, living room, bedroom, and bathroom. The kitchen area was on a raised wood platform, and at the end of the L-shaped kitchen counter was a toilet. Although this was clearly the kitchen of an immodest chef, two even more peculiar conditions immediately caught my eye. In the foreground, I could see smoke coming out of the chimney pipe connector on the

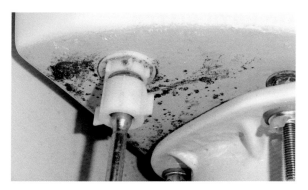

FIGURE 8.1. If a toilet is flushed several times, on humid summer days the temperature of the toilet tank and water within can be below the dew point of the bathroom air. Water will then condense on the outside of the tank below the water level in the tank. Homeowners may wipe the sides of the tank dry, but rarely if ever do they clean or dry the tank bottom. Then mold grows on the moist dust. Sometimes, as is the case here, mold also grows in the dust on the wall behind the tank.

building's oil furnace. The furnace exhaust was supposed to be going into the chimney, but the pipe had been purposely disconnected so that the exhaust gases would keep the unit warm. In the background, smoke was coming out of the toilet bowl. It was a scene from hell and smelled like it. The apartment reeked of burning oil. It was hard to believe someone lived there. Had the combustion gases from the furnace contained carbon monoxide (CO), the tenant wouldn't have been living there for long.

The "smoke" from the toilet turned out to be steam, which is formed when liquid water is heated and evaporates as vapor. When the vapor hits the colder air, it condenses into droplets that remain suspended. You can't see water vapor in the air even though it is there all the time, because it is a gas and just mixes invisibly with the other gases in air. But you can see steam droplets because they reflect light. When the droplets evaporate, they become vapor again and disappear from view.

Apparently, whoever "renovated" the basement had set the water heater's thermostat to "scald" and inadvertently (unless he was hoping for a second source of heat) attached the toilet tank to the hot water rather than to the cold water. The flush lever was stuck and the tank's flapper valve was open, so boiling hot water was running continuously into the bowl. Steam was billowing from the toilet bowl into the cold basement air. That's one toilet I wouldn't have wanted to use, that's for sure!

THE WAX RING

A toilet bowl is usually secured to the floor by two bolts. If the floor isn't perfectly flat, or if there is too much or too little space between the toilet bowl and the sewer pipe flange, the toilet may rock. A wax ring under the toilet creates the watertight seal between the toilet and the sewer pipe. This ring is all that keeps flushed water in the piping. If a toilet moves from side to side at all, the seal is broken and water can leak out, soaking into the floor around the toilet and dripping onto the ceiling below to produce a circular stain with mold. If there is a bathroom rug present, the water produces an environment in the rug where mold can grow. If the situation gets bad enough, the toilet can start to tip as the wood under it decays. If the wood rots so much that the floor gives way, the pipe underneath it may not be strong enough to support the toilet; then the "throne" may find its way into the living room below!

A disrupted wax ring seal also lets sewer gas enter the room—a most unpleasant smell. Even if you can barely detect the gas, it can cause nausea and headaches. The source of sewer gas is often difficult to locate, since the emission can be intermittent. Air always flows from higher pressure to lower pressure. When the air pressure in a bathroom is greater than the air pressure in the sewer pipe, air will flow from the bathroom into the pipe. If the air pressure in the sewer pipe is greater than the air pressure in the bathroom, sewer gas will flow from the pipe into the room. Several factors can cause the air pressure in a bathroom and sewer pipe to change. When a bathroom exhaust fan is running, the air pressure in the bathroom will be reduced. Wind direction at the exterior can either raise the air pressure in a sewer pipe (when exterior air flows down the pipe) or reduce the air pressure in the sewer pipe (when exterior air flows over the top of the pipe). If a toilet's wax ring is intact, such pressure differentials won't result in the flow of sewer gas into a bathroom, but the water level in a toilet may fluctuate.

If you have a loose toilet, a wax seal that isn't airtight is the most likely source of sewer gas. In older homes, however, there may be a broken or open vent pipe in a wall. One client removed the garage roof and demolished a room in her house before discovering that the source of a sickening odor was a broken vent pipe leaking sewer gas into the bathroom wall.

SINKS

Common sources of water leaks in sinks are worn valve packings (the seals around the stem for the hot and cold water valve handles) and leaks around the base of the faucet. Water leaking into the vanity below can cause rot and odor. Many vanities are packed so full of cleaning supplies and other items that a leak at the sink trap or pop-up lever arm escapes notice. To check for leaks, lower the pop-up, fill the sink with water, drain the sink, and then look underneath with a flashlight and mirror.

Even small amounts of water, if continually applied, can rot a finished wood floor or other wood surface. A vanity should be flush with the back wall and installed with a watertight backsplash; otherwise, water may drip down the back, rotting the wall and the vanity. In addition, if a vanity is installed almost flush with the bathtub or close to it, you won't be able to see water dripping from a tub or shower. When kept consistently damp (from tub overflow), these vanities can be sources of musty odors. If the mold growth is disturbed, spores will become airborne. If vanities are chronically wet, they can even decay owing to macrofungal growth (see chap. 2).

Odorous biological growth can occur in sinks without vanities. Occasionally, a musty odor will come from the sink, particularly an older wall-hung model. This is the result of microbiological decay of nutrients (such as soap and dust) in the overflow; you can treat this condition with dilute bleach (one part bleach to sixteen parts water) or with a 9 percent peroxide solution (see chap. 24).

Microbial growth in a sink overflow caused one man to close off his half bath on the first floor of his townhouse. He was embarrassed to have his friends use the bathroom because it contained a terrible odor. He thought he'd have to tear out the entire bathroom, but I found that the sink overflow was full of mold and bacteria. He cleaned out the overflow with dilute bleach and an old toothbrush, and the odor disappeared (see chap. 24 for further discussion of the use of bleach and alternatives to bleach).

SHOWERS AND TUBS

When using a shower curtain, be sure all the water stays inside the tub or shower enclosure. Sometimes it helps to watch when someone else takes a shower so you can see where the water is dripping or spraying out. Even small leaks can cause problems. If the floor is tile, the water will probably evaporate. Water can leak underneath tile, though, if there is loose caulking or grout. Soon the tile will loosen, and the situation will worsen. Water can also pool under curled linoleum edges and rot the subfloor beneath. Push on the flooring near a tub to see if there's decay below; if the floor bends (or your finger goes through), you have a problem.

In one apartment a simple grout crack led to long-term concealed leakage of shower water under a tub. This leak had serious health consequences, for the water soaked into the plywood subfloor under the wall framing and spread to the adjacent bedroom of an asthmatic child. For months the carpeting in the room had been secretly soaking up the daily deluge. The moisture led to the growth of *Aspergillus* mold on the subfloor and in the pad and carpet dust, and mites and other microarthropods flourished. Unfortunately, the child played in this corner of her bedroom; she wheezed when she inhaled the spores and mite fecal material that aerosolized as she jumped on the carpet.

Even when properly used to keep water inside a tub or shower area, shower curtains can become covered with biological growth, especially at the bottom edges, and they can become a source of odor. Shower curtains should be replaced periodically, particularly if they don't have adequate time to dry or if they start to smell. I recommend using an inexpensive shower liner (inside the curtain) that can be discarded and replaced when it gets discolored with microbial growth.

Many people prefer shower doors, but these too must be kept clean. They can accumulate malodorous slime in the tracks, which is not easily removed. The frame must also be watertight. If caulk is not properly placed between the metal track and the tub's porcelain, water can leak out. In addition, when the shower door frame is installed, the vertex of the angle (where the ends of the vertical and horizontal pieces meet) must be embedded in caulk, because water pools at the ends of the lower track. Putting caulk at the inside of the corner or at the edge of the frame after it has been put in place will not provide a sufficiently watertight seal.

When Connie and I purchased the last home we lived in, the seller mentioned at the closing that her family didn't use the shower in the third-floor bathroom much because the kids had more fun in the tub. The tub enclosure had sliding glass doors. Our daughter was fifteen years old at the time and preferred to take showers—long and hot! One day Connie noticed a spreading ceiling stain in the hallway beneath the bathroom.

She ran up the stairs and shouted through the door, "Turn off the shower!" When I looked closely at the tub, I found that the lower corner of the shower door track was caulked only on the inside. In fact the frame was loose, and water from the shower was sneaking out over the edge of the tub, draining down through the joint between the tub and the tile floor, and pooling on the ceiling beneath. To stop the leak, I removed all four pieces of the metal frame and caulked the wall and tub sections back into place. I also caulked the floor joint.

Sometimes even the best shower curtain or door won't prevent water from escaping, because people are careless once they've finished showering. We had a houseguest one summer who insisted on stepping out of the third-floor tub soaking wet and dripping on the cloth bathroom rug. In addition, she left the bathroom door closed for the rest of the day. This became a little tug-of-war between us; I would open the door whenever I could, and she would close it. She felt it was impolite to leave a bathroom door open, even if no one was inside.

Within two weeks the entire third floor of the house began to reek from the bacteria growing on the wet nutrients in the bathroom rug. The sour smell reminded me of an old dirty sponge. Wet towels can also acquire that smell if they don't dry out fast enough, so it's always a good idea to hang towels to dry, preferably outside the bathroom during humid weather. But bacteria can cause more than odors. One client wheezed in his house, especially in the bathroom. On the tile floor next to the tub was a small cloth bath mat. He told me he washed it regularly, yet I found that the material was severely contaminated with bacteria. Whenever he stepped onto the rug, particles (digested skin scales, bacteria) became airborne and from there settled with other dust onto bathroom surfaces. The client's wheezing subsided after the bath mat and all the dust on the walls and floor were eliminated.

WINDOWS IN TUB ENCLOSURES

In an older home, windows inside a tub or shower enclosure can cause a particular problem, especially where a tub on legs has been replaced by a built-in tub with a shower. It is extremely important to cover such windows adequately with waterproof curtains to protect them from the shower water, or the windowsill and even the entire wall can rot. Leave this kind of window uncovered after showering to allow for drying. Windows within tub and shower enclosures, as well as shower doors, should be glazed with safety glass in case someone slips and falls against them. Safety glass shatters into many small fragments, whereas normal plate glass breaks into long, sharp shards.

On winter days I have seen icicles coming out of exterior walls under bathroom windows. At one home with such icicles, I suspected concealed wall decay behind asphalt siding, and I recommended that the siding be removed near the bathroom window. Underneath and to the right and the left of the windowsill, the wood siding and the wall structure behind it had been turned to dust by macrofungal growth. Even if you replace an old wooden sash window with a vinyl one, the wood structure is still vulnerable to water that may leak around the window frame.

Water has a mind of its own. It can seep insidiously behind loosened wall tile in the tub enclosure or leak intermittently from the tub overflow (the opening at the bottom of the metal escutcheon plate around the pop-up control below the faucet). If the overflow seal is ineffective but only a small amount of water leaks past, you may have only paint blisters or a minor stain on the ceiling beneath the tub. Damage can be substantial, however, if someone fills the tub to the level of the plate and then climbs in.

How can you avoid a tub overflow disaster in your home? Check the escutcheon plate; it should not move at all. If the plate is loose, don't fill the tub to the level of the plate, because the water will rise when you get in the tub, and water will overflow. Have the plate secured in place; just tightening the two plate screws may not be adequate if the gasket (seal ring) is broken or out of position. (The escutcheon plate may have to be removed to properly position the gasket.)

I once inspected a residential building that housed faculty apartments. Water was pouring down into the basement onto stored books that had been covered in plastic to protect them from the deluge. The building's maintenance personnel had traced the origin of the leak to a bathroom on the second floor. They were about to open up the tiled bathroom walls to find a pipe leak but thought I might be able to figure out which wall should be opened up. Using an infrared camera, I couldn't find any temperature differentials in the walls that would suggest the presence of moisture. I looked carefully around the tub area and noticed a ring of soap scum that was above the escutcheon plate. It ended up that a visiting professor from England preferred baths to showers. He liked to soak in a hot bathtub, so he kept refilling the tub with hot water to levels above the leaking escutcheon plate. He lowered the level of water in the tub when he took a bath, the loose escutcheon plate was repaired, and the problem was solved (fig. 8.2).

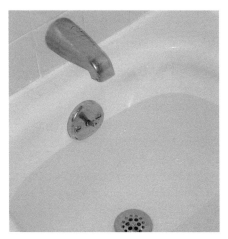

FIGURE 8.2. This bathtub has a ring of soap scum above the level of a leaky escutcheon plate. I filled the tub to a level just below the plate, then pushed a plastic trash bin into the tub to raise the water level above the overflow opening at the bottom of the plate. Instead of going into the drainpipe, water poured down to the bathroom below. The soap scum ring on the tub wall illustrates the water level maintained by the visiting professor when he bathed.

SHOWER HEAD SLIME

We had a mold problem in our stall shower at the shower head that I hadn't at first noticed. One day I looked up at the shower head and observed black tentacles extending more than an eighth of an inch from each hole. Naturally, I took a sample and observed it with a microscope. The black bioslime consisted of an ecosystem containing slimy bacteria and mold. The microorganisms were growing at the interface of air and water. Since the shower head was constantly rinsed during use, dust did not seem to be a likely source of nutrients for the bioslime. I assumed that the source of the nutrients was the water itself: microscopic bits of plant material that cannot be removed owing to the cost at the water filtration plant that takes the water from our river and supplies it to homes. We had an expensive filtration system for the incoming water installed that removed the nutrients for the mold and bacteria. The shower head problem went away.

AN UNWELCOME DECORATION

The most common complaint I hear about bathrooms is that there is mold growing on the ceiling. Warm, moist air from showering is less dense than the air around it, so it rises to the ceiling, where water condenses on the cooler surface. To minimize condensation, be sure there is adequate insulation above the bathroom ceiling.

I inspected one bathroom in which mold grew only on one small area of the ceiling above the tub. There was a two-inch gap between two batts of fiberglass insulation in the attic, immediately above the moldy bathroom ceiling. The homeowner happened to have a piece of two-inch sheet foam insulation, so I cut a piece to fit tightly over the gap. The mold growth never reappeared in the problem area. If you can't retrofit insulation, it may be easier to install sheet foam insulation and a new drywall ceiling. If mold grows on the walls, insulate them as well (fig. 8.3).

INDOOR RAIN

You may notice after you take a shower that water condenses on the mirror (that is, it turns from a vapor to a liquid). In fact, water condenses on all surfaces in a bathroom, particularly on cold surfaces such as exterior walls, uninsulated ceilings, and windows. Accumulations of water on wooden window sashes can lead to mold growth and wood decay (see chap. 2).

One couple who called me had been renting an apartment from the young man's parents. He had asthma, and his girlfriend was an attorney. During the first winter they noticed mold growing on the walls of the apartment. The mold growth was most abundant in the

Mold can grow on tile grout in tubs and showers, on wall surfaces, and in rugs. Given a damp environment, biological growth can flourish on just about anything organic, including skin scales, soap film, dust from cornstarch body powder, cellulose or glue from wallpaper, caulk, and the resins in paints.

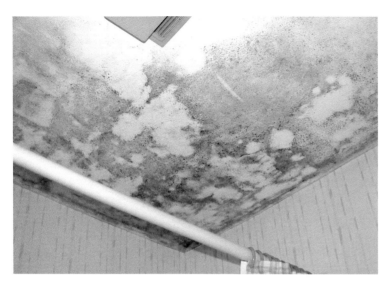

FIGURE 8.3. This moldy bathroom ceiling was in an apartment rented by several college students. They obviously didn't worry too much about cleaning, and the moisture from multiple showers in the bathroom led to mold growth in the dust on the ceiling. Mold can grow even on a surface coated with mildewcide paint, which protects the paint film from mold but does not prevent mold from growing on dust that accumulates on the painted surface.

outside-corner closet, but mold was also growing on the wall next to their bed.

They washed clothing in the bathtub and hung it on the shower curtain rod to dry. They took long, hot showers. When they went to work, they turned down the thermostats on the baseboard electric heaters to save money. They also kept the shades pulled down on the new insulated glass windows, which had wooden sashes. The shades kept the heated air away from the windows, so they stayed cooler than the rest of the air in the apartment (which wasn't that warm to begin with). The window glass was below the dew point of the apartment air, and moisture then condensed on the new windows. Before long the window rails, which sat submerged under condensed moisture, began to rot. The father's ire was roused, the son's asthma flared, and the young lady's legal instincts sought someone to fault for the moldy clothing she had discarded from her closet. But in turning down the heat and creating conditions of excess moisture in the apartment, the couple was responsible for the mold growth and wood decay.

There is always lots of moisture in bathrooms, for obvious reasons, but inadequate ventilation makes the situation worse. If the excessive moisture is a long-standing condition, biological growth is more apt to occur. Keep your bathroom clean and dry, and both you and the room will benefit.

After someone takes a shower, the shower curtain or doors should be left partially open to allow airflow to evaporate the water remaining on the tub or shower walls. Most bathroom exhaust fans do not create sufficient airflow to remove all the moisture in the air and on the walls, so I also recommend that people leave the bathroom door open after a shower. An oscillating table or tower fan can increase airflow in the room, which will speed up drying of surfaces. Keep the fan where it can't be knocked over easily and plug it into an outlet protected by a ground fault interrupter (GFI). (Don't use a fan before you disinfect a surface with existing mold, though, lest you stir up spores with the airflow.)

Building codes require at least a window or exhaust fan in every bathroom, primarily to reduce odors. In most cases this means having separate ducts to the exterior for each fan. In one condominium this was not the case. The owner was complaining about fabric softener odors and lint in the bathroom. The bathroom exhaust shared a hose with the dryer exhaust. When the dryer was operating, it vented into the bathroom, because the hose between the bathroom and dryer was shorter than the distance between the dryer and the outside. There was thus less resistance to the airflow from the dryer to the bathroom than from the dryer to the exterior. To solve the problem, the owners installed a separate vent hose for the dryer.

Another one of my clients who had allergies noticed that whenever he was in the bathroom and the exhaust fan was turned off, he began to cough. Why did this happen? This bathroom was on the first floor. Warm air rises, and in the winter, warm house air leaked out (exfiltrated) from the uppermost levels. Cold air infiltrated at the lowest levels to replace the air that had leaked out. In this bathroom the seal at the vent kit (the outside end) of the exhaust hose was not airtight (few are), so when the exhaust fan was turned off, cold air leaked through the exhaust hose into the room. Since the inside of the hose was at a lower temperature than the moist air passing through it from the bathroom when the exhaust fan was on, condensation occurred inside the hose, and mold grew on the dust inside. Air continued to enter the house through the mold-lined hose, carrying mold spores with it. In the end my client disconnected the exhaust fan, blocked the duct, and no longer coughed when he was in the bathroom. Instead he installed a window, which ventilated the room just fine.

If you have an exhaust fan in your bathroom, check the vent to be sure the damper opens when the fan turns on and closes when the fan is off. I also recommend an exhaust with a squirrel-cage blower rather than a propeller fan, as it has greater capacity.

MINIMIZE DUST

If you limit the amount of dust on surfaces in your home, you will reduce the nutrients that microbes need for growth.

One condominium owner was plagued by dust in her home that she thought came from a yearlong renovation project in the unit above hers. She said the dust deposits were heaviest in the bathroom. She wanted to sue the condominium association, and she called me to help her gather evidence for her case. When I examined the bathroom air sample with a microscope, I discovered that the dust contained mostly cornstarch and short, fibrous cellulose lint. It's easy to guess that the cornstarch came from body powder, but where do you think the lint came from? Toilet paper fibers. My advice? Tear the toilet paper only at the perforations, buy body powder made from talc and not cornstarch, which is biodegradable, and forget the lawsuit.

Any floor heat or air conditioning supply can accumulate dust. In areas prone to moisture, such as the bathroom, the dust can become moldy, particularly if the supply duct is in a cold attic, basement, or crawl space. In one home the cornstarch on a wall register got damp and moldy, and when the heat was on, spores blew into the bathroom.

Mold that is growing on a bathroom heat or air conditioning supply register can be a significant risk to someone who is sensitized. But is the mold you see on the ceiling or on the tile grout a health risk? The danger depends on the number of spores you inhale. Surprisingly, mold that is growing on the ceiling may not result in exposure to mold spores, because the spores do not regularly become airborne. The type of black mold that often discolors grout grows mostly beneath the surface of the material, and these spores also do not readily become airborne. Just the same, because mold can be a source of odor and spores, I recommend that people disinfect moldy bathroom ceilings and tile grout with dilute bleach (see chap. 24) or with any suitable cleaning agent.

UNHEALTHY CLOUDS

We think of water as a transparent fluid (unless it contains particles that reflect or absorb light). Now and then you might find bits of rust or minerals from the tap in your glass, so you throw out the water and draw a fresh glass. But water, whether it is piped into your home or bottled, comes from an ecological system that contains living things like fish, plants, snails, and insects. If the water is from a reservoir, pigeons, geese, and other birds may fly overhead, and ducks, dogs, or even people may enjoy a swim. All these living things periodically leave their "signatures" in the water.

Legionnaires' disease is a sometimes lethal form of pneumonia caused by a type of bacteria (*Legionella*) that grows best in warm water and is a common organism. People have acquired Legionnaires' disease from hot tubs after breathing bacteria aerosolized from the warm, frothy water. A recent study identified household showers as potential source of the bacteria. As far as I know, as of the writing of this book, no incidences have been reported where the *Legionella* bacteria in a home shower led to Legionnaires' disease.

D. Hayes-Phillips et al., "Factors Influencing Legionella Contamination of Domestic Household Showers," *Pathogens* 8, no. 1 (February 2019): E27.

When water is stratified (layered by temperature), the warmer water at the surface, closer to the air, has more dissolved oxygen than the colder "stagnant" water below. Different microorganisms thrive at different water depths, depending on their need for oxygen and nutrients. As the layers of water mix during fall and spring "turnover," organisms are stirred and dispersed. (Surfaces of bodies of water get colder in the fall and warmer in the spring, resulting in increased convective water movement.) Water that is drawn from the reservoir during these biannual turbulent periods contains organisms that are different from the microorganisms drawn during "quieter" times of the year. Among these organisms may be algae, molds, and even disease-causing agents such as bacteria and amoebas.

In industrialized countries, a water treatment plant between the water supply and the tap works to keep people healthy. Treatment plants filter and chlorinate water and are successful in removing most serious health threats, but they cannot remove everything or prevent growth after the water leaves the plant to make its way into our pipes. Microorganisms continue to flourish, particularly on the walls of water pipes and fixtures. When we shower, water from the shower head is broken up into droplets, some of them small enough to be inhaled. Most of us can tolerate this because our lungs and immune systems protect us. For individuals weakened by immune disorders, smoking, or old age, however, water containing biological growth may cause disease.

Radon, a radioactive gas that causes lung cancer, is another threat to health. Where underground radon levels are high, well water contains the gas and carries the dissolved radon with it when it enters your home. When you shower, most of the radon gas bubbles out of the water and into the air, and you can breathe it in. Cities are required to test public water for radon, but homeowners are not.

If you use well water, it's a good idea to purchase a test kit and have the water tested. It is estimated that for every 10,000 picocuries of radon radioactivity per liter in tap water, there will be about one picocurie in the air. (The EPA guideline for home exposure to radon in air is four picocuries per liter of air.)

SOME RECOMMENDATIONS

CLEANING

- Keep shower doors clean. Remove slime from the tracks, and clean those areas with a dilute bleach solution (see chap. 24) or with any suitable cleaning product.

- The bottom of a toilet tank can acquire mold growth; clean this surface on a regular basis.

- Mold odors from a sink overflow can be eradicated with a dilute bleach solution (one part bleach to sixteen parts water; see chap. 24).

- Moldy bathroom surfaces can be cleaned with a dilute bleach solution or with any suitable cleaning product.

- While cleaning moldy bathroom surfaces, wear a NIOSH N95 two-strap mask and operate an exhaust fan in the bathroom window. If the room does not have a window, operate the ceiling exhaust fan.

- Bathroom rugs should be cleaned regularly and replaced as needed.

MISCELLANEOUS

- If you use well water, test the water for radon as well as other contaminants.

- Use bath powder made of talc rather than cornstarch, which is a nutrient for microorganisms.

MOISTURE LEVELS

- If mold tends to grow on your bathroom walls or ceiling, avoid drying clothes or towels in the room.

- Keep the bathroom door open, operate the exhaust fan, and leave the bathroom window open (weather permitting) for an hour after showering.

- Operate a small oscillating fan to mix bathroom air and speed drying of surfaces.

- Use a squeegee to remove water from shower walls.

REPAIRS AND RENOVATIONS

- Repair any loose wall or floor tiles.

- If you are renovating your bathroom and want to minimize the chances of mold growth, insulate the bathroom walls and ceilings with sheet foam.

SINKS

- If your sink leaks, have it repaired.

- Don't store too many goods in the cabinet under a bathroom sink; use plastic bins for storage.

- If your sink is installed in a cabinet, be sure to clean the cabinet kickspaces on a regular basis (see chap. 9).

TOILETS

- If a toilet is loose, the wax ring must be replaced.

- If condensation occurs on the outside of your toilet tank, put a tray under the tank to collect the water.

TUBS AND SHOWERS

- If you have a shower curtain rather than a shower door, install splash guards at the ends of the tub.

- Keep the shower curtain inside your tub or shower enclosure.

- Replace shower curtains periodically.

- Be sure that your shower doors are watertight.

- Windows in shower enclosures should be made of safety glass.

- Cover windows in shower enclosures with waterproof curtains.

- If the escutcheon plate on the tub overflow is loose, the seal is leaking. Be sure that the screws are tight and the rear seal is intact and positioned properly.

- Drip a while or dry yourself off before stepping out of a shower or tub.

VENTILATION

- Be sure the bathroom is ventilated by a window, an exhaust fan, or both.

- The vent kit (the outside end) of your bathroom exhaust hose should be airtight when closed but fully open when the shower exhaust is running.

ROOMS WITH WATER— THE KITCHEN

9.

We want to be certain that we prepare and cook foods safely, and that no unwelcome life forms enjoy the food along with us or are part of our meal.

COOKING

STOVES

A woman had experienced chronic headaches for all of the twenty years she had lived in her home. She loved to cook and spent a great deal of time in the kitchen. She called me because she realized she always felt a little better when she spent extended time away from the house. I first sampled for gas sources in the basement with my TIF8800 combustible gas detector. The clocklike ticking remained constant there, but as I ascended the stairs to the first floor, the pulse began to increase. The closer I got to the kitchen stove, the faster it ticked. As I moved the detector along the back of the stove, it screeched with its characteristic siren sound. I soon found that gas was leaking from piping concealed in the wall behind and under the stove.

A representative from the gas company was fearful enough of an explosion that he cut off the gas to the kitchen and laundry. On the following day a plumber cut holes in the basement ceiling and walls and found three significant leaks in the gas piping joints. The woman's headaches diminished once the pipe joints were repaired. Her husband had never smelled the gas or had any headaches at all. The house had been built on fill, and the only thing that bothered him was that the house had sunk about six inches at one end. It's possible the settling had stressed the pipes and caused some of the leaks.

Even in the absence of leaks, you must be careful with gas appliances. Most gas stoves have a spark ignition coil to light the top burners and an electric glow plug to light the oven. If the automatic spark does not operate properly when a burner is turned on, gas will pour out around the stove. If ignition is then initiated (or if you try to light the stove with a match), the gas/air mixture can ignite and produce a large flame. Accidents like these are also likely to occur with propane gas because it is denser than air and hangs around the stove. Utility-supplied gas is lighter (less dense) and thus rises and dilutes faster.

Older gas stoves lack automatic ignition mechanisms and instead have pilot lights that burn day and night. Occasionally, pilot lights can cause disasters. My next-door neighbors renovated their entire first-floor condominium. The walls were sparkling, and they had only the floors to refinish before the project was complete. Workers sanded the floors in the entire unit, vacuumed up all the sawdust, and applied a sealer coat of lacquer that contained a highly volatile solvent. The fumes filled the apartment. Because they were denser than air, the fumes were concentrated in the space close to the floor. When the invisible cloud of solvent reached the oven pilot light, the vapor ignited. There was a *whoosh!* and the entire floor was ablaze. The fire flashed back to the open bucket of lacquer, setting it on fire too. The foolish floor sander tried to extinguish the flames by pouring the burning lacquer down the bathtub drain rather than covering the bucket with a plate or metal pot cover.

Fortunately no one was injured, and the burning floors self-extinguished once the volatiles had burned off. If there are solvents or any type of chemical fumes in a home, turn pilot lights off and keep the windows open. (A pilot doesn't produce much gas, but turning the gas to the appliance off altogether will stop gas leakage.) After the solvent vapors have cleared, it's safe to light the pilots or turn on the gas.

CARBON MONOXIDE

Pilot lights on older gas stoves can produce significant amounts of carbon monoxide (CO). In addition, if there are minor gas leaks in the kitchen piping, the hot pilot light thermally decomposes the gas/air mixture in the room air to produce CO. Other odorous chemicals are also produced, resulting in a characteristic odor that I often associate with kitchens in older homes. (When homes are painted with oil paint, the hot gas flame of a pilot light or burner thermally decomposes the solvent vapor and can produce a pungent, irritating odor.) Whether you have an older or a newer gas stove, a poorly adjusted flame on a burner or in the oven can produce significant amounts of CO. Gas ovens should be tested periodically for CO and should never be used to heat a home.

One woman who was renting her apartment called me because a peculiar odor in her unit was making her nauseated. She had been able to live there for only one week; in fact, on the day she moved in, she called the gas company and the fire department because she was so worried about the odor. They found no problems and even questioned her mental health. The building owner recommended she install a portable air filter.

I could detect the odor of combustion gases as soon as I entered her apartment, so I went out to my car to get my Bacharach Monoxor II CO detector. At 800 parts per million (ppm), CO can cause loss of consciousness and death within hours; the maximum allowable short-term exposure in a home is 9 ppm (unless there is a source of combustion gases, the level of CO indoors should be zero). Fortunately, the level of CO was low, 5 ppm, but it was enough to be of concern. (The level in the uninhabited apartment should have been zero!) The gas pipe that supplied her cooking stove was in the basement. The pipe had not been properly threaded into a fitting, and a large amount of gas was leaking from the joint and rising up into her kitchen through the hole for the pipe. I told her to call the gas company and request an immediate service call. A technician came and was so alarmed that he turned off the gas supply in the basement.

When electric ovens are on the self-cleaning cycle, the temperature in the oven can be as high as 900°F. This high temperature causes thermal decomposition of the residual food bits in the oven, resulting in the production of CO. If you have ever experienced nausea or headache in a closed kitchen during the oven's self-cleaning cycle, CO may have contributed to your symptoms. To whatever extent possible, keep the kitchen doors and windows open and the exhaust fan on when your oven is self-cleaning.

Carbon monoxide is formed when oxygen and carbon combine in the presence of heat. When we pour lighter fluid (kerosene) on charcoal and light the fluid, the fluid heats, turns to vapor, and burns with a flame. The charcoal then heats up in the flame, and the oxygen in the air at the charcoal's surface combines with the carbon to produce CO. It is the CO gas that burns with a flame after the lighter fluid has been consumed. Only burning vapor or burning gas produces a flame.

Some people love the taste of grilled foods, but a charcoal barbecue should never be used in the kitchen or anywhere indoors. Not only does this present a fire hazard, but glowing or burning charcoal (which is mostly carbon) produces large amounts of carbon monoxide.

A candle illustrates this process. The wick is covered with wax, which we light with a match. The match flame melts the wax on the wick and heats the liquid wax, creating a vapor that then ignites into a flame. The heat from the flame melts the wax in the candle, which the wick then soaks up. The heat turns the wax into vapor, and on it goes.

BLACKENED FOOD

It's easy to overheat foods. Occasionally, burned foods can create air quality problems. Years ago our teenage son offered to prepare a spaghetti dinner using his special sauce recipe. Unlike most of us in the family, he likes hot, spicy food. He began by heating oil in a large cast-iron frying pan. He added freshly chopped jalapeño peppers. Next he cut up an onion and threw it into the hot oil. Grease spattered. Shortly afterward I heard a loud commotion in the kitchen. My son was coughing and his face was flushed. He had overheated the frying pan and found the clouds from the cooking vegetables so irritating that before I entered the kitchen, he shoveled the mixture into the disposal. When I entered the room I also started coughing, even though the cooking had stopped. Connie rushed in and immediately felt a burning sensation in her lungs. We turned off the stove and threw open all the windows to air out the room.

I asked our son what had happened. He was not forthcoming because he wanted to keep the peppers a "secret." He said he had burned the onions, which then filled the room with smoke. I took bits of the leftover onion skin from the cutting table and looked at them under the microscope. I found several types of mold growing, including *Stachybotrys*, the mold that produces trichothecene mycotoxins. I had no idea whether the mycotoxins could have caused our distress, but since we were all affected, I was concerned enough, even though it was evening, to call a mycologist (a specialist on molds).

Imagine my embarrassment when my son finally admitted there had been jalapeño peppers in the pan. These peppers contain a highly irritating chemical, capsaicin, as you may have discovered if you have ever chomped on one. Capsaicin is an ingredient in some pepper sprays that police use for personal protection. When the peppers were fried, some of the irritant dissolved into the oil. Oil in a hot pan can be aerosolized when water (including moisture from some foods) is added to the pan. When water boils, it changes from liquid to vapor. One teaspoon of liquid water becomes a thousand teaspoons of water vapor, because vapor takes up more space than liquid (the molecules in vapor are farther apart). As water or moisture in some foods begins to boil, the moisture turns into water vapor bubbles surrounded by oil. When the bubbles break, the oil splatters into small droplets and is dispersed into the air.

Even before food is added to the pan, any kind of overheated fat can thermally decompose and produce noxious smoke that contains acrolein, another pungent, irritating chemical. Worse, the smoke can erupt into flames. Never pour water on such a fire; the ensuing spattering only makes the flames worse. The simplest way to instantaneously extinguish a grease or oil fire is to remove the source of oxygen by covering the pan.

I put this concept to good use when in graduate school and living with two other chemistry graduate students. I had never made French fries before and decided to try making them. I heated up about two quarts of cooking oil in a pot and threw in a handful of potato slices that were still dripping wet from rinsing. The oil frothed up immediately; some of the oil hit the flame on the stove, and the oil droplets caught fire. The flames rose to the ceiling and could easily have burned the rented home to the ground. The three of us stared at the conflagration for a bewildered moment when I remembered the trick about covering the pot to cut off the air to the flame. I grabbed a plate and covered the pot; the flame was extinguished immediately.

EXHAUST SYSTEMS

Cooking smoke consists of water vapor and droplets of water and grease. If the grease droplets are small enough, they remain suspended in the air and are carried by convection currents to walls, ceilings, windows, and shelves. The droplets coalesce into a sticky film after they collide with surfaces. On vertical surfaces the yellowish film may not be apparent, though it makes blue walls look green. On horizontal surfaces, like the top of the refrigerator or window rails, the film is visible because house dust sticks to it.

Grease droplets can also be deposited in rooms adjacent to the kitchen. One dining room had a ceiling light fixture with five small lightbulbs. Five yellow stains above the fixture mirrored the arrangement of the lamps. When the fixture was on, warm air rose from each bulb by convection, carrying droplets of grease that stuck to the ceiling directly above the bulbs.

In another home the new owners were plagued by the odor of curry every time the heating system came on. The former owners had loved to fry foods with curry powder. When the heat was on, the warm radiators created a current of air, drawing kitchen air across the outside of the cast-iron radiator pipes. Droplets of grease containing fragrant curry seasonings were carried along with the air, and they collided with the radiator pipes and stuck. Whenever the radiators became warm, they would reintroduce the aroma into the house air. The new owners washed the radiators with detergent and TSP (trisodium phosphate, a cleaning agent), and the curry smell went away.

Since the smoke and steam produced in cooking can create IAQ problems, I always recommend stove exhaust fans. Be sure to get one that has a squirrel-cage blower and not a propeller fan (propeller fans do not have adequate capacity). It's also extremely important that exhaust fans be vented to the outside; otherwise, the cooking fumes are blown right back into the interior air. To find out if your exhaust is working properly, check the exterior vent when the fan is on to be sure the damper opens. Sometimes these dampers stick shut or become blocked with the nests of birds or bees.

PANTRY PESTS

Unwelcome life forms such as mice, cockroaches, ants, flour moths, storage beetles, and mites might lurk in your pantry. Body parts and fecal material from any of these creatures can be present in infested foods. It is always possible that someone will develop an allergic sensitivity after eating contaminated foods over a long period.

Flour moths are small (about 10 millimeters, or 0.4 inch), grayish-brown slow-flying insects whose larvae live on grains such as flour and cereal, as well as in baked products such as cookies, crackers, pretzels, and other snack foods, including nuts and raisins. It's easy to acquire a flour moth infestation. If you borrow a box of crackers from an infected house or buy grains or dry pet food from a moth-ridden supermarket, it's likely you will import eggs and larvae into your home. The eggs hatch into larvae with big appetites. When mature, the larvae find hidden places to pupate into moths.

I first became aware of flour moths when I saw them flying in large circles around my pantry. I didn't do anything about them for some time. Then one day I walked into the pantry to see a jungle of writhing larvae dangling from threads stuck to the ceiling. It was like a scene from an Alfred Hitchcock movie.

I opened a box of crackers, and it was full of crumbs stuck together by fine threads. Inside a bag of flour, the white powder was writhing and full of fine filaments of larval silk. I ended up throwing out everything but the canned goods, and these I washed, because larvae were pupating behind the paper labels. The larvae were even in cracks between the shelves and the wall, so I realized I could never kill them all. I abandoned the pantry and kept the door shut for about two weeks. I checked every day and was able to kill the newly hatched moths because they flew so slowly. Finally, after a few weeks, new moths stopped appearing, so I knew the nightmare had come to an end. If you have a moth infestation, don't use pesticides. Be patient and take a more cautious approach.

REFRIGERATORS

DRIPS

Because gas stoves contain fire, people approach them with caution and respect. The same cannot be said of refrigerators. One client was awakened in the middle of the night by an enormous crash. He turned on the lights and wandered around trying to locate the source of the noise. When he got to the kitchen, he realized in his sleepy stupor that something was missing. Where the refrigerator had been there was now a gaping hole in the floor. He looked down and there was his refrigerator, lying in the basement. The rotted floor under it had finally failed—the victim of years of leakage from the icemaker's water line.

In another home, water from a refrigerator leaked between the flooring and the plywood subfloor. Moisture ran along the plywood, causing decay in the kitchen and dining room. Both floors had to be replaced. Leakage from these lines can be subtle. Occasionally, I have found oak flooring buckled in front of a refrigerator, one of the few obvious signs of a refrigerator leak. Obscure water seepage can be detected with a Tramex moisture meter. If you don't have a meter, you should check with a flashlight under the refrigerator and at the icemaker's water line for signs of leaks.

REFRIGERATOR MOLD MUNCHIES

Even refrigerators that don't have water lines can harbor mold. Frost-free refrigerators have a drip tray at the bottom or behind a panel in the back that collects water. The water drains from the freezer section during the defrost cycle or from the bottom of the refrigerator section when liquids are spilled inside. The drip trays in most homes also collect a considerable amount of house dust and bits of food.

At one point I coughed intermittently in my own kitchen. I never understood why until one day I realized that my coughing always began shortly after the refrigerator compressor started. I removed the grille at the bottom and looked inside. Somehow a pearl onion had bounced along the floor and ended up in the drip tray. The onion was fuzzy with a thick beard of blue-green *Penicillium* mold. Every time a refrigerator compressor turns on, room air is drawn over the coils that dissipate the heat from inside the appliance. By design, this air is used to evaporate water that accumulates in the drip tray, but sometimes all the water does not evaporate. When my refrigerator's compressor turned on, air blew over the moldy onion and spewed spores into the room.

Ever since then, I've been careful to keep the drip tray clean, and people with asthma or allergies should do the same. If the drip tray is

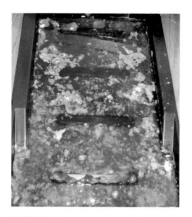

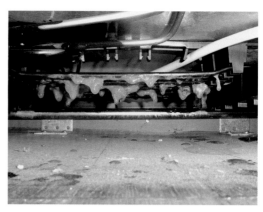

FIGURE 9.1A. I removed this drip pan from the bottom of a refrigerator. The pan was full of water and floating clumps of bioslime consisting of bacteria and other microorganisms.

FIGURE 9.1B. The refrigerator coils above this drip pan had been immersed in the pan water and were decorated with hanging globs of bioslime, drooping from the coils and dripping onto the dusty floor beneath the refrigerator after the pan was removed. Airflow from the compressor over the bioslime could have released allergens.

behind a panel at the back of the refrigerator and built into the metal bottom, it cannot be removed, so just clean the tray in place as best as you can (figs. 9.1A and 9.1B).

The refrigerator coil is another item to keep clean. If you have pet allergies and a previous resident had a pet, it's especially important to clean the coil. The dust that accumulates on the coil and around the refrigerator itself can remain allergenic for years. In general, it's a good idea to roll out your refrigerator once a year so that you can clean the top, bottom, and sides. If your refrigerator has a water line, be sure not to disconnect the line when moving the appliance.

Refrigerator doors can be a source of mold and odor if the gasket seal is poor or broken and food falls into the spaces. In damp weather, moisture condenses on the cooler gasket surface: combine the nutrients and moisture, and voilà! Mold. Try to keep the gaskets clean, and if they are damaged, replace them. So much moisture had condensed on one refrigerator gasket that it was covered with mold, and mites were happily foraging on the crop. Another place where you can find mold growing is at the bottom of the trap door for the ice chute. Check the condition of the door with a mirror and flashlight.

MOLDY FOODS

It makes sense to keep the inside of your refrigerator free of moldy foods, but many foods like cheeses include molds intended to be eaten. The white skin on Brie and Camembert, for example, consists primarily of *Penicillium* hyphae and spores. Blue cheese is made by fermenting milk curds with *Penicillium roqueforti*, which sometimes contains *P. crustosum* (another species of *Penicillium* mold produces a nervous system toxin that can kill animals when they eat grain contaminated with this mold). People who are allergic to mold may react to such fermented foods. Moldy foods (fruit, bread, or discolored cheese) should not be eaten by people with allergies. Keep in mind that moldy food, even when being thrown out, can emit allergenic spores, either on the way to the garbage or while in the garbage can. Carefully place moldy food in a bag, seal the bag, and remove it from the kitchen.

People with food allergies can be so sensitized that just being in the same room with someone eating a food such as peanuts or walnuts can make them ill. Particles from the nuts become airborne, and the sufferer inhales them.

UNPLUGGED REFRIGERATORS

Remember to always leave the refrigerator door open if you unplug the appliance. Whatever food is left inside (including food that is spattered on the walls, not all of which you can readily see) will be fodder for mold and bacteria, so get rid of it and clean the appliance's internal surfaces.

Don't leave an unplugged refrigerator with an open door in a space where children may play. It's tempting to hide inside an appliance like that and close the door!

SECOND REFRIGERATORS

I've inspected many properties in which a second refrigerator is located in the garage or basement. For some reason, people don't often think of keeping this appliance clean because it's not in the kitchen. If you have a second refrigerator, treat it with the same care as you do the refrigerator in your kitchen.

SMELLY GARBAGE

Some people get headaches or feel sick when they smell rotting foods, so garbage should not be kept indoors for long (for this discussion, garbage includes compost). Disposals can also smell, particularly in hot weather, because they retain foods that are being decomposed by bacteria or mold. When you use your disposal, be sure all the food is ground up. In addition, you can pour a dilute bleach solution (one part bleach to sixteen parts water) into the disposal to eliminate bad smells (see chap. 24). After adding the bleach solution, be sure to run water through the disposal for a few moments and step back from the sink when you first turn the disposal on, in case some bleach solution splashes out of the appliance.

SMELLY SPONGES

The conference room in a law office had been abandoned because whenever the attorneys met there, they experienced headaches and nausea. This is not a lawyer joke; there actually was a problem. The moment I entered the room, I could smell the unpleasant odor. I took air samples and checked surfaces, but I couldn't find the source. The last item to check was the enormous, oval-shaped mahogany conference table. The only thing on the table was a Yellow Pages book. I picked up the phone book and sniffed the top. There was no odor at all, but the bottom side that had been against the tabletop had a powerful odor of dirty sponge. I had one of the lawyers repeat this test. She sniffed the top of the phone book and smelled nothing. When she smelled the bottom, she blurted out, "That's it! That's the smell!"

The lawyers often met over lunch, and afterward someone always wiped the table with a sponge from the kitchenette in the corner. The guilty sponge must have been full of bacteria, which were then spread over the table in a slimy, odoriferous film. When the film dried, the smell remained. A chemical called butyric acid—a by-product of bacterial growth—causes this type of odor. In the stomach, enzymes digesting fats convert them to butyric acid; when we throw up, the smell of our vomit is similar to the odor of a dirty sponge (fig. 9.2).

Butyric acid can be neutralized by a base (acid and base, when mixed in the right proportions, may produce a substance in water that is neither acidic nor basic). I sprayed and wiped the table three times with a window cleaner containing ammonia (a base), and the odor was gone. I called the next day at lunch hour, and once again the conference room was in use. I reminded them to wipe the table with a clean sponge!

Soaking a smelly sponge in diluted ammonia will eliminate odor and kill bacteria. If you find the odor of ammonia objectionable, a little baking soda in water will also neutralize butyric acid. If you use a baking soda solution to clean a surface, be sure to rinse and dry the surface thoroughly afterward. Ammonia is a gas dissolved in water, so when the water evaporates, the ammonia goes with it. Baking soda is a solid, and when the water in a baking soda solution evaporates, crystals of soda remain behind, so the surface has to be rinsed and then dried.

Sponges help contain water, but because of their open-celled structure, they soak up food and become sources of bacteria and odor. One type of bacteria that grows in dirty sponges is *Pseudomonas*; some species cause illnesses in people and animals.

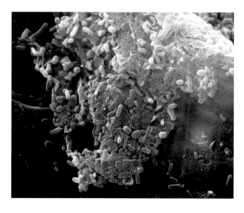

FIGURE 9.2. I wet an old, damp sponge with some milk and let it sit at room temperature for a few days. When the sponge started to stink, I cut off a piece and took it to the scanning electron microscope (SEM) lab. The micrograph shows the skin scale being digested by different species of bacteria, some oblong and some round (4,000× SEM).

If you suspect a surface is generating an odor of some kind, try the aluminum foil/paper towel test described in chapter 23.

LEAKY SINKS

If your kitchen sink has a long-standing leak, whether around the faucets, behind the backsplash, or in the pipes underneath, then the counter and the cabinet can rot and smell. Nearly every sink sprayer I have seen has leaked from the fitting in the spray handle. When this happens, the water runs down the hose and drips into the base cabinet. It's a good idea to move stored goods periodically to check for leaks.

You should use as little water as possible throughout your kitchen, even when wiping counters, so that moisture does not seep into the countertop (most often particle board made from sawdust) and cause swelling and cracking. These spaces can become catchalls for food bits, and when moisture is added, they become a haven for pests and microbes.

DISHWASHERS

My new dishwasher could have burned my house down. When the appliance was first installed, it had a strong plastic odor that I found irritating. The odor got worse when the dishwasher was running, particularly on the dry cycle. I assumed the plastic was off-gassing and that the odor would go away with time, but it remained for months. One day in the middle of the dry cycle, the dishwasher ground to a halt. A repair person came out and took off the front panel and unscrewed the electric junction box cover. He discovered that the wires had not been secured properly by the wire nuts. The poor electrical connection led to arcing and heating. The plastic wire nuts were melted almost beyond recognition. If you detect a strange odor coming from your dishwasher, trust your instincts and call for a repair.

When dishwashers are in good working order, water in the wash cycle is splashing around inside the machine. The interior is open to the kitchen through an air vent in the door. The splashing creates minute droplets that can exit the machine with airflows. The droplets contain small amounts of detergent that can be irritating to those who are sensitized. If my clients say this bothers them, I suggest that they stay out of the kitchen when the dishwasher is on or try another detergent (but only use a detergent that does not create soap suds and that is formulated specifically for dishwashers).

I also recommend that in the summertime people rinse dishes and cutlery thoroughly before placing them in the dishwasher or that they use the "rinse and hold" cycle if the dishes will be sitting in the machine for a while before the complete wash cycle. Don't let water sit in the bottom of the dishwasher. Bacteria will grow in the food bits, and the dishwasher will start to smell rotten.

HEATERS

A couple thinking of purchasing a luxury unit in a complex on a wharf jutting out into a harbor asked me to inspect the property. Because the building was literally "on the water," it was constructed over a crawl space rather than a full basement. While inspecting the exterior, I noticed that several screened covers to the crawl space vents were missing. Inside the unit, someone had placed plastic from a garbage bag between the heat register and the floor to prevent air from blowing out.

The register was in the kitchen floor right next to the sink, a poor location for such a heat supply. One could easily imagine all sorts of food scraps falling into it. Curious about the condition of the duct, I removed the register and then the plastic beneath it. I noticed that the fiberglass insulation inside the duct was chewed, and then I realized what was happening. The plastic flexible ducts for the unit all ran through the inaccessible crawl space; rodents had access to the crawl space from the wharf because of the missing vent screens, and they had chewed through the ducts, attracted by the food that fell into the registers. Can you imagine peeling carrots at the sink and looking down to see an unwelcome guest nibbling on the scraps? I recommended that my clients replace all the flexible plastic ducts in the crawl space with metal ones and that they try not to drop food into the registers. In addition, they could move the register away from the sink (and ask the condo association to replace the crawl space vent screens).

In homes with forced hot-water heat rather than hot-air heating, a heater may be installed in the kickspace under the kitchen cabinets because there is no room for baseboard convectors or radiators. A blower forces air across coils containing hot water and then blows the air out of the kickspace. Food often gets into the space and can never be cleaned out unless there is an access panel at the bottom of the cabinet. I sampled the air coming out of the blower in one home and found large numbers of mold spores. In another house I found a layer of mouse droppings almost an eighth of an inch thick around the blower.

Another problem with a kickspace heater can be the source of makeup air. When the blower is operating, it usually draws air from

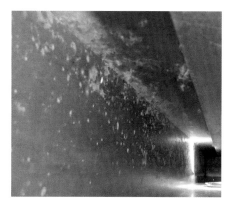

FIGURE 9.3. I often find moldy dust on dirty kitchen kick plates in the cabinet kickspaces, which rarely get cleaned. Dust and food spatters accumulate on these surfaces. Floor cleaning products, high humidity, or spilled liquids can provide moisture for mold growth in the dust.

beneath the cabinet or wherever else it can get it. Often this air comes from a moldy basement through holes around the pipes rising through the bottom of the cabinet. If you have a kickspace heater in your kitchen, make sure there is an access to the blower for cleaning and that there is a way for air from the kitchen to flow into the kickspace. You may need to seal around the pipes from the basement.

MOLDY CABINET KICKSPACES

People who keep their countertops and cabinet faces sparkling clean often don't think about cleaning the kickspaces at the foot of kitchen cabinets. These surfaces collect dust and can acquire mold growth when dampened with moisture from spilled food, mopping, or high humidity. Check kickspaces beneath your kitchen cabinets on a regular basis, HEPA vacuum away accumulated dust, and then damp-wipe and dry the surfaces (fig. 9.3).

SOME RECOMMENDATIONS

CABINET KICK SPACES
- Keep cabinet kickspace surfaces as clean and dry as possible.

CARPETING
- I don't recommend wall-to-wall carpets in areas where food is prepared and served. If you have a rug in your kitchen, keep the rug clean and dry; hard flooring is always preferable, however.

COOKING

- If you have a gas stove, be sure there are no gas leaks.

- Always be sure the ignition is on when you turn on a gas burner.

- On older gas stoves, be sure all the pilot lights are lit.

- Never use flammable liquids around pilot lights.

- Once in a while, put a carbon monoxide (CO) detector in the kitchen when you are baking with a gas oven.

- Keep the room door and windows open when operating any stove on the self-cleaning cycle.

- Have an adequate vented exhaust fan with a squirrel-cage blower over the oven and stove. To be effective, the fan should vent to the exterior.

- To minimize cooking odors in the kitchen and the rest of the house, keep the walls and other surfaces free of grease.

- Don't use a gas stove as a source of heat.

- Never use a charcoal grill inside the house.

DISHWASHERS

- If you find the air irritating when you operate your dishwasher, consider changing dishwasher detergents.

- Liquid dishwashing detergents do not contain particles that can be aerosolized.

- Don't let water sit in the bottom of your dishwasher.

FIRES

- If a fire starts in a pan, cover the pan rather than throw water on the fire.

KICKSPACE HEATERS

- The area around a kickspace heater should have an access panel and should be kept clean.

- The makeup air should come from the habitable space rather than from the basement or crawl space.

ODORS

- Get rid of your garbage quickly.

- A dilute bleach solution (one part bleach to sixteen parts water) will remove smells from a disposal (see chap. 24).

- A mild ammonia solution or baking soda in water will remove a rotten sponge odor from a surface.

- Smelly sponges can be soaked in a mild ammonia solution to remove the odor.

- Never mix bleach with ammonia; doing so creates chloramine, a toxic gas.

PANTRIES

- Keep grain foods tightly sealed in plastic.

- If you see a flour moth in a supermarket, don't buy grain foods there.

- If you have a flour moth infestation, clean the surfaces of solid food containers (such as cans) and either get rid of flour goods and grains or encase them in tightly sealing plastic bags, to see if any larvae emerge over time. Remember to clean all shelves and countertops.

REFRIGERATORS

- If your refrigerator supplies ice or cold water, check the water line for leaks by looking behind the refrigerator with a bright light.

- Keep drip trays clean.

- If you move your refrigerator for any cleaning work, be sure you don't disconnect a water line, if present.

- Replace broken gaskets.

- Keep the refrigerator coils dust-free. HEPA vacuum the coils periodically, using a suitable vacuum cleaner attachment.

- Clean the tops, bottoms, and sides of a refrigerator on a regular basis to remove biodegradable dust.

- A second refrigerator in your garage or basement must also be well maintained and kept clean.

10.

ROOMS WITH WATER— THE LAUNDRY

Having a washer and dryer in the house is a great convenience, but if we aren't careful, the machines can make the air in our homes dirty even as they're making our clothes clean.

WASHING MACHINES

LEAKS

Referred by her concerned pulmonologist, a retired woman called me because she was facing a third bout of lung surgery for aspergillosis: a disease in which *Aspergillus* mold actually grows in the lungs. The first floor of her home was open to the basement, where she spent several hours each day working on hobbies. The woman cleaned the basement using a shop vacuum; such machines are notoriously leaky and spread many particles into the air. She also did her laundry in the basement. Behind the washer and dryer I saw a large piece of plywood with dark stains at the bottom. The water supply to the washing machine had a slow leak, and the water had been soaking into the plywood. The dryer hose was partially disconnected, so air from the dryer blew against the plywood.

I took samples of the dust from the stained plywood, and I could see with a microscope that it consisted almost entirely of *Aspergillus* mold. There were even *Aspergillus* spores in the dust on top of the insulation on the steam pipe. The leaking exhaust from the dryer blew the mold spores into the air, and some went into the woman's lungs with her every breath. Once the problem was solved, she began to recover. Her pulmonologist prescribed steroids and canceled the surgery. She felt so much better she took a cruise around the world.

Another homeowner with allergies had symptoms whenever he was near the laundry area that was in a closet off a carpeted second-floor hallway. The carpet extended beneath the washer and dryer. I took Burkard air samples in the house and found that the air in the hallway contained many more mold spores than the air in the rest of the house contained. The washing machine had been leaking unnoticed, and mold was growing in the damp carpet. The man's symptoms subsided after he fixed the washing machine, replaced the hall carpet, and had a vinyl floor laid in the laundry area.

I heard about one man who operated his washing machine and forgot to turn off the plumbing valves when he went away for the weekend. The washing machine was located off his bedroom on the second level of his condominium. While he was gone, the washing machine hose burst and flooded his unit, causing extensive damage to the second and first floors and basement. This is why I recommend using laundry hoses covered with stainless steel mesh and turning off the water supplies when a washer isn't in use.

When laundry appliances are installed on the first or second floor rather than in the basement, a floor drain piped into a basement sink should be added, if possible, to handle any leaks. Occasionally, these drains are piped into the house drain system, but the drain must have a trap to prevent sewer gas from entering the house. A trap can function only if there is water in it, however. If you have a drain of this kind, pour a cup of water into it about once a month to keep odors out of the house.

MOLDY MACHINES

Front-loading washing machines are prone to developing mold problems, resulting in musty odors. If you own such a machine, clean the exterior and interior of the door gasket now and then, with either a dilute bleach solution (one part bleach to sixteen parts water) or a product suitable for the purpose (see chap. 24). Keep the door and detergent dispenser drawer open between loads to help keep these surfaces dry. Even top-loading washing machines can develop strong odors. Although the tub may look clean, the outside of the inner tub and the inside of the outer tub can become moldy (figs. 10.1 and 10.2). A washing machine has to be dismantled to clean these surfaces—work best done by a professional.

The space around the agitator shaft can fill with wet lint that can be degraded by bacteria and mold. To clean this area, a homeowner can remove the agitator and clean the inside and outside of the shaft. If the shaft in your washing machine has a basket at the top to capture

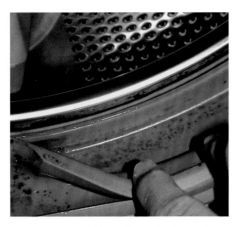

FIGURE 10.1. Mold growing on the door gasket of a front-loading washer. Water often sits at the bottom of this location, and the chronic dampness leads to the growth of odorous mold. The washing machine door and the detergent dispenser drawer should be left open between loads, and the bottom of the gasket should be dried after use.

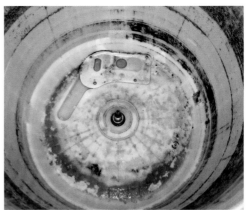

FIGURE 10.2. A family was concerned about a musty odor coming from their washing machine. They ran a few loads with bleach, but doing so did not eliminate the odor. They dismantled the machine, removing the agitator from the inner tub and removing the inner tub from the outer tub. They sent me several photos of the parts they had removed. Pictured here is the outer tub full of mold; the bottom of the inner tub was also covered with stinky mold.
PHOTO BY MIKE NEEDHAM; USED WITH PERMISSION.

lint, this too should be cleaned out periodically. If the machine has an "extra spin and empty" cycle, use it when you've finished washing all your clothes or bedding. This will help empty any water left over under the drum.

FROM DIRTY TO CLEAN

How you handle the clothing before and after it's washed can also affect indoor air quality. Dirty clothes often go into a hamper, but some people let dirty clothes accumulate on the basement floor if the laundry area is on that level. Either way, if some of the dirty clothing is damp, bacteria may start to grow on skin scales or on the cellulose fibers in cotton within hours, particularly in warm weather. If the clothes are left long enough, mold may begin to flourish (fig. 10.3).

In a basement of one property I was inspecting, the lighting was poor, but I could see large piles of laundry on the floor. The scene reminded me of a mountain range except that the air wasn't fresh. When I looked more closely, I could see mushrooms (macrofungi; see chap. 2) growing at the bottom of some of the piles on the damp basement floor; the soiled clothing must have been there for months. The mother had gone on strike and refused to continue washing her children's clothing. I wouldn't suggest wearing any of those clothes again!

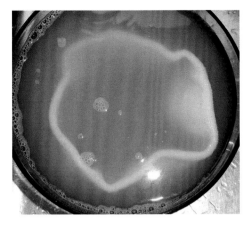

FIGURE 10.3. I decided to wash my sweat band in a bowl of detergent water. After I placed the band in the water and stirred it around, the water became murky. The discoloration of the water is due to the release by the detergent of all the skin scales that were trapped in the fabric.

LAUNDRY CHUTES

Some homes have laundry chutes, and the clothing ends up on the basement floor waiting to be washed. Don't leave the piles of dirty clothes there too long, particularly if the basement is damp. I also have a safety concern about laundry chutes. There should be a secured door on a laundry chute to prevent a child from falling in. I heard about one family in which an older child dropped the youngest child down the chute as a joke. Luckily he landed on a pile of clothing—the very pile I just recommended that you not accumulate.

After clothes are washed, it's not a good idea to leave them wet for too many hours because bacteria may start to grow. If this happens, you can rewash the clothes with some ammonia in the water, but never mix ammonia with bleach.

DETERGENTS AND FABRIC SOFTENERS

BUBBLES

Detergents and fabric softeners contain chemicals (including fragrances) that some people find irritating to inhale. When a washing machine is operating, small amounts of these chemicals enter the air. As the water is agitated, bubbles float to the surface because they are less dense than the liquid. When a bubble reaches the surface, it pops through, and the thin water film at the top of the bubble (the cap) breaks. The surface of the water beneath the cap springs up and ejects a droplet of soapy liquid.

Some of these droplets enter the air even though the washer lid is closed. When the machine refills after emptying, the water displaces air that contains droplets, and even more potential irritants are emitted into the room. Some of these droplets are so small they become suspended in air, where they and the laundry chemicals they contain may be inhaled. For this reason, people with allergies and asthma should avoid using perfumed detergents and liquid fabric softeners.

One of my clients had a laundry closet in a hallway outside her child's bedroom. The boy had asthma, and his symptoms seemed to increase on washday. I recommended that the family do the laundry when the son was in school, because the droplets released persist for only a short time. They quickly evaporate and dry, and the residues settle out of the air or leak out of the house with airflow, which can be increased by opening a window.

ENZYMES IN DETERGENTS

In the late 1960s, Procter and Gamble (P&G) started incorporating an enzyme (subtilisin) in its laundry detergent in order to assist in removing bloodstains from clothing. Enzymes are chemicals that all living things use to digest and synthesize proteins, carbohydrates, and fats necessary to sustain life. Enzyme names usually end in "ase." Lipase enzymes digest fat, amylase enzymes digest starch, cellulase enzymes digest cellulose, and protease enzymes digest protein (protease is manufactured by a genetically modified bacteria called *Bacillus subtilis*).

Soon after introducing subtilisin (a protease) into the detergent formulation, P&G started to notice that in some plants there was an unusual increase (up to 50 percent)[1] in allergy and asthma symptoms in its workers. The cause of the workers' symptoms was determined to be inhalation of the enzyme dust in the factory air. P&G then took steps to reduce the dust. (I believe that most detergents today are liquid because manufacturing these detergents results in far less worker exposure to the detergent dust from powdered products containing enzymes.)

When the news of this occupational health issue was publicized, some scientists and homeowners became concerned that exposure to this allergenic component in some laundry detergents might cause comparable rates of sensitization among consumers. Karen Sarlo, a biochemist at P&G, conducted a study of the effect on guinea pigs of exposure to enzymes and concluded that consumers were not at risk of developing sensitization to protease.[2] In 2012, the *Journal of Immunology* published an article that stated: "Detergent enzymes have a very good safety profile, with almost no capacity to generate adverse acute or chronic responses in humans. The exceptions are the limited ability of some proteases to produce irritating effects at high concentrations, and the intrinsic potential of these bacterial and fungal proteins to act as respiratory sensitizers, demonstrated in humans during the early phase of the industrial use of enzymes during the 1960s and 1970s."[3] Yet a number of our clients told us that some of their allergy symptoms abated when they stopped using laundry detergents containing enzymes.

The original enzymes were not stable in hot water, so the bacteria that made the enzymes were bioengineered to produce enzymes that were more stable at higher temperatures. Still, washing clothing in hot water destroys much but not all of the enzyme activity. Any residual enzymes left in the clothing or bedding being washed will more than likely be eliminated when these materials are dried in a hot dryer.

But what about people who use cool or cold water to wash and air fluff or clotheslines to dry clothing? One of our clients did his laundry on Saturdays, using a cool-water wash and drying the laundry on medium to low heat. After folding the laundry, he experienced such serious allergy symptoms that he spent the rest of the weekend in bed. Our daughter has always hung her laundry to dry rather than use a dryer. When she went to Puerto Rico as an AmeriCorps volunteer, she started using a laundry detergent containing protease. Her asthma symptoms worsened but then abated when she switched to a non-enzyme-containing detergent. I experimented with enzyme-containing laundry detergent by washing some clothes in cold water and drying them on the air fluff setting. I sent the lint from the lint screen to a laboratory to test for enzyme activity. The lab found a low level of protease activity in the lint.[4]

If you wash your clothing in hot water and use a hot dryer for drying, you may not risk exposure to active enzymes. If you use cool or cold water to wash and a cool dryer or hang your clothes up to dry, however, you may be at an exposure risk to active enzymes on the clothing lint that you inhale and in the clothing or bedding that touches your skin. Unfortunately, many popular detergent brands (including "organic" ones) contain enzymes, and sometimes more than one kind of enzyme. Typically, the only detergents that do not contain enzymes are generic brands, but always check the ingredient label. If there is no ingredient list on the bottle, choose another brand. I recognize that millions of people wear clothing and sleep on bedding washed with enzyme-containing detergents but only a small percentage of these people become sensitized. If you or someone in your household is one of the unfortunate few who are sensitized, switching to a non-enzyme-containing detergent seems a sensible step. Most of our clients have a variety of allergies, so as a precaution I always recommend that they avoid using any laundry detergents that contain enzymes.

Why are enzymes so problematic? Possibly because anytime a microorganism infects a body, the microorganism secrets enzymes to digest its surroundings (i.e., you!). It is therefore essential that the human immune system detect the presence of foreign enzymes; in fact, many of the most significant allergens are enzymes produced by plants and animals.

SOFTENERS AND FRAGRANCES

After our first child was born, I began to wake up in the morning with irritated eyes. Within a few months my eyes would be swollen shut each morning. After a year or so this condition cleared up. My eyes swelled up again when our second child was born. Connie finally figured out what was happening. When our children were infants, she added a liquid fabric softener to the wash to make their clothes fragrant and soft. Unfortunately, she washed their clothes with some of our own, and soon our shirts, pants, and sheets picked up the chemicals in the fabric softeners—chemicals to which I was sensitized.

I am glad to see that there are more unfragranced laundry products available now than when we wrote the first edition of this book. Still, some companies advertise "natural" products that are supposed to be nontoxic but are nonetheless fragranced. For asthma and allergy sufferers, even "natural" scents can be irritating. The individual chemical components of both natural and synthetic fragrances can cause health symptoms. "Overall, 34.7% of the population reported health problems, such as migraine headaches and respiratory difficulties, when exposed to fragranced products."[5] Many of the volatile organic compounds (VOCs) in fragrances affect the nervous and respiratory systems.[6]

DRYERS

Dryers should always be vented directly to the outside or they will spew excess moisture and lint coated with laundry chemicals into the house. In addition, gas dryers may exhaust carbon monoxide.

VENTING A DRYER INSIDE

In an attic of one home, I found a serious moisture problem caused by a dryer that was venting into the house. The front of the house faced south, and the rear faced north. When I looked at the south-facing roof sheathing, the plywood looked fine. On the north side it was a different story. The sheathing was soaking wet, and water was dripping from the tips of all the shingle nails protruding through the sheathing to the inside of the attic.

The owner had three children and had just done her fourth load of laundry for the day. A year earlier the family had finished the basement where the laundry was located. To save money, their plumber suggested they vent the dryer into a lint trap in a closet under the basement stairs rather than vent the dryer to the exterior. (A lint trap is a plastic device that is about half-filled with water and that looks like a barrel with holes in it. The device does not contain all the lint, but what lint it does contain becomes damp and then can support mold growth.)

Warm, moist air from the closet was less dense than cooler air and thus rose up around plumbing pipes to the unheated attic, where vapor condensed onto the cooler, sunless north side of the roof. Fortunately, this condensation had been occurring for only a year; had it gone on for two or three more years, the entire roof structure on the north side would have been covered with mold and possibly even macrofungi.

One afternoon I was inspecting a multifamily house and was in the basement while one of the building occupants was doing his laundry. The dryer exhaust was venting directly into the basement, and there was a layer of lint on everything. I heard a commotion from the other side of the basement and saw flames coming out of the dryer. The terrified man turned off the dryer and managed to extinguish the fire. Lint had built up in the air intake, close to the gas flame, and had ignited! It's therefore a good idea to check the bottom of the dryer in the vicinity of the gas flame and clean as needed.

At a single-family property located on an island off the Massachusetts coast, a couple had designed their home to make it as "green" and energy efficient as possible. Unfortunately, part of the home was built over an inaccessible crawl space. Their dryer was venting into the crawl space, introducing moisture and biodegradable lint into the space. I detected a musty smell as soon as I entered the part of the house over the crawl space. Even though the couple never went into the crawl space, air carrying mold spores was flowing from the crawl space into the rooms above. To solve this problem, they had to create an opening into the crawl space from the outside, have the crawl space professionally remediated, and then vent the dryer directly to the exterior.

A newly renovated million-dollar duplex condominium contained a living room, dining room, and kitchen on the upper level. The bedrooms were partially below grade (below ground level), with direct access to a private city garden at the rear of the property. Faucets were gleaming, carpets were plush, and appliances all top-of-the-line, but the builder had taken a shortcut when he vented the dryer.

To vent the dryer to the outside, the builder would have had to go through a brick wall. To avoid this expense, he vented the dryer into a small storage area under the front masonry steps. To handle the excess moisture, he included a dehumidifier as a feature in the price of the condominium. The dehumidifier drained into a sewer-ejection system (into which the toilets on the lower level also drained), but the system was leaking. The new owners were getting some features they hadn't expected!

THE SICKENING LAUNDRY ROOM

One woman called me because she had headaches now and then when she did the laundry. The laundry was in their basement boiler room. When the boiler was operating, a fan turned on to bring in outside air for combustion. At the exterior wall, the boiler's vent pipe exhaust was about 18 inches away from the boiler's fresh-air intake duct. Both ducts were at an interior corner of the home near the ground, where there was a large overhang at the roof. The geometry of this setup trapped the combustion products in the area close to the exterior wall and fresh-air intake. The combustion products from the boiler contained a high level of carbon monoxide, and this gas was sucked in by the "fresh-air" intake and blown into the boiler room. When the boiler was operating and the woman was doing laundry in the room, she was exposed to carbon monoxide. Connie was with me on this appointment, because we were on a trip and the house happened to be on our way to our destination, so we agreed to go to the property. The woman was so relieved to know that she hadn't been imagining things that, as Connie and I were leaving, she lunged forward and hugged Connie with tears in her eyes.

HEAT AND DRYERS

Occasionally, a water heater or boiler will be placed next to a dryer in a small mechanical closet. In such an arrangement, the dryer can cause backdrafting if the closet has a solid door and there is no other source of makeup air. In one such mechanical closet with the door shut, I tested for combustion spillage with my TIF8800 combustible gas detector at the vent pipe of a water heater. When the dryer was off, there was normal draft at the vent pipe, but when the dryer was running, it sucked the makeup air it needed from the water heater's vent pipe, and combustion gases filled the closet. In the best of all worlds, dryers should not be placed in small spaces next to combustion equipment (unless the equipment is direct vented, bringing in its own combustion air directly from outdoors). If you have such an arrangement in your home, a louvered door will supply combustion air from the house to eliminate the backdrafting.

I investigated a home for a man who was chemically sensitive. The recently renovated master bathroom contained an unvented gas dryer and an air return for the heating and cooling system. When the dryer and the heating and cooling system blower were operating at the same time, combustion products, fabric softener, and lint were circulated throughout the condominium. I encountered a similar situation involving allergies in another single-family home. The first thing I noted when I entered was that the house smelled like a laundromat. We pulled the dryer away from the first-floor wall and discovered that the exhaust hose took an unusual route. Instead of venting directly to the outside through a wall, the hose had been fed through a hole in the floor. Unfortunately, the return duct for the heating and cooling system was in the basement ceiling directly below the hole, and the installer had cut holes for the dryer hose through the top and bottom of the return duct. The hose then exited the building from the basement.

In this case the exhaust hose had become disconnected from the dryer. The holes in the floor and the sheet metal of the return duct were bigger than the hose itself, leaving gaps. Whenever the heat pump and the dryer operated simultaneously, air from the laundry room was sucked in through these gaps. Then fabric softener and detergent chemicals exhausting from the dryer were drawn into the return duct and from there were circulating throughout the house. Lint was also being drawn into the duct.

To relieve his allergies, the man had installed an expensive, central electronic air cleaner (refer to part IV), but there was so much debris in the return air that the electronic power module for the cleaner had burned out several times. He had also replaced the air conditioning compressor twice because the evaporator coil had clogged with lint.

The solution? Install a dryer vent that exhausted to the exterior and did not pass through the return duct.

COLD VENTING

Dryers should not be vented for great lengths through cold spaces. I was in the four-car garage of an expensive seven-year-old house in which the laundry was next to the garage. The dryer had to be vented at the opposite gable end of the garage attic. The many sections of metal vent pipe rested on the joists above the garage ceiling and traveled through the unheated attic. The warm, moist air from the dryer cooled as it traveled through the piping. As water condensed inside the pipes, it leaked out the joints and dripped onto the garage ceiling and down the rear walls, creating stains about every six feet where the sections of pipe connected.

I heard about a similar situation where a flexible dryer vent hose went through an unheated attic. The hose drooped and formed loops inside the bays between the ceiling joists. Again, water condensed within the hose as the moist air traveling through it cooled. This type of plastic hose is watertight, so instead of leaking out, the moisture formed puddles at the bottom of each loop. The lint provided nutrients for mold growth in each of these little ponds, so when the dryer was not running, air carrying mold spores back drafted through the dryer and into the house, aggravating the owners' allergies.

AIR-DRYING

Some of us hang our clothes inside or outside to air-dry. In households where occupants have allergies or asthma, clothing should not be dried where the air is full of allergens. Be careful to avoid moldy basements or pollen-laden trees. And a word of caution: it's a fire hazard to hang clothes within three feet of furnaces, boilers, or water heaters. Never use a boiler or furnace vent pipe to dry anything!

SOME RECOMMENDATIONS

DRYERS

- If you or anyone in your household has allergies or asthma, don't use fabric softener sheets, particularly those with fragrance added.
- Always vent a dryer to the outside and be sure that the dryer exhaust hose is intact (there should be not be lint piles behind your dryer).
- Unless sloped correctly, dryer vent hoses should not travel for great lengths through cold spaces.
- Avoid placing a dryer in a mechanical closet that also contains the water heater or furnace that takes combustion air from the closet. If you have such an arrangement, have a louvered door installed.
- Keep the area near the flame of a gas dryer as lint-free as possible.
- Don't hang clothes to dry indoors where there are allergens in the air (such as in a moldy basement).
- If you are allergic to the pollen of some trees that grow near your home, don't dry your clothing outdoors.

WASHING MACHINES

- Regularly check your washing machine for leaks and repair any you find.
- When the washing machine is not in use, close the water supply valves.
- Use water hoses covered with stainless steel mesh.

- If the laundry room is not in the basement, consider installing a drain and waterproof flooring under the washer. Put a floor water alarm near the washer to detect leaks.

- Do not put a carpet on the floor of your laundry area.

- Try to avoid laundry detergents that contain fragrance and enzymes for a while, to see if the allergy or asthma symptoms that you or others in your household experience abate.

- Don't let damp clothing sit around.

- If your washing machine develops an odor, clean any lint that may have accumulated around the base of the agitator or in the basket at the top.

- Keep the lid of your top-loading washing machine open between loads.

- If you have a front-loading washing machine, keep the front door and laundry-dispenser drawer open between loads; regularly clean the inside of the door gasket.

- Musty odors in a washing machine can be minimized after doing a load by placing a 200-watt ceramic heater inside the empty machine (for a few hours only). Never place the heater inside the machine if there is visible water or clothing in the drum. Leave the washer's lid or door open at least six inches. Obviously, unplug and remove the heater before loading the machine with any clothing or turning the machine on. Other people who use your washing machine should exercise similar cautions and never put clothing in the machine or operate the machine when the heater is inside.

11.

BEDROOMS

Even if you sleep as little as six hours a night, you still spend a quarter of your twenty-four-hour day in your bedroom. If you sleep eight hours a night, you spend a third of your twenty-four-hour day in your bedroom. Add a nap to these numbers, and you spend even more of your day in the room. People spend a lot of time in bedrooms, so controlling the quality of the air in these rooms is essential for maintaining health. In families with allergies or asthma, it is vital.

I am constantly amazed at the particles I find in bedroom air. These particles may make you cough when you get into bed, or they may make your asthma or allergy symptoms worse when you get up. In such circumstances many people feel they need to wash the sheets or blankets more frequently than usual. You could spend your entire life cleaning floors, windows, shelves, and books, as well as laundering the bedspread, and you would still be coughing if the mattress or even one throw pillow was full of dust mites, mold, bacteria, or yeast. To solve the problem, the source of the irritating dust must be identified and eliminated.

MITES

Before I started looking at air quality problems, I had no idea how big a hazard dust mites could be. I found out when my son, in eighth grade at the time, was hospitalized in the middle of the night with his first asthma attack. Even though we were always conscientious about changing sheets weekly and washing blankets and quilts every month, I decided to test all the beds in the house for dust mites. I vacuumed each mattress for several minutes, using a filter cassette (made for the purpose) on the end of the vacuum hose that trapped most of the dust and prevented it from going into the vacuum bag. I sent each filter cassette containing the dust to a laboratory for analysis. Fewer than 2 micrograms of mite allergens per gram of dust is considered low; over 10 is considered at significant risk for asthma. The concentrations of mite allergens in each of our mattresses were outrageously high, with more than 30 micrograms of allergens per gram of dust. This is why I always recommend that people put dust mite allergen-control covers on mattresses and pillows.

If any family member has asthma or dust mite allergy, all mattresses, box springs, and pillows throughout the house should be encased in mite covers. It's not enough for people to cover the mattresses and pillows in the bedrooms, because dust mites can also flourish in couch pillows, the mattresses in sofa beds, and futon couches. I recommend that these too have allergen-control covers. Some people think waterbeds can't harbor dust mites because the mattress is essentially a sealed plastic bag. It's true that mites cannot imbibe the moisture contained within the plastic, but the thick mattress pads used on water beds can contain a high level of mite allergens. A detailed discussion of mites and dust-mite encasings appears in chapter 2.

FEATHERS

Down bedding can be a particular problem for more than one reason. First, the species name for dust mite is *Dermatophagoides pteronyssinu*, Latin for "skin eating, feather loving," because anything that contains down can become a haven for mites. Second, the feathers themselves can break up into small, sharp, airborne fibers that can be inhaled. The first time I saw down fragments under the microscope, I thought, "These could be irritants." I foolishly put my face into the sleeve of my down parka, compressed the material, and inhaled. The pressure forced the down fragments into the air I inhaled, and I coughed deeply and painfully for several hours. And third, feathers can be a source of bird-bloom particles. See chapter 3 for a detailed discussion of the possible consequences (including the respiratory illness hypersensitivity pneumonitis) of exposure to these particles.

One woman I know spent her winter holidays in a friend's basement apartment, sleeping in a guest bed that backed up against a brick wall. It was cold in the apartment, and she pulled the comforter over her face to keep warm as she slept. After her first night there she woke up with a mild rash on her face and neck. She applied soothing creams, but in the days that followed her skin turned red and mottled.

In the last few days of her visit her chest felt tight. She and her friend thought the down comforter might be bothering her. As soon as she replaced the comforter with a cotton quilt, her rash faded and her chest discomfort subsided.

In another situation, two elderly sisters lived together. Every October the older sister began having respiratory symptoms. The younger sister always gave the older one her extra pillow so she would be more upright in bed to ease her coughing. This routine went on for years, until the older sister got worried about the increasing severity of her annual bouts with bronchitis. I found that her symptoms began each year when she put a down comforter on the bed as the weather turned cooler. She knew she was irritated by feathers, but she never realized that her own comforter was down because it was encased in a cotton cover. But there's more to the story: the pillow her sister lent her was also filled with down! The cotton coverings did not prevent the release of irritants. Once she got rid of the down comforter and pillow, she got rid of her bronchitis.

In my experience, many people who cough when they go to bed or when they first get up find relief when they get rid of their down pillows or comforters. Wool can also be a problem, so I suggest using bedding made of cotton or synthetic materials. We discuss surrogate allergens in detail in chapter 3.

BEDROOM "GUESTS"

Earlier in the book we discouraged you from allowing pets in bedrooms. Animals don't have to be alive to carry contaminants. Stuffed animals can be full of mites and dander if they are in the bed and serve as miniature pillows. Even the filling of new stuffed animals can be allergenic. (One case in the medical literature described a toy animal stuffed with soybeans, and the child was sensitized to the stuffing.[1])

The parents of one small child with asthma and dust mite allergy had done everything possible to prevent him from experiencing symptoms in his bedroom, but nothing seemed to alleviate his wheezing in the room. The little boy hated taking baths, so his mother used to encourage him by making a game of wiping his favorite stuffed bear with a damp washcloth and then drying the bear with a towel. He slept with the bear every night, so seeing the bear be brave about water gave the little boy courage. Unfortunately, I found a massive dust mite infestation in the bear, because it had been dampened again and again and because the bear's fur had collected the little boy's skin scales. The parents secretly replaced the infested bear with an identical one

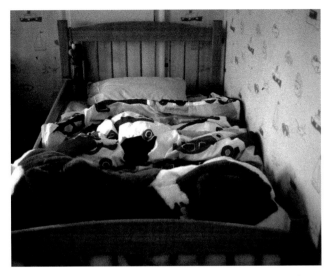

FIGURE 11.1. Well-meaning parents damp-wiped this stuffed bear in order to entice their son to bathe. Due to the moisture from the damp-wiping, the bear became infested with dust mites, and the boy suffered asthma symptoms in his Spartan bedroom until the bear was secretly replaced with an identical new one.

that they never again wiped down! The boy's asthma symptoms in his bedroom abated (fig. 11.1).

EXCESS MOISTURE

Bedrooms can become mold greenhouses if too much moisture is present. Moisture can be introduced in unexpected ways. One teenager with asthma went off to college and was relatively symptom-free. When she returned home on vacation and went to bed the first night, her asthma symptoms flared up. It might seem that the air in the entire house was contaminated or that the girl's symptoms were caused by emotional upheaval, but the truth is that during high school she had showered every night before going to bed and then placed her mop of wet hair directly on her pillow. The pillow she slept on at home for at least six hours each night was covered with mold.

Taking long showers in a bathroom next to a bedroom and operating a portable humidifier in the room can raise the relative humidity (RH). As the RH rises, more moisture is present for mites and microarthropods. Carpeting laid on concrete can also acquire mite infestations. The carpet is cooled by contact with the concrete, and then air within the carpet fibers or in contact with the fibers will be cooled in return. Microbial growth can ensue when the RH is over 80 percent.

In one family, an infant suffered from bouts of wheezing, month-long colds, and ear infections. In the baby's bedroom I found barely visible colonies of pale yellow *Aspergillus* mold growing on the bottoms of the dresser, bed, and table. (After gently waving a notebook to disturb dust, I found that the concentration of *Aspergillus* spores in the bedroom was thousands of times higher than in the outside air.) The parents ran a humidifier in the baby's room, so the RH levels were excessive.

One woman who constantly ran two steam humidifiers in her bedroom all winter started having severe allergy symptoms. The moisture had condensed on the cold exterior wall of the house. Behind the peeling wallpaper, I found the plaster completely black with mold. Dust hung like vines from the box spring beneath her bed, and when I looked at a sample of the dust with a microscope I found mites nibbling on the mold-covered dust balls. In the home of another client with a chronic cough and a diagnosed mold allergy, a bedroom humidifier ran all night during the winter.

TYPES OF ROOM HUMIDIFIERS

There are four types of room humidifiers: ultrasonic, evaporative pad, steam, and warm mist. Some are more conducive to IAQ problems than others are.

ULTRASONIC HUMIDIFIERS

An ultrasonic humidifier, also known as a cool mist humidifier, uses sound energy to convert liquid water directly into microscopic droplets that are suspended in an airstream blowing through the unit. I don't recommend this kind of humidifier, because whatever minerals, bacteria, or algae that are in the water to begin with can be aerosolized.

Before I knew better, I was using an ultrasonic humidifier in our bedroom. This worked fine for a while, but I suddenly started coughing in the bedroom when the humidifier was on. I took some of the water, centrifuged it to collect suspended solids, and looked at the solids with a microscope. To my utter amazement there were small (about 5-micron) round microorganisms with tails darting around in the water. I discovered much later that these were motile fungal spores (*Chytridiomycota*). Another type of *Chytridiomycota* called *Phytophthora infestans* caused the infamous Irish potato famine.

EVAPORATIVE PAD HUMIDIFIERS

Most evaporative pad humidifiers contain an evaporative cellulose (paper) mesh pad. Water from the reservoir evaporates into air

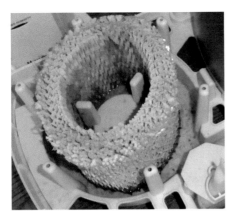

FIGURE 11.2. This moldy portable humidifier was from a home in which the occupant suffered from headaches and sinus problems. Portions of the cellulose humidifier pad (called a "wick") were coated with bacteria and mold growth. The pads should be replaced regularly, and antimicrobial chemicals should be added to the water as directed by the humidifier manufacturer.

that the fan draws across the pad. I have seen the pads of several such humidifiers covered with mold and bacteria. In four homes the pads were black with potentially toxic *Stachybotrys* mold (fig. 11.2).

An evaporative pad humidifier is prone to biological contamination for two reasons: first, the cellulose pad itself can serve as a nutrient, and second, the mesh pad acts as a filter, capturing biodegradable particles (such as skin scales and cornstarch from body powder) from the air. I believe humidifiers with cellulose evaporative pads should be banned because they are so prone to contamination. There is at least one European portable evaporative humidifier that uses a large set of plates that rotate in a water reservoir. If you use one of these, always use the water treatment additive solution that comes with the unit, as it prevents microbial growth in the water.

In one home, a mother and her daughter had been suffering from continuous respiratory problems for most of the winter. The worse their symptoms became, the longer they operated their evaporative pad humidifier. I found high levels of actinomycetes (filamentous bacteria) in the air and on the pad. The family stopped using the humidifier and cleaned up house dust, and within two weeks mother and daughter were well again.

STEAM HUMIDIFIERS AND WARM MIST HUMIDIFIERS

Steam humidifiers and warm mist humidifiers both boil water and emit only water vapor; minerals and other contaminants remain behind in the water reservoir. In a warm mist humidifier the "steam" is mixed with and cooled by room air as the vapor leaves the unit. The vapor condenses to small droplets of visible "steam" that quickly evaporate back to invisible water vapor. Steam humidifiers produce much more moisture than warm mist humidifiers

Actinomycetes are soil bacteria but grow the way mold grows, with very fine hyphae and very small spores. Exposure to one species of actinomycetes is a recognized cause of hypersensitivity pneumonitis.

and can result in excess RH, so of all the kinds of humidifiers available, I prefer the warm mist type (preferably one with a humidistat). In any case, the RH should be monitored.

MEASURING THE RELATIVE HUMIDITY

If you use a portable humidifier or have a central humidification system, you should monitor the RH with a thermo-hygrometer, available in most hardware stores. The RH should never exceed 40 percent (under 35 percent on very cold nights). A humidistat shuts a humidifier off when the RH in the room reaches the set point. Few steam and warm mist humidifiers have humidistats. For portable steam or warm mist humidifiers without a built-in humidistat, the RH can be controlled by plugging the unit into an outlet adapter (which can be purchased in any hardware store) that is an on-off timer. With the timer, the humidifier can be turned on and off in intervals (usually thirty minutes). If the RH is too high, reduce the number of "on" intervals.

CLOSETS

Cedar walls or mothballs in bedroom closets emit chemicals that can irritate people who are sensitized to them. In addition, most mothballs are pesticides (either napthalene or p-dichlorobenzene), which can be harmful to anyone's health. An ordinary closet can be a source of mold and mite contamination, particularly if it is in a shaded outside corner of the house or is cantilevered (overhanging an exterior wall). The temperature of such an outside wall or floor may be below the dew point, causing condensation to form. Mold and mites find a welcome home in such locations. If the RH is high enough, mold can spread to shoes, clothing, stored boxes, and carpeting. As people remove their clothing and shake it, allergens become airborne and flow into the bedroom.

A physician referred a patient to me who was having difficulty controlling his asthma symptoms, which occurred wherever he went. I found mold growing in his closet and mite fecal pellets in his clothing, including the jacket he wore to work. In another home in which the master bedroom was partially below grade, the closet in the room had an exterior wall. The occupants kept the heat low when they were at work. They also kept the closet door closed, so the RH was high inside the space. The clothing inside the closet was covered with mold.

WALL-TO-WALL CARPETING

I have found dust mite droppings and other allergens in many bedroom carpets. Even with the most thorough vacuuming, you can never remove all the dust and allergens from carpeting. Since we spend so much time in our bedrooms (shedding all those skin scales), for people with allergies or asthma, I recommend solid flooring such as wood or laminate, since hard surfaces like these are easier to clean.

COOLING THE AIR WITH WINDOW OR THROUGH-WALL A/C UNITS

People often use window air conditioners to cool the air in their bedrooms. Air conditioners increase our comfort by cooling air and removing moisture, but because nearly all air conditioners have inadequate dust filters, biodegradable material accumulates on the cold, damp cooling coils. Within days, mold, bacteria, and yeast can start to grow in the dust on the coils. In dirty air conditioners the mold can spread to the interior walls of the unit and even to the blower, growing until every speck of dust is consumed and converted to hyphae and spores. The air movement from the blower may then circulate by-products of these organisms. Even if the organisms themselves aren't circulating, the odors they produce fill the air inside the unit and pass into the room with airflows, alerting people that an IAQ problem is brewing.

Some people leave window air conditioners in place for years. This is asking for trouble. If you find that running your air conditioner makes your allergy or asthma symptoms worse, have the unit cleaned and disinfected. If you have allergies or asthma, window air conditioners should be removed and cleaned and disinfected at the beginning of every cooling season. If your bedroom has a through-wall air conditioner, it may have to be cleaned in place (see chap. 24).

Sometimes, window air conditioners can leak condensate water. In one home, a child developed asthma symptoms because the water from an improperly sloped window air conditioner dripped onto the carpet under his desk in his bedroom, causing mold growth. As he sat at his desk to do his homework, his feet disturbed the moldy dust in the carpet fibers, and he breathed in the spores.

We discuss maintenance of and filtration for portable rather than window air conditioners in chapter 20.

SOME RECOMMENDATIONS

BEDS

- I recommend that you install allergen-control covers on all pillows and mattresses in your home (see chap. 2). Cover the mattresses on sofa beds and futon couches as well.

- Wash sheets weekly in hot water.

- Wash blankets at least monthly, and tumble them weekly in a warm or hot dryer for about twenty minutes.

- Wash quilts a few times a season, and be sure to dry them thoroughly. Tumble them weekly in a warm or hot dryer for at least twenty minutes.

- If you do not encase pillows, tumble them at least monthly in the dryer and replace them periodically.

- Wash and thoroughly dry thin mattress pads monthly.

- If a friend offers you a mattress, refuse it with thanks. Secondhand mattresses may be contaminated with mites.

- Avoid down quilts or pillows (see chap. 3).

- If you are sensitized to wool, avoid using wool blankets on beds.

- Don't overload beds with pillows and stuffed animals.

- Stuffed animals that you or your child can't part with can be tumbled in the dryer weekly.

CARPETING

- Avoid having wall-to-wall carpeting in bedrooms; use small, washable rugs instead.

CLOSETS

- If the odor of a bedroom cedar closet bothers you, either remove the cedar or seal the walls with aluminum foil and aluminum foil tape.

- Keep your closet as clean and dust-free as the rest of the bedroom.

- Don't store too many items in exterior closets (closets that face the exterior). Keep goods up off the floor and away from cold walls.

- Don't store goods on a closet floor that is concrete or that has carpeting laid on concrete.

- To facilitate the flow of heated air into exterior closets, keep the closet doors ajar, install louvered doors, or get closet heaters made for this purpose (don't use space heaters that present fire hazards).

CLOTHING

- Wash or dry-clean clothing frequently.

- Frequently worn but rarely cleaned items of heavy clothing such as winter jackets and coats should be tumbled periodically in a warm or hot dryer.

- Dry cleaning kills mites and destroys some mite allergens.

MOISTURE

- Don't go to bed with damp hair.

- If you use a portable humidifier, monitor the relative humidity with a thermo-hygrometer. Keep the relative humidity below 40 percent in the winter (preferably under 35 percent on very cold nights). (We discuss central humidification systems in chap. 18.)

- I only recommend warm mist humidifiers.

- Follow the manufacturer's directions about cleaning and maintaining humidifiers.

- When using a portable humidifier, keep the door to the room closed to prevent loss of the moisture.

PESTICIDES

- I don't recommend using mothballs or pesticide sprays inside a home, especially in a bedroom.

PETS

- Keep dogs, cats, rabbits, hamsters, and other pets out of your bedroom (see chap. 5).

- People with asthma should not have fish tanks in their bedrooms.

- People who own pets should not lie on the bed of anyone who has asthma or allergies.

12

ATTACHED GARAGES, BULKHEADS, PORCHES, AND DECKS

Conditions in an attached garage as well as in a bulkhead and on a porch or deck can have a negative effect on our indoor air quality.

ATTACHED GARAGES

People think of an attached garage as an exterior space, but as far as the flow of air is concerned, an attached garage is part of your living space, particularly if you have finished rooms above or next to the garage. Your exposure to irritants and allergens in a garage will be even greater if you enter and exit the house through that space.

To prevent airflows from a garage into adjacent rooms, the door from the garage to the house should be made airtight with gasket material, and there should be no openings in the garage walls or ceiling, particularly if there is a room above. (An airtight ceiling, required for most attached garages, will also prevent smoke from spreading if there is a fire.) It is also important to keep the garage as clean and allergen- and contaminant-free as possible.

PESTS

Garages are prone to pest entry because overhead garage doors don't always fit tightly at the bottom or sides (see chap. 5). Decayed trim at the door casing may present another entry point for pests. And there should never be exposed fiberglass insulation present, because mice love to nest in the stuff (fig. 12.1).

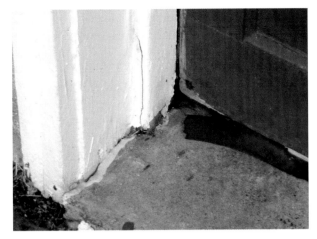

FIGURE 12.1. Rodents can enter homes through an overhead garage door, as there are often openings or gaps at the bottom edge of the door or at the bottom of decayed exterior trim boards. Generally, the rodents chew through decayed wood or flexible rubber or plastic gaskets. Once in the garage, rodents may find openings to enter the home.

Don't store open containers of birdseed or other food goods in your garage that may attract mice. We have made that mistake. Connie likes to have bird feeders at the edge of our yard. Once she spilled a few tablespoons of birdseed on the garage floor when she was filling up a bird feeder. She left the garage door open while she went to hang the bird feeder up on a tree branch. When she returned, she entered the house through the garage and closed the automatic garage door. As she was working in our adjacent kitchen, she heard some rustling in the garage. When she opened the door between the kitchen and the garage, she saw a chipmunk feasting on the spilled birdseed. She opened the garage door and shooed the animal back outside. From then on, she filled the bird feeders in our driveway and not in the garage, and she stored birdseed in a tightly lidded plastic box. Chipmunks are one thing; mice are another, and mice seem to like birdseed, too.

STORAGE

Storing anything in an attached garage can cause trouble. If people sometimes keep garbage or old, moldy furniture in an attached garage, odors can enter the house. Items that are leaning up against cool concrete walls and boxes sitting on the concrete floor can acquire mold growth. Don't clutter your garage with goods; remember, the more goods that are present, the more surfaces there are for the collection of dust, and the more nooks and crannies there are in which rodents can hide and nest. Keep goods in tightly lidded plastic bins and use rolling metal shelving to keep stored goods up off the floor.

MOLD

There's plenty of biodegradable dust in most garages to provide fodder for mold growth. Humid outdoor air, rain or snow on vehicles, or water seeping through the foundation or under garage doors can supply the moisture that mold requires for growth.

I often find mold growth at the back of overhead garage doors because these surfaces can be cool, resulting in condensation due to elevated relative humidity (RH). Generally, the mold growth is black and darkest near the bottom of the door, although if you have a diesel engine vehicle, the discoloration could be due to soot. It's hard to prevent mold growth like this, but it will not decay the wood (see chap. 2) and can be wiped away with a dilute bleach solution (one part bleach to sixteen parts water) or with a detergent and water solution (see chap. 24). Newer overhead garage doors are insulated and less prone to condensation and mold growth.

The moisture that mold requires for growth can be introduced into a garage when someone drives a car into the space on a rainy day or when the vehicle is covered with snow that melts in the garage. If you live in a climate with snowy winters and park your car inside your garage, large snow buildups often stick to the insides of the wheel wells and then melt and cause puddles that spread on the floor and soak into the walls, leading to mold growth and wall damage. Brush snow off your car before driving it into the garage. If snow starts to melt on the garage floor, sweep the snow and water to the outside.

If your driveway slopes down to the garage, rainwater may flow into the space. If you have a drain in front of your garage door, watch the drain during a heavy rain to see if the drain is functioning as it should. Clear the drain out as needed. When the weather is particularly warm and humid, consider operating a dehumidifier in the garage to keep the RH at no more than 70 percent (but do not operate a dehumidifier in cold weather because the coil can become covered with ice and cease to function).

THE DRIPPING GARAGE

I inspected a home for a fellow who was highly allergic to mold. When I arrived, he greeted me and led me into his kitchen, where he was preparing his lunch. On the table was a large cardboard box full of dozens of bottles of vitamins, vegetable extracts, and other health remedies.

He and I walked around the home, and when I came to the laundry, I noticed that the dryer hose was venting directly into the garage. I looked in the garage and was met with an amazing sight. Water was dripping down the glass windows of the overhead door, because the heat from a dryer can evaporate as much as 20 pounds of water from a load of laundry: the difference between the weight of a wet load and a dry load. Lint was stuck to every surface, and mold was growing on all the walls. The man was exposed to mold spores every time he went into the garage.

GARAGES "UNDER"

Some houses I have inspected had "garages under," meaning that they were at the basement level of the house and had one or two walls that were below grade or partially below grade. And below-grade spaces are prone to developing high RH conditions. Such garages can also suffer from water intrusion. In many townhouses that I have inspected, the bottom level consists of a one-car garage and an adjacent office. The driveway often slopes down sharply from the street. This design begs for water problems. One townhouse was built between two asphalt parking areas that sloped toward the property. All the drainage and roof water from several adjacent homes ran onto the pavement in front of the steep driveway and down into the garage. In one storm the owners had more than three feet of water in the garage and the adjacent basement office.

Even with more level adjacent grading, these steep driveways can collect rainwater during heavy rains. And it's often easy for water to move from the garage into another room or space on that level, where it wets carpeting and creates conditions conducive to mold growth and mite infestation. If you are living in a townhouse with a sloping driveway leading to your garage, you can install a drain with a powerful sump pump at the bottom of the driveway. Check the drain during a heavy rain to be sure it is functioning as intended. You might also consider getting rid of the basement office space or at least replacing the wall-to-wall carpeting with vinyl (if possible, use low volatile organic compound adhesive) or ceramic tile.

A more drastic option that I have seen is to change the garage into basement space by replacing the overhead door with a foundation wall and filling in the driveway with soil. Just be sure that the new lawn is graded away from the house for water control.

EFFLORESCENCE

You may see feather-like white patterns on your garage walls if they are concrete. These patterns are probably efflorescence rather than mold growth. Efflorescence is a crystalline mineral pattern that occurs when moisture migrates from the exterior through concrete to the interior. Some of that water dissolves the cementitious material in the concrete. When the water evaporates on the garage-facing side of the wall, the crystalline mineral matter is left on the surface. Efflorescence is not mold, but its presence nonetheless is evidence of moisture intrusion from the exterior. If you live in a region where roads are salted in winter, you may also see white patterns on the floor and concrete wall from crystallized salt (fig. 12.2).

FUMES

Paints, varnishes, and pesticides can be sources of volatile organic compounds (VOCs). Gasoline-powered equipment can leak. A gasoline-powered mower or snowblower, if started in a garage, will introduce combustion products, typically high in carbon monoxide (CO), into the space. Don't leave your car running in an attached garage, because CO can rise to rooms above. Individuals with chemical sensitivity should not park the car in an attached garage. If you must keep a car or any gasoline-powered equipment in the garage, start the equipment with the overhead garage door open. Allow time for the garage to air out before closing the door, and if this isn't adequate, install an exhaust fan on a timer.

Starting a car inside an attached garage is probably one of the largest sources of low-level carbon monoxide in homes.

Many newer homes have the electrical panel in the garage. Occasionally, the cables from a panel go through a large opening in a garage ceiling, providing a pathway for auto exhaust and gasoline fumes (as well as rodents). Such gaps should be sealed.

MECHANICAL SYSTEMS

I was inspecting a newly constructed townhouse condominium in a three-unit building. To my amazement, the hot-air furnace for each of the condominiums was suspended from the ceiling of the underground garage, hanging in the middle of what I expected would be a twice-daily "rush hour" cloud of CO. As is generally the case, the filter access at each furnace was open, so whenever a furnace blower operated, it drew in garage fumes. I recommended building an accessible, airtight enclosure around the furnaces (with an intake for combustion air).

BULKHEADS

Sometimes people use plywood doors and ordinary trim to construct a bulkhead (a projecting framework with a sloping door giving access to the basement from the exterior). Such bulkheads are prone to decay from moisture and pest infestation. I prefer to see people use a solid metal bulkhead. It's also important to have an airtight interior

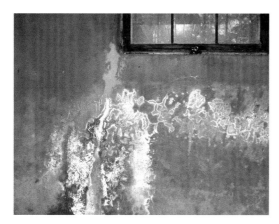

FIGURE 12.2. Roof water ponded on the ground at the exterior of this partially below-grade garage wall. Water entered the concrete at a vertical crack and along the exterior of the wall where it met the ground surface. Minerals in the concrete were dissolved in the water but crystallized into white efflorescence on the concrete at the interior when the water evaporated.

door at the bottom of the bulkhead stairs, because spaces around and in the metal bulkhead doors offer rodent entry pathways.

A relative of ours had a mouse problem. Her home is in the middle of a field, and in the past she often saw field mice scurrying around inside her house. Once I was sitting in her living room, and a field mouse walked boldly across the fireplace mantle, stopping in the middle to stare at me. Whose house was this, anyway? Clearly, the mouse claimed ownership! The basement had a bulkhead that lacked an interior door, and the spaces around the bulkhead door were invitations for mice to move in.

Keep the stairs and space at the bottom of the bulkhead stairs clear of leaves and other biodegradable debris, because moisture can accumulate in such areas, leading to mold and decay. There should also be cementitious material or a vapor barrier at the floor of the bulkhead, because exposed soil releases moisture and contains microbial growth.

PORCHES

I've seen a lot of three-season porches with mold growth on the underside of the ceilings. This makes sense when you think about it. Unpainted wood has nutrients on the surface, and painted wood may have some biodegradable dust on it. At night the roof loses heat to the universe owing to radiational cooling, and the ceiling beneath cools. (Radiational cooling occurs when heat moves from higher temperatures to lower temperatures.)

It's difficult to prevent mold growth like this, but installing a ceiling fan on a porch will help to mix the air, and installing insulation above the ceiling will reduce the heat loss due to cooling of the roof. I would avoid using cushioned furniture and rugs on the porch, as they can become moldy. Solid furniture surfaces can be cleaned and sealed (see chap. 24).

Some people convert an outside porch into an interior, habitable room. If such a space originally extended beyond the foundation, the new room may be built over soil and have exposed fiberglass insulation between the floor joists. Such spaces are prone to pest infestation. Fiberglass insulation should never be exposed to the exterior. If you have exposed fiberglass present, replace it with new fiberglass and cover it with plywood. Make certain that there are no openings through which pests can access the fiberglass. Cover any exposed dirt with a vapor barrier; if you install a lattice skirt around the crawl space, line the interior of the lattice with insect screening. Taking these steps will help prevent rodent entry and keep your "new" room warmer in the heating season.

I've inspected many such "porches turned into year-round living" spaces, and many of them developed horrible odor problems. In one case, the owner had installed fiberglass insulation under the floor joists and covered the insulation with drywall. Unfortunately, the drywall was not a tight fit, so there were spaces at the edges. Mice had no problem going through these spaces and nesting in the fiberglass insulation. The drywall had mouse urine stains, and the fiberglass was full of mouse carcasses and droppings. The owner had turned his porch into an office. He was a computer technician and did much of his work at home. Since his office was nearly uninhabitable, it caused a great disruption in his life. He had the space professionally remediated, and had the dirt covered with a vapor barrier. He called me several years later because the odor had reappeared. He'd made the mistake of again insulating beneath the floor joists with fiberglass accessible to the outdoors, and generations of mice had moved back in.

Even if you didn't change your porch into a more indoor habitable space, be sure that there are no spaces between the porch and your house that could invite mice in. All those warm and dry wall cavities! Mouse heaven.

DECKS

Unless you have a wide roof overhang (about two feet), you must have a gutter above a deck, or large amounts of water will pour from the roof onto the deck, and from there it will splash up onto the siding or, worse, onto the threshold of a door leading from the house to a deck.

I knew of one condominium association that consisted of six buildings, each containing twelve townhouses. Each townhouse had decks in front of the building. The buildings backed up against a mountain and faced northeast, so they took quite a beating weather-wise. (In New England where Connie and I live, severe, windblown weather often flows in from the northeast.) When the buildings were more than twenty years old, the condominium association decided to do some siding repairs and replacements. As the work began, extensive decay was found on the joists attaching the decks to the buildings, and in some units decay was found on the subflooring right inside the sliding doors leading to the decks.

The association hired a general contractor to inspect the decks. Many of them needed extensive repairs, and some even had to be replaced. Meanwhile, the association had the contractor rope off the decks, because some of them were so tentatively attached to the building that had four or five people stood on them, the decks would have fallen off. What had caused this near-catastrophe? The build-ings had been constructed in a hurry, and important details had been left out, like pan flashings beneath the sliding door installations. The joints between the vertical sides (casings) of the slider openings and the thresholds were not watertight, so water entered the framing.

If roof water or wind-driven rain wets the threshold of an exterior door, on a dry day add a small amount of water from an eyedropper to the joint between the threshold and the vertical casing. If the water sits there, you are in luck. If the water is sucked into the joint, hidden decay may be present.

SOME RECOMMENDATIONS

ATTACHED GARAGES

- Make sure the door from the house to the attached garage is airtight.

- Seal any wall or ceiling gaps between your garage and any adjacent space (including a room above the garage).

- Don't store vehicles that leak gasoline in an attached garage. If possible, keep the mower and snowblower in a separate shed.

- Don't store gasoline, pesticides, or fertilizers that contain pesticides in an attached garage.

- Don't let the car idle in the garage, even if the overhead door is open.

- If you're chemically sensitive, don't park the car in the garage.

- Minimize moisture levels.

- If you use your garage for storage, put goods up off the floor and away from cool walls. Rolling metal shelves are best for storage; whenever possible, keep possessions in tightly lidded plastic bins.

BULKHEADS, DECKS, AND PORCHES

- Use metal bulkhead doors.

- Be sure a bulkhead has an airtight interior basement door.

- If your house doesn't have an adequate overhang (about two feet), prevent roof water from splashing onto a deck by installing a gutter above a deck.

- Don't install accessible fiberglass insulation under porches.

- Don't vent a dryer exhaust into a crawl space (see chap. 15) or your attached garage. It's also best to avoid venting a dryer under a porch or deck.

PESTS

- There should be no holes in the walls or ceilings in your attached garage that would allow rodents to enter the house.

- Don't store open containers of birdseed or other possible "mouse food" in your garage.

- Minimize storage in your garage; the more surfaces there are, the more places there are for rodents to hide.

THE EXTERIOR

13

It's impossible to separate your home from its environment, no matter how tight your house is, but if you understand how problems starting at the exterior evolve, you can reduce the flow of contaminants from outside your house into your indoor air.

RODENTS

One family asked me to find out how mice were getting into their home. The basement was littered with exterior debris like leaves, acorns, and shells of sunflower seeds from the backyard bird feeder. The family never realized that at the back of the house there was a gap of about an inch between the sheathing and the foundation sill (the wood resting on the foundation). The previous owner had attempted to stop up the opening with fiberglass, but the rodents carrying in their pilfered seeds bypassed this obstacle with ease.

The lesson here is to avoid having spaces between the top of the foundation and the sill and not to leave other foundation holes open. For example, if you've had an oil pipe removed, fill the opening with mortar if it's in the foundation. If you can't easily see the sill or look under the edge of the siding, carefully check the perimeter of the foundation with a mirror and a flashlight, especially where two foundations meet at right angles or at the sides of the front stoop where it contacts the house. Also be sure to check for openings around basement windows. Seal any gaps or openings you find with masonry, wood, or metal mesh and foam as appropriate.

TERMITES

Termites are worrisome pests because they can cause structural damage. If used indoors, the treatments intended to combat these insects can also impair indoor air quality. Avoid the use of pesticides whenever possible. The first step in your battle against these pests is to understand what termites are and how they live.

Termites can be found in most states, and as our climate warms, the march of termites continues ever northward. The common termite lives several feet under the surface of the ground. A subterranean termite colony includes workers, soldiers to protect them, and a queen to lay eggs. Some colonies consist of several connected underground nests. Termites travel concealed in dark spaces or in tubes called "shelter tubes" or "mud tubes" about a quarter of an inch wide (though they can grow to over an inch), which termites construct from sand and a secretion that serves as glue. Shelter tubes protect termites from predators such as carpenter ants.

Shelter tubes can be found inside or outside wood or rising up from cracks in foundation floors or walls. When interior wood beams or joists are heavily infested with termites, you may see tubes hanging down from the structure. The longest tube I ever saw ran up a foundation wall from the floor to the ceiling, and the widest was about three inches (figs. 13.1 and 13.2).

When you find sand inside decayed wood, termites almost certainly caused the damage.

Worker termites destroy wood by chewing it, but it is the protozoa (microscopic single-celled animals) in their guts that supply the enzymes (cellulase) to digest the cellulose from the chewed-up wood. Termites are drawn to wood decayed by macrofungi (see chap. 2), and the fungal fragments and wood fibers that the termites ingest provide them with necessary nutrients. Some mold volatile organic compounds (MVOCs) may function like insect pheromones, attracting the termites. It may be small comfort to those who find termites in their homes, but it's worth noting that workers are commuters. They live in the soil and travel back and forth to your home to destroy it (though Formosan termites, recent invaders in the South, nest inside walls).

Traffic inside shelter tubes can resemble rush hour on a freeway. Worker termites are about 5 millimeters (0.18 inch) long, but you will probably never see one crawling about, because they are as shy as they are completely defenseless. Workers are soft, move slowly, and have no claws or stingers for protection. They look like a grain of rice with two antennae and six tiny legs. The soldier termites that protect them are much more formidable; they are about 8 millimeters (0.3 inch) long and have large mandibles. If you break open a mud tube, the soldiers rush to the opening to defend the workers.

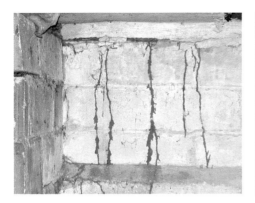

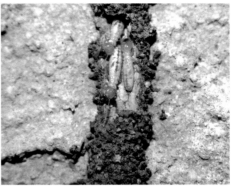

FIGURE 13.1. Termite tubes on a block foundation wall. Connie and I were looking for a smaller home after our children graduated from college and moved out. One of the houses the broker showed us had a major termite problem. There were multiple shelter tubes rising up the foundation into the wood sill that had been partially destroyed. We did not make an offer on this home!

FIGURE 13.2. I discovered this termite tube on a condominium inspection. The tube ran up the stone foundation. I broke the tube open and saw worker termites rushing up and down the tube. They obeyed American traffic rules, up on the right and down on the left.

Untreated wood in the soil or in direct contact with soil invites termites. Wood house trim, basement windowsills, and wooden steps should not be in direct contact with the dirt. Termite tubes can even be found on stockade fences when the pickets are set in the soil. A woodpile sitting directly on the ground may invite termites, particularly if the wood is decayed. Even mulch made from wood chips can attract termites. In large numbers, termites pose a serious threat to your home because they hollow out beams, joists, and studs from the inside. They usually leave behind the outer layer of structural wood, but by the time the pests have finished their meal, the remaining material may be no thicker than a coat of paint. One home inspector described a time he vigorously "probed" the main beam of a house to show the buyers how decayed it was. For the sake of drama, he bashed the beam with a hammer, and he was horrified when the entire bottom splintered open, spewing live termites onto the broker and his buyers.

For decades, termite treatment has consisted of creating a chemical envelope around the foundation. The chemical is injected into the soil at high pressure, and the soil bearing the pesticide creates a barrier against termite intrusion. To prevent termites from entering the foundation wall on the inside, pesticide is often also injected into the soil beneath the basement floor through holes drilled about every 46 centimeters (18 inches) into the concrete at the perimeter. If a nest is under the middle of a basement floor in a home, perimeter treatment alone may not be effective. In this case the pest control operator (PCO) will probably suggest injecting additional chemicals under other areas of the floor.

Although thousands of homes are treated safely for termites every year, problems can occur. First, all the chemicals used are toxic. Chlordane, for example, is one of the many pesticides that in the past were used to combat termites. The soil around and under many slab-on-grade houses was treated preventively with chlordane. In some such homes with heat ducts in or below the concrete slab, people became ill because vapors from the soil diffused into the ducts.

In some homes with dirt crawl spaces, pesticides were "broadcast sprayed" onto the soil and wooden floor structure because that was easier than crawling under and injecting it into the dirt. When chemicals are applied in this way, a great deal of surface area is exposed and soaked. The pesticide evaporates slowly for years, and the vapors saturate the air in the crawl space. Unfortunately, the air pressure in most crawl spaces, particularly in the winter, is higher than that in the rest of the house, because air exfiltrates at the upper levels of a home and infiltrates at the lower levels. Then contaminated air flows from a basement or crawl space into the living areas. I have been in homes with crawl spaces that had been treated with chlordane where the basement or even the entire house reeked of termiticide.

Most pesticides have to be diluted with water, and the mixture is typically applied as an emulsion (small drops of oil dispersed in water). After the emulsion is pumped into the soil, the water eventually evaporates, and the oil droplets spread out onto the soil particles and become immobile on their surfaces. Before the water dries out, however, the pesticide emulsion can be carried with rainwater into a basement with a leaky foundation. In older homes with stone foundations, even properly applied pesticides can flow from the surrounding soil into the basement in the form of vapor. The pesticide may also enter the basement if an unexpectedly heavy rain occurs shortly after the chemical is injected into the soil.

I believe people can become chemically sensitive if exposed to pesticides, so I recommend my clients use a newer treatment that consists of bait systems in which traps containing small amounts of relatively nontoxic chemicals are installed at the outside perimeter of a home just beneath the surface of the soil. These traps contain levels of chemicals that are primarily toxic only to termites. In theory, the termites carry the chemicals back to the nest and poison it. As a preventive treatment, you can also have a sodium octaborate solution (prepared from disodium octaborate tetrahydrate) applied to the wood structure of a crawl space, back porch, garage, or in locations where wood is close to grade. This chemical is not volatile but is soluble in water, so its effectiveness is reduced on wood that is exposed to the weather.

DIY DISASTERS

Wasp sprays, ant sprays, and mothballs are readily available in supermarkets and hardware stores. Advertisements about mothballs and insect sprays give us the impression that these chemicals affect only bugs, but that's not so. In one case a woman sprinkled an entire box of moth crystals into the soil of a crawl space under her front porch. Air flowed from beneath the porch and infiltrated the basement, and from there it rose into the rooms of her house, carrying pesticide vapors throughout the living spaces. She felt that she was becoming ill from the fumes, so she hired an inept handyman to clean out the crawl space. He buried more of the moth crystals than he removed, and the vapors continued to infiltrate. Eventually, she became chemically sensitive, sold the house, and moved. Another homeowner decided to cure an insect infestation on his own by pouring quarts of chlordane all around the hollow-block foundation of his house. The young couple that later purchased the man's home became so ill they had to sell the property.

One family called a pest control company because they saw a carpenter ant in the kitchen. Instead of ants, the PCO found evidence of old termite activity and recommended treatment. It just happened that on the day of the treatment, the city had temporarily shut off the water to the street for pipe repairs before the technician had finished diluting the pesticide. The PCO went ahead with the treatment anyway, inserting a long metal wand around the house at about two-foot intervals and pumping the incompletely diluted chemical into the soil.

The house had an old leaky stone foundation. Concentrated pesticide from the soil outside dribbled down the foundation walls and into the basement, and the family was forced to move out. To help eliminate the pesticide fumes, they operated their powerful whole-house attic exhaust fan for two months in the vacant house. They left the door from the house to the basement open so that the airflow created by the fan would draw the pesticide fumes from the basement into the attic and outside. This wasn't a great idea, because fumes were distributed throughout the house. To make things even worse, the depressurization of the basement air caused combustion gases full of carbon monoxide to backdraft from the furnace into the home.

Every time the family entered the house, no matter how briefly, they became nauseated and suffered headaches.

The husband thought he could correct matters by "rinsing" the chemical from the soil with dishwashing detergent, and he poured dozens of bottles of this detergent onto the ground between the shrubs and the foundation all around the house. Then he generously hosed the dirt. The bath didn't seem to help, so he purchased pumping equipment and injected hundreds of gallons of concentrated bleach into the soil in an attempt to destroy the pesticide. The bleach combined with the soap and other materials in the soil to create a toxic cloud of gas, forcing people in surrounding homes to evacuate. Then the man called me. Should he inject hydrogen peroxide into the ground, he asked, to eliminate the chlorine bleach? I was flabbergasted by the story and astounded that he was willing to inject still more chemicals into the soil.

CHEMICALS AND PARTICLES FROM NEIGHBORS

If you are considering moving into a new home and you or a member of your household is chemically sensitive, keep in mind that the appeal of the well-manicured lawn next door or the golf course down the street may be due in part to pesticide applications. It's worth a little research before committing yourself to the property. If a neighbor's pesticides bother you, at least plan to be away during applications. If there is or used to be a gasoline station, a buried oil tank, or a light manufacturing operation next door, chemicals that were dumped or leaked from underground storage may have migrated through the soil to your property. This can result in toxic basement vapors.

If you are living in a house or are considering moving into a house that you think has a peculiar chemical odor in the basement, do your research and believe your nose. Don't let other people convince you that you're imagining things, and be suspicious of overpowering room deodorizers or potpourri. You can also purchase a test kit containing activated charcoal that adsorbs air contaminants (we discuss some testing methods in chap. 23). The kit is left in the basement for several hours and then returned to the lab for analysis.

A young family purchased a newly built home next to a gasoline station. They called me because there was an odd odor in the finished basement where their children played. Using my TIF8800 combustible gas detector, I discovered a strong odor entering the basement at a crack in a closet; the odor seemed to be that of gasoline. The homeowner notified the city, and city technicians did testing that confirmed that high concentrations of chemicals from gasoline were entering the basement. A neighbor's house was also tested, and similar results were found. The gasoline station was shut down, the tanks removed, and a soil vapor extraction system set up to suck fume-laden air from the ground under and around the station and burn it.

Pesticides are powerful chemicals; read the instructions of the label carefully. Don't apply them yourself if they require professional application, and be sure to use licensed, qualified workers.

The system ran for over five years. To prevent fumes from entering the homes, radon systems were installed. The families were able to remain in their homes, and the corner lot where the garage stood is now a block of stores.

Mold from neighboring properties can also be bothersome. For example, if you are downwind from a mulching facility or even a neighbor's compost pile, vast clouds of spores can be carried in air that intermittently flows toward your property and into your house.

VEGETATION

I have seen much damage to buildings caused by trees and shrubs. In several homes, leaves in contact with house trim or siding deflected streams of rain onto the wood, causing rot. Dead leaves from overhanging branches can clog gutters, and a falling branch can damage a roof or skylight. Plants growing up against the siding also slow the drying of surfaces after it has rained. I always recommend that people prevent plants from touching their homes and allow enough space for inspection between the foundation wall and plantings, so they can keep an eye out for moisture issues or signs of pest activity.

People who are sensitized should be careful when handling vegetation. One of my clients developed hives while collecting cuttings from a shrub. Another man who didn't know he had allergies experienced asthma symptoms immediately after dumping a barrel of moldy leaves over a fence.

If you have allergies to certain plants, try to avoid growing them on your property. If you live in a wooded area, you may have to be particularly careful about poison ivy, which can cause a rash when touched and even when burned. Many people have had serious reactions when upwind neighbors burned poison ivy. Even if you aren't sensitive, avoid burning poison ivy, because someone who lives in your neighborhood may be vulnerable.

WATER

If not properly channeled away from the walls and the foundation, rain can fuel mold growth both inside and outside your home. Let's start at the top of a house and follow the various courses water may take as it makes its insidious attack on your property.

CHIMNEYS

One spring I received a call from a man who in the past year had had the exterior of his home repainted and new asphalt shingles installed over the old roof. After the first winter, stains and large water-filled blisters appeared in the paint film on the clapboards at the front of the house between the windows of the two second-floor bathrooms. The contractor thought moisture from the bathrooms was the culprit, but the owner thought the contractor's poor prep work was at fault.

With a Tramex moisture meter, I detected elevated moisture content in the roof shingles above the stained and blistered area. I suspected that water might be getting in under the shingles from the chimney. Carrying a hose, I climbed onto the roof, where I found a large crack in the mortar cap at the top of the horizontal portion of the oversized chimney. The chimney was made of brick but coated with stucco. Shortly after I directed a small stream of water into the crack, moisture exited the stucco at about the middle of the vertical side of the chimney. I then knew that water was entering the crack, sneaking down the chimney between the brick and the stucco, and running unseen down the roof on top of the old shingles and beneath the new ones. Before the water reached the edge of the roof, it leaked behind the fascia board in the soffit and into the wall behind the clapboards. The moisture behind the clapboards passed through the wood as vapor and then condensed behind the paint film. The accumulation of water had blistered the film. I advised the owners to install a leak-proof chimney rain cap, which is a metal or masonry cover supported about a foot above the flue opening.

Flashing at the bottom of that chimney would have prevented the water from getting under the roofing. Chimney flashings are usually made of lead and are embedded in the mortar used to hold the bricks together. Normally, the lead is bent flat against the brick, and each piece overlaps its neighbor. The chimney flashings at one home I inspected were bent upward and made the chimney look like a top hat. The tenants told me why.

Apparently, a raccoon had been living in the chimney on top of the damper of the unused fireplace. When the landlord discovered the animal, he covered the flue with metal mesh to prevent her from climbing down the flue. The raccoon was undeterred; she was so infuriated that she bent all the chimney flashings up into the air in an effort to get back into her old home. She then found an area of the roof sheathing around the chimney that had decayed and made her new home inside the attic. Water leaked in around the hole, flowed down the chimney brick, and caused severe mold growth in the room below.

When I'm inspecting homes, I always find that old chimneys with rain caps are in surprisingly good condition. If you have a chimney, it's a good idea to have a rain cap with an animal screen at the sides as well as proper lead flashing at the base. It also makes sense to cover a chimney's shoulder with slate to protect the mortar from erosion. (A chimney's shoulder is the sloped portion, designed to accommodate the fireplace.)

ROOFS

Obviously, if your roof is leaking, you should have it repaired. Don't assume your roof won't leak because it's new. The old-style organic felt asphalt shingles lasted twenty to thirty years, but the newer fiberglass asphalt shingles may last only fiften to twenty years. In thousands of homes, premature failure of this newer material owing to manufacturing defects has led to roof replacements in as little as three years. Fortunately, manufacturers have corrected the shingle formulations, and this type of premature failure is no longer occurring. If you are replacing your fiberglass asphalt shingles, try to get organic felt rather than fiberglass shingles, but check that the fire rating complies with your local building codes. (Other roof coverings are available and may be more suitable for specific climate conditions.)

Look around your attic with a bright flashlight during a heavy rain to check for leaks. On rare occasions, animals can chew holes in a roof, or falling branches may cause damage. Never allow a branch to touch your roof, because movement caused by wind can lead to abrasion and holes. I also encourage people to cut away tree branches overhanging the roof, because falling leaves and branches can clog or damage gutters.

Other roof problems can be created by design errors. In one home the family began to detect a powerful smell of mold after they completed a second-story addition, designed by an inexperienced architect. All the roof water from the addition and from about a third of the original roof was channeled into a valley and from there to a narrow section of gutter, which did not have the capacity to handle the water. Some of the overflow cascaded down the wall and entered the wall cavity through a gap around an exterior light fixture, and mold started to grow.

In homes without gutters, an adequate roof overhang is essential to keep water away from the walls and the foundation. Overhangs are particularly important for homes with hardboard siding and no gutters, because hardboard (a composite of sawdust and glue) absorbs moisture and swells at the cut ends and nailheads, leading to decay.

FLASHINGS

Ice damming is a source of water damage at the outside of a house and is caused by heat loss from the attic to the roof. When wind

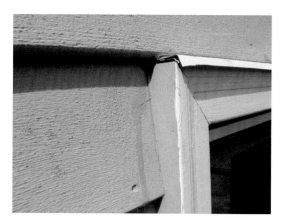

FIGURE 13.3. This window drip-cap flashing bends up instead of down. I placed some water from a squirt bottle on top of the metal flashing. Instead of dripping off the front edge of the flashing, the water traveled to the end. Some of the water dripped down the clapboard, and some of the water flowed into the open miter joint of the window casing. I removed the window casing and found that the casing and stud behind it were wet and rotted.

drives rain against a house or when ice damming occurs, water can enter wall cavities through cracks in siding or gaps in trim. Wooden or plastic window and door frames and wood trim can protrude from the siding of a building and can catch rainwater at the top edge. For this reason a window or door is often installed with a drip-cap flashing that is supposed to shed water (the flashing is just an L-shaped piece of aluminum).

If the flashing is sloped toward the building, it can channel water to the two ends of the flashing and from there into the joint between the vertical trim and siding and into the wall cavity. I have seen numerous new homes in which this condition has caused paint peeling and severe concealed decay and, in some cases, indoor musty odor. Be certain your drip caps are pitched correctly. Water should flow off the drip cap all along the edge, not just at the ends (fig. 13.3).

WALL CAVITIES

One young family was concerned about a musty odor in their baby's corner bedroom, which they had vacated out of concern for their child. Owing to poor roof design, a large amount of rainwater was flowing down a valley onto a small soffit corner with a narrow gap between the vertical corner boards just above the baby's bedroom. I lifted the carpet in the outside corner of the baby's bedroom and saw that the underlayment had a water stain; I checked the moisture content of the drywall in the corner, and it was elevated. The homeowner gave me permission to cut a small hole in the drywall. I found that the insulation and sheathing were wet. Water had been entering the baby's wall cavity from the soffit. Fortunately, the home was still under the builder's warranty (one year in Massachusetts), and the problem could be repaired from the exterior. The builder replaced the insulation and siding and made the leaky soffit watertight.

When another couple arrived to tour a house that was on the market, the owner was baking cookies. The price, location, and condition of the house as well as the inviting cookie odor convinced the couple to buy the property. During the home inspection, the different but still fragrant odor of plug-in floral air freshener welcomed them. The masking odor should have cautioned the couple as well as their home inspector, but in this case no warning flag was raised. After the couple moved in and pulled the plug on the fragrance emitters, they noticed a strong musty odor. They eliminated all the old carpeting and gutted and remodeled the kitchen and bathrooms, but the odor persisted. Soon the husband, who had allergies, began to experience symptoms.

When the musty smell became a stench, the couple called me. I walked around the outside of the house, and one of the first things I noticed was a large mushroom poking out of the hardboard siding on the shaded end of the building. I made several recommendations to improve the air quality inside the home, but my main concern was determining the condition of the concealed materials where the wall seemed to be decaying. I suggested that the couple hire someone to conduct exploratory wall surgery.

A few months later I received a thank-you note telling me what had happened. There had been extensive decay at the back of the soaked hardboard siding, and macrofungi and microfungi (see chap. 2) had spread throughout the building paper between the siding and the sheathing. The couple ended up residing the house with vinyl. During the removal, the dumpster outside the house (containing all the decayed hardboard siding and building paper) smelled so strongly of fungi that the couple could not remain in the house. In addition, several neighbors complained about the odor. Once the dumpster was removed and the house resided, the owners were able to move back into their "home sweet home."

MOLD GROWTH ON THE EXTERIOR OF A BUILDING

A number of people have called us because they are worried about mold growth on the outside of their homes. It's common to find mold

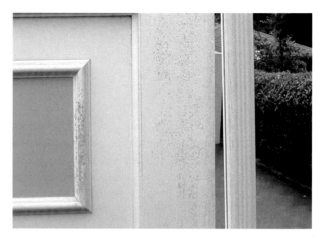

FIGURE 13.4. Wood trim with mold colonies. Mildewcides in exterior paint prevent fungi from growing in the paint film, but fungi can still grow on the nonvisible plant material (pollen, tree sap, etc.) that sticks to exterior siding and trim, including vinyl siding (and even the metal downspout in this photo). Mold often grows on the bottoms of overhangs, exterior porch ceilings, and soffits.

(microfungal) growth on the outside of buildings. Such growth may be unsightly but rarely has an effect on indoor air quality. Some people power-wash the cladding (siding) to get rid of the mold. Mold growth will return, however, because nutrients (pollen grains, mold spores from outside mold growth) and moisture will always be present. In addition, with certain kinds of siding, power-washing can force water up under the cladding and dampen the sheathing, potentially leading to microfungal growth. If the sheathing gets soaked and remains wet long enough, even macrofungal growth can occur (fig. 13.4).

GUTTERS AND DOWNSPOUTS

Most homes should have gutters, which sit at the edge of the roof. If they are properly positioned and well maintained, gutters can prevent many moisture problems. They must be kept clean and be wide enough to handle water flow, pitched correctly, and watertight at joints. Downspouts should also be kept clean. There should also be adequate overhang at the edge of the roof so that if the gutters overflow, water will run directly to the ground from the roof edge rather than down the sidewall. The metal drip-edge flashing at the roof overhang must also be at the right angle to direct the water into the gutter and not behind it.

Despite their positive features, gutter systems are a common cause of water damage. Gutter joints and end caps often leak, causing paint to peel on wood trim below. Even the order in which the downspout

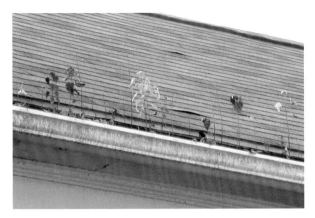

FIGURE 13.5. This gutter is growing tree seedlings. I took this photograph in the fall. I assume that the gutter was full of nutrients, because these tree seedlings were flourishing. I didn't have to look into the gutter to know that it hadn't been cleaned for some time!

sections are connected is important. Most of the water flowing within a downspout clings to its inside walls, and when the joints are reversed (the crimped "male" end of the section facing up instead of down), a lot of water leaks out of the joints. In one home with reversed downspout joints, water leaked out and flowed down the outside of the downspout until its path was thwarted by the bracket that secured the downspout to the house wall. At that point the water was diverted toward the wall, where it flowed down the trim and soaked the wood. Termites moved in to complete the destruction.

Stand outside your house during a heavy rain and observe the gutters. If you see water dripping behind the gutters, leaking out of joints or end caps, or flowing on the outside of the downspouts, you have a problem. In a house that Connie and I used to own before we downsized when our children moved out, a gutter filled with leaves couldn't handle the water during a heavy storm, and the water streamed down the outside of the house to a kitchen window. Although the window was closed, the storm window was open, and the space at the bottom of the window filled with water, which leaked through the walls and into the basement. It was quite a mess, and it all happened because I hadn't had a chance to clean out that gutter.

In another building the owner never cleaned the gutters. When the gutters filled and overflowed, the curvature of the gutter channeled the overflowing water at one end into a stream that sprayed against the vertical corner trim boards of the house. Years of water entry caused severe concealed decay of the entire corner structure. Repairs entailed replacing the corner posts of the walls (a major structural repair) as well as large sections of the siding (fig. 13.5).

Cleaning gutters is a tiresome chore and one that few people do often enough, including me. Clogged gutters are far more likely if you have tree branches overhanging your home. Some people install gutter screens to keep out debris. In New England at least, such screens are rarely effective, because the ice that fills gutters every winter dislodges them. People who are not physically active should hire someone to clean gutters. I know of two homeowners who broke their backs falling from ladders while doing this job.

When gutters aren't working properly for one reason or another, moisture problems are likely to follow. In one wood-framed medical office that I inspected, the gooseneck had fallen off so the downspout was not connected to the gutter. Water flowed out of the gutter down the side of the building and entered the wall cavity through a crack in a windowsill. The entire wall cavity was full of mold. I was called to investigate because the examining room had to be abandoned after several patients complained of asthma symptoms.

A quick way to see if roof or grade water is entering your basement is to use a hose to flood the area near a downspout close to the foundation. On a few inspections I've done this kind of testing. In one home I turned the water on and asked my client to go into the basement and shout when/if the water began to appear. I heard him scream as soon as he went down the stairs. A little sooner than I had expected, a sizable puddle had formed in the corner under the oil tank. The heavily rusted legs of the oil tank spoke silently of numerous earlier "baths."

GUTTERS AND GRADING, GRADING AND GUTTERS

When land slopes toward the house, water runs toward the foundation. In a heavy rain, moisture soaks into the soil at the foundation and can leak into the basement, particularly if there are cracks in the masonry walls. Proper handling of roof and grade water is particularly important with older stone foundations, which are often full of gaps. If you have a stone foundation, it's a good idea to keep the mortar intact. No matter what kind of foundation you have, clogged or missing gutters allow water to pond close to the house, and then the water can migrate into the basement.

WATER DISPERSAL

Properly working gutters and downspouts take the water to grade (to the ground), but it must still be directed away from the house to avoid basement moisture. If the soil outside the foundation is graded properly away from the building, then a downspout extension or a splash block should provide adequate dispersal. But if the grading is level or slopes toward the house, other measures must be taken (my advice is to regrade wherever possible). Many homeowners have the mistaken notion that if they can't see the water, it isn't a problem. They simply bury the downspout in soil at the corner of the house without providing any piping to carry the water away, which often results in excessive foundation moisture.

Many people install dry wells, which are usually nothing more than reservoirs in the ground filled with crushed stone, although plastic barrels with pipe fittings are also used. Water from the downspouts is conducted through a pipe beneath the soil surface into the excavated area or barrel. Dry wells work for a time, but ultimately they become clogged with fine organic and inorganic material and cease to function effectively. When water can no longer be dispersed below grade by a dry well, the water backs up, ponds around the foundation, and finds its way into the basement. I recommend that people use a subsurface dispersal system where the pipe end discharges to daylight; this way you can see water coming out. (Just don't direct the water to the side-walk or to your neighbor's driveway!) A subsurface drain consists of a PVC schedule 40 pipe that conducts the water away from the down-spout and foundation to an area where it will not cause problems for you or your neighbors. The pipe must be pitched so that water drains out by gravity flow, and the end should be open to the air, not buried.

Some home designs are more prone to wet basements than other designs. For example, if the footprint of your house is U-shaped, the water from one side of each of the three roof gables may flow toward the interior of the U. If the grading is level, as it often is, excessive moisture soaks into the soil. In such cases more extensive methods of water dispersal must be in place. These may include installing sub-surface drains (either with or without dry wells), creating a deeply sloped concrete or paved patio, or sloping the land away from the building.

ON AND UNDER THE GROUND

If, despite your best efforts, you have a buildup of water on the ground around your foundation, what can you do to minimize basement moisture? Be sure your basement walls are watertight. Have major cracks professionally evaluated and sealed. Do all you can to have your land graded away from the house.

If your house backs up to a hill and the land around the house slopes toward the foundation, you can create a swale or moat behind the house that will channel water away from the foundation. If the wood siding doesn't have several inches of clearance from the soil, rainwater flowing down the hill can rot the siding. To avoid this problem, dig a trench several inches deep around the foundation, line it with a waterproof membrane adhered to the foundation, partially refill the trench with crushed stone, and hold back the soil on the other side of the trench with a retaining wall made of treated wood or masonry. Keep the trench narrow enough so that water from the roof edge or an overflowing gutter will fall to the ground beyond the retaining wall.

When the soil is eroded next to a house, it is almost impossible to prevent water from dribbling in around a leaky foundation. One way to minimize this type of water intrusion is to install a foundation skirt at the sides of the home where needed. (You shouldn't need a retaining wall with a foundation skirt.) Excavate around the perimeter about 15 inches down and about 30 inches out. The bottom of the trench should be sloped away from the foundation and smoothed. A waterproof membrane (a deflection skirt) installed at the bottom of the trench is folded up a few inches against the foundation and secured to it. You can even put crushed stone or a perforated drainpipe buried in crushed stone inside the trench. A layer of soil and filter fabric can cover the trench. This arrangement prevents surface water from flowing directly down the foundation wall, and if the trench has perforated pipe, water can be carried away from the building downhill to a remote site.

In locales with cold winters, foundation skirts can be particularly useful. If you live in New England or anywhere else with severe winter conditions, you may have noticed that snow tends to melt on the ground near foundations because of the heat loss from the basement. In the middle of the cold months the ground elsewhere may be frozen several feet down from the surface and thus will be impermeable to water. If water ponds at the side of the house owing to ice damming or a winter rain, it will seep into the warmer soil near the foundation and may leak into the basement. A foundation skirt provides a barrier that will prevent water from sinking down along the foundation. A foundation skirt can also be useful when the grading around a house can't be sloped away from the foundation.

Even if you have proper grading and a subsurface drainage system, if you don't maintain the wells around the basement windows, you may still get water in the basement. Always be sure that water from downspouts flows away from window wells. The soil in the wells should be several inches below the window, particularly if the sill is wood. I have seen many termite infestations begin in buried wooden trim around basement windows. If you don't mind plastic covers, you can install one over a window well to keep the rain out. Be careful to keep the space clean and free of leaves and other materials that can degrade, or you may end up with a musty odor around the window, which can be carried by air infiltration into the basement. If you are really sick of maintaining window wells and having water enter the basement from a window, you can always raise the level of the lower masonry and install glass blocks. Check your local building code, though, to find out the minimum number of windows required in a basement.

SOME RECOMMENDATIONS

GRADING

- Make sure the soil around the house is graded away from the foundation.
- If your house is on a hill, divert water away from the foundation with a swale.

GUTTER SYSTEMS

- Check gutters and downspouts during a heavy rain to be sure they don't leak.
- Keep your gutters and downspouts clean.
- Wherever possible, use subsurface dispersal for roof water and install the pipe so that water discharges to daylight downhill from the house or at the edge of a deep landscape furrow.
- If moisture leaks through your basement walls after it rains, clean the gutters, extend the downspouts, correct the grading, and then, if all else fails, install a foundation skirt.
- If you don't have gutters, be sure you have adequate roof overhang (at least two feet).

MOLD GROWTH

- If you are bothered by mold growth on the overhang outside your house or on a ceiling of an outside porch, you can clean such a surface and then spray it with an antimicrobial product. The product will not be washed off by rain the way it would if applied to an exterior surface that is exposed to the weather.

PESTICIDES

- When pesticides are necessary, hire a professional to apply them.

- When considering moving into a new home, believe your nose and take chemical odors seriously.

- If your home has a lingering chemical smell, consider purchasing a kit to test for volatile organic compounds (VOCs).

- If you have a dirt crawl space that you suspect contains chlordane, I recommend having the soil tested by a lab; you may have to remove soil and have a vapor barrier and concrete floor installed.

- If the wood structure in a crawl space was broadcast sprayed with a toxic, semivolatile, persistent pesticide such as chlordane, even the wood may have to be replaced or sealed.

- If you are constructing a home with a crawl space, consider using pressure-treated wood in the space, or treat the wood with borate to minimize the threat of termite infestation.

- A sodium octaborate solution is an option for preventative termite treatments for wood that is not exposed to weather.

PESTS

- Don't allow untreated wood (including piles of firewood) to remain in contact with soil.

- Seal any openings at the exterior that could be rodent pathways; use mesh and foam, masonry, or wood as appropriate.

VEGETATION

- Do not allow trees or shrubs to touch any part of the house. Wherever possible, maintain at least 18 inches of clearance between the house and plant growth so you can keep an eye out for pest activity or siding decay.

- Don't let tree branches extend over your gutters or roof.

- Don't burn poison ivy or oak.

- Keep leaf debris out of window wells, and keep the soil level several inches below any wood.

- If you have allergies or asthma, it's a good idea to wear a fine-particle mask and gardening gloves when handling plants, raking, or digging in dirt.

WATER

- Inspect the attic, basement, and exterior of your house during a heavy rain to watch for leaks.

- Be sure drip-cap flashings above windows and doors are pitched correctly (away from the siding).

- Consider installing a rain cap with an animal screen at the top of your chimney.

- Cover your chimney shoulder with slate to protect the mortar from erosion.

- If you have hardboard siding, keep it painted, and never let roof water flow over it.

14.

INDOOR AIR QUALITY IN MULTI-UNIT BUILDINGS

As we discussed earlier in the book, air flows in a building from the bottom to top and out, especially in the heating season (warm air rises). Air also flows from spaces with higher air pressure to spaces with lower air pressure.

You may think that you live only in your own unit, but air flows throughout your building, moving through even small gaps and cracks. This means that the air that you inhale in common areas and even in your own home may contain allergens and odors from other units and spaces in the building. If you live in a multi-unit building or are considering moving into one, the information throughout this book will be helpful, but in this chapter we discuss indoor air quality issues that are primarily relevant to multi-unit residential buildings.

MOISTURE

Structures with different shapes and sizes have different problems. In a one-story building with a flat roof, any room could be affected by a roof leak. In a building with a gable roof, a roof leak might only affect one area. In a single-family home with a kitchen and one or two bathrooms, those two or three rooms can be sources of interior moisture. In a multi-unit family residence with eight apartments, there are eight kitchens and at least eight bathrooms, which means at least sixteen rooms that are moisture sources. Like a single-family building, however, a typical multi-family building has only four exterior sides and a roof.

In cold climates, a multi-family building has an increased potential of having moisture condensation in exterior wall cavities, which can lead to mold growth. If the cavities remain damp for long enough, there may be sheathing decay (see chap. 2). That is why it's important in such a building that all the cooking stove and bathroom exhausts vent to the exterior. This will also help to control odors.

Moisture can also come into a building from the exterior. In one expensive garden-level condominium, the basement master bedroom opened onto steps leading to a private urban garden. The scene was bucolic. One could lie in bed and look through the sliding glass door onto a pastoral scene. Unfortunately, water cascaded down the steps and flooded the landing below whenever it rained heavily. The threshold of the sliding door was at the same level as the patio, and water simply flowed into the bedroom, soaking the carpet. In another garden unit, roof water from two properties collected in a narrow alley between them and soaked into the old brick foundation walls. From there the water ran along a concrete floor beneath the carpet, soaking the concrete, the jute pad, the carpet, and the carpet dust. Carpeting below grade that gets wet should be replaced; hard flooring is preferable in such spaces.

HEATING AND COOLING

Some apartments or condominiums in larger buildings have hot-water baseboard convectors. I've taken samples from hundreds of these convectors, and it is rare that I don't find allergens such as pet dander particles, mold spores, and insect parts in the dust on the convector heating fins. When people move into a new apartment, they don't think about having hot-water baseboard convectors cleaned, but it's likely that such convectors contain allergens collected over time and from previous occupants. Some of those allergens become airborne when the heat is running and air flows by convection through the fin tubing. Some older buildings have radiators for heat. Radiators as well as radiator covers can also collect allergenic dust.

There should be no dust on radiator surfaces or on the fins in baseboard heating convectors.

Some multi-unit residential buildings (as well as most schools) have univents installed at exterior walls to supply heating (and often cooling). A univent must be serviced on the recommended schedule and have pleated media filters that are airtight at the perimeter so that no air can bypass the filter. Another type of heating and cooling unit is called a vertical stack fan coil (figs. 14.1 and 14.2).

Every vertical stack fan coil I have inspected was highly contaminated with mold. I inspected one high-end apartment in which the

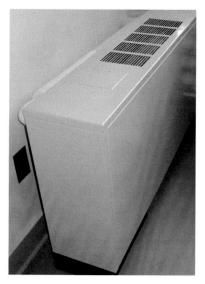

FIGURE 14.1. A univent is a type of heating and/or cooling unit that is usually found at an exterior wall under a window. The supply air exits from the grille at the top; the return air enters at the bottom, where the filter is located. The front panel can be removed for inspecting the interior where the heating or cooling coils and blowers are located. There should be no dust at the interior.

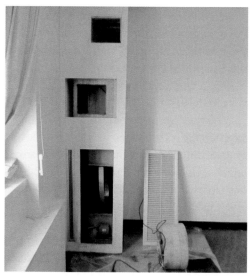

FIGURE 14.2. A vertical stack unit undergoing remediation. The ductless heating and cooling stack unit is concealed within the drywall "bump out" at an exterior wall. The larger opening at the bottom is for the return (air intake) grille that has been removed and is leaning against the wall; the opening in the middle was cut into the wall in order to clean the supply duct. The top opening is for the supply grille, which has been removed. This type of unit is often found at a shared internal wall where it supplies conditioned air to two adjacent rooms.

occupant was experiencing asthma symptoms. The unit was heated and cooled by several vertical stack fan coils that probably had not been serviced in years. Each unit was contaminated with mold, and every time a unit turned on, airflows carried mold spores into the air in the apartment, and from there into the woman's lungs. Unfortunately, most of these units are built into walls and cannot be accessed for proper cleaning. If such a unit has to be thoroughly cleaned or replaced, drywall must be removed. Fortunately, most people are not affected by mold spores, but if you have mold sensitivities or are concerned about your indoor environmental conditions, I encourage you to be cautious about moving into an apartment with this kind of mechanical system.

One of my saddest stories concerned a fellow who was renting an apartment on the first floor of a multilevel building. Each apartment had an exterior mechanical closet off a balcony. I found that contaminated moldy water leaked from the mechanical closets in the floors above him into his mechanical closet, which had mold growing on the walls. His bedroom and dining area shared a wall with the mechanical closet, and floor water from the closet flowed unseen under carpeting in these two rooms. There was mold growing in the carpeting, which he regularly disturbed with foot traffic, causing allergenic spores to be aerosolized. He developed several serious health conditions typical of exposure to mold spores and became so hypersensitized that he moved out of the apartment.

He began to withhold rent in the hopes of getting some type of acknowledgment of his situation as well as some recompense. The landlord hired a respectable environmental testing company that sampled the air when no one had been living in the apartment for months. In addition, samples were taken of the carpeting in a location where there was no mold growth present. The company reported that there were no mold issues in the apartment.

The judge would not hear the case unless my client's doctor came to testify that my client's symptoms were due to mold exposure. The doctor wouldn't testify, so there was no judgment against the landlord, and my client was forced to fork over all the rent money that he had withheld. He was by then so hypersensitive to indoor environmental contaminants that he was unable to live or work in any typical indoor space. He spent subsequent years living in a bus that he had converted into a space that he could tolerate.

One condominium owner told me she could smell mold in her unit on the third floor of a 90-year-old building with hot-air heat. This seemed curious, since it's unusual to have mold odor on the top floor of a building. When I walked into her unit, I readily agreed about the strong mold odor, which seemed to be coming out of one of her heat ducts. We went into the basement and determined that the duct leading to that register passed through the ceiling of a storage area belonging to another unit owner. The basement had flooded several times because of sewer backups, and all the stored goods were covered with mold. The odor in the storage area was overpowering—a stronger version of the smell on the third floor. When the heat was off, air from the storage area was drawn into the system by convection through the space in the chase (vertical shaft) around the heat duct and several gaps in the loose duct joint. The odor disappeared when the moldy furniture was removed and the duct and chase were sealed.

In buildings heated by hot-air systems, there can be a constant "passive" (convective) airflow through the entire duct system, even when the blower is off. Flows from the basement to the other rooms can increase if the ducts leak.

SMOKING AND COOKING ODORS

We get a lot of calls from people who want air testing done because they smell cigarette smoke or cooking odors from other units in the building. Sometimes the odors come from an adjacent unit, and sometimes they waft from a unit several floors below. This problem is difficult if not impossible to eradicate because of the omnipresent airflows in a building, which carry these odors. There are some steps you can take, though, to try to isolate your apartment from such airstreams.

To determine the source of odor infiltration, you could put a window fan on exhaust in a window (with all other windows closed) and sniff at floor, wall, and ceiling openings (including electric switches and outlets) to see where the odor is strongest. Then you can seal such gaps as needed. You can also try to increase the air pressure in your apartment by operating a window fan or two on supply (not a great option in cold weather, though). Another option in a building with a whole-building exhaust system (and there are no "on/off" switches in your unit) is to temporarily cover the operating kitchen and bathroom exhaust grilles when the odor infiltration seems strong. This can increase the air pressure in an apartment and make air infiltration from a hallway less likely.

You can't really ask other building occupants to stop cooking. If the stoves in the various apartments have exhaust fans that vent to the exterior, you can ask the occupants to use the fans when they cook or bake. If you smell cigarette smoke in your unit and are concerned (and rightly so) about exposure to secondhand smoke, you can ask people to smoke outside (but not near the entrance to the building!). At present, unfortunately, people have a right to smoke in their own homes. In the end, you may just have to move. First, though, seek legal counsel to find out your rights in this situation.

COMMON AREAS

HALLWAYS

In some buildings, a gap under an entrance door leading to an apartment is purposeful to allow "fresh" air into the apartment from a hallway that has a fresh-air supply. The apartment's kitchen and bathroom exhausts pull in the hallway air.

As you walk down the hallway to get to your own front door, you are exposed to any hallway contaminants or allergens that may be present, particularly if there is carpeting. If there is a gap under your front door, hallway air can flow into your apartment. If you see any conditions in the hallway that concern you, report these conditions to your association, property manager, or maintenance personnel. Add a sweep or gaskets to your front door as needed to make it airtight.

BASEMENTS

If the basement in your building smells musty or if you see visible mold growth, report the condition to the association, property manager, or maintenance personnel. The space may have to be cleaned or even professionally remediated, and then the relative humidity may need to be more adequately controlled in the future. Many buildings contain private storage spaces in the basement for occupants. If the basement in your building smells musty, say "no, thank you" to that storage option.

ELEVATORS

As an elevator goes up and down in the elevator shaft, it increases the air pressure above the elevator's car by pushing air into a smaller space. The air pressure below the car is then reduced, and air from the basement and from other levels below the moving elevator flows upward. This air can carry mold spores from the basement, cooking and cigarette odors from other units, or combustion products from an underground garage up to your level of the building. Often there is even water at the bottom of the elevator shaft containing moldy debris. The bottom of the elevator shaft should be kept clean and dry. The shaft should also be isolated from any crawl space, if present.

GARAGES

In large buildings with basement parking garages, soot from automobile exhaust (particularly from cars with diesel engines) may enter hallways through airflows up the elevator shaft. If air for the common hallway gets into an apartment under the unit's entry door, the carpeting there may develop a long, tongue-shaped soot stain. If you live in an apartment or condominium and your light carpet backs up to your unit's front door, you may have noticed this discolored "welcome mat." (Even if your building doesn't have an underground garage, you may still find soot patterns on your carpeting, because the soot from vehicular traffic on the street migrates from the exterior into the building.)

Along with the soot, combustion products from vehicles' gas engines may be carried on airflows from a basement parking garage into habitable spaces above. In a building with a basement garage and an elevator, the elevator entry door should not open up directly into the garage but rather be located in a vestibule with an airtight door.

LAUNDRIES

One woman called me because she kept smelling laundry product odors in the entranceway and hallways of her building and sometimes even in her own apartment. She lived in a six-unit building with a common laundry in the basement. Other occupants in the building were using fragranced laundry products that the woman found irritating and that kicked up her asthma. She lived on the third floor, and sometimes (especially on weekends, when people were home and doing their laundry) she was wheezing by the time she arrived at her own front door. She was about to look for a new place to live when she called me as a last resort.

She told me that there was a small gap beneath her front door, so air from the hallway flowed into her apartment. She and I discussed her options, which included making her front door more airtight, but there was really no way to assure that she would ever solve this problem so long as other building occupants used laundry products that caused the woman's symptoms. I suggested that she explain her situation to her neighbors and offer to buy them fragrance- and enzyme-free laundry detergents. She took my advice, and all the other building occupants agreed to the plan. The woman was then able to enter the building and walk to her apartment without holding her nose and breath. In the end, this solution was less expensive and a lot less troublesome than if she had been forced to find a new place to live.

MAINTENANCE PRACTICES

Maintenance practices can make or break the indoor air quality (IAQ) in a building. If the heating system is inadequately maintained or the carpeting in a common hallway is contaminated with microbial growth, the IAQ will be compromised, potentially affecting the health of occupants in the building.

I once inspected a condo in a three-family building. My client was interested in purchasing the second-floor unit, which was spacious and recently renovated. The building exterior was in good shape, and there was a large yard with a common vegetable garden in back of the building. My client was excited about living there, but she also had allergies and thus wanted to know whether there could be potential IAQ problems in the building. Luckily, the building had hot-water heat, with cooling supplied by window air conditioning units owned by occupants (we discuss cleaning heating and cooling equipment later in the book). I explained to my client how to clean the baseboard convectors before she moved in and how to properly maintain and store window air conditioners.

I was impressed with conditions in the unit; it was clean, and the renovation had been done well. When she and I descended to the basement, however, we found a moldy and unkempt space full of stored goods. It even appeared as if former occupants had left their goods behind when they moved out. I cautioned her about moving into the building until the basement was cleared of moldy goods and then remediated. She approached the association's board members (consisting of representatives from the other two condominiums in the building), who were sympathetic but told her that they had no plans to clean up the basement. After all, they were not experiencing any health problems living in the building, and they didn't want to assume their shares of such an expense. If she moved into the building, the chances were that any motions she raised to have the basement remediated would be voted down, because she would only have one vote in a group of three. In the end, she reluctantly walked away from the apartment and ended up buying a small single-family home in which she would have much greater control of indoor environmental conditions.

MOVING IN

If you move into a multi-unit building, you may inherit a refrigerator or carpeting. Refrigerators can be sources of bioaerosol (see recommendations for cleaning refrigerators in chap. 9). Consider getting rid of any wall-to-wall carpeting, as it is likely to contain allergenic dust. If you cannot get rid of the carpeting, thoroughly HEPA vacuum the carpeting (using a vacuum with high-efficiency particulate arrestance filtration). Then treat the carpeting slowly with steam vapor from a steam vapor machine (see chap. 24). Test a corner of the carpet first to be sure that the steam won't damage the fibers. Don't accept freebies such as beds or upholstered furniture, because such pieces may contain dust mite infestations and even mold.

It's always a surprise to me when people thinking about moving into a multi-unit building only consider conditions within a particular unit, and yet the IAQ (as well as rents and condominium fees) are affected by the conditions and maintenance practices in the entire building, including its mechanical equipment.

Connie grew up in Vermont near the base of a mountain and a timeshare resort. One of the timeshare buildings had been split up into quarter-share, half-share, and full-share ownership portions, meaning that people could buy a three-month, six-month, or full-year occupancy of a unit in the building.

It took some time for all the timeshare slices in that building to be sold. As far as we know, not one prospective buyer thought to have the whole building inspected. Eventually, the exterior of the building had to be resided, and the roof and heating system needed to be replaced. Guess what? The timeshare fees were raised considerably to cover these expenses. A timeshare building in which the ownership shares represent one week has a large ownership base. In this building, however, the timeshare portions were longer, so the ownership base was smaller. As a consequence, the fees each owner had to pay rose considerably.

If you are considering moving into a multi-unit building, do not just look at conditions within the unit in question. Inspect the basement and common areas. Ask about maintenance practices and plans for future capital work.

Multi-unit buildings are political communities in which owners or tenants negotiate with each other, board members, and property management/building maintenance personnel. But as far as airflow is concerned, the unit you are considering as your future home has no walls, so be your own advocate to protect your health.

SOME RECOMMENDATIONS

- If you have a vertical stack fan coil, remove the top supply grille and check the interior of the supply plenum for dust and mold with a mirror and flashlight. Owing to humid conditions in the plenum from A/C use, mold often grows in the dust.

- Insist that any univents in your apartment be maintained on the recommended schedule; there should not be visible dust at the interior or on the coils. Use a MERV-8 pleated media filter that is airtight at the perimeter.

- Fins in hot-water baseboard heating convectors should be cleaned thoroughly prior to your occupancy or shortly after you move in (see chap. 24).

- Radiator surfaces (including spaces between the sections) should be cleaned annually before the heat is turned on for the season.

- Do not store window or portable air conditioning units in a moldy basement (unless sealed in plastic).

- Window and portable air conditioning units should be cleaned before the start of every cooling season (see chap. 24).

- Bathroom and kitchen exhausts in a multi-unit building should vent to the exterior.

- If you are considering moving into a multi-unit building, look at the entire building and not just the one unit.

PART III.
BELOW AND ABOVE

UNFINISHED BASEMENTS AND CRAWL SPACES

15

Like many people, you might not enjoy going down into your basement or crawl space and breathing the air down there. Like it or not, however, air from below-grade spaces enters your lungs no matter where you are in the house. Many air quality problems are caused by legions of unseen organisms growing in a basement or crawl space. If below-grade spaces are teeming with life, by-products of biological growth will find their way into living spaces. It's therefore vital to pay attention to environmental conditions below grade.

UNFINISHED BASEMENTS

Depending on a home's construction, 30 to 50 percent of "fresh" house air may come from a basement, especially in the winter.

THE MOLD FARM

I was asked to investigate a 200-year-old home because the owner had severe mold allergies and was suffering from sinus trouble and respiratory symptoms. The interior was one of the cleanest I had ever seen. There were hardwood floors with few rugs and little furniture. Most people might consider this Spartan, but because of her allergies to dust and mold, the owner believed this decor (or lack thereof) was necessary.

The basement was an entirely different story. One side of the basement developed a stream in heavy rain, and moldy leaves and other debris littered the whole basement. The house had steam heat, and pipes went from the basement up to the radiators on the first floor. There were gaps around the pipes, and when the heat was on, moldy warm air rose from the basement into the rooms above.

I demonstrated this air movement with a nontoxic smoke pencil, which I use to track airflows. I released puffs of smoke at cracks in the basement ceiling and in the gaps near the heat pipes. Standing on the first floor, the owner was enveloped in clouds of white smoke that billowed up through the openings. It was dramatic enough that she was convinced. Once the family cleaned the basement and crawl space and sealed the gaps around the pipes, her symptoms abated.

SPIDERS

There is a hidden ecology in a damp basement. Mold grows on surfaces, and microarthropods such as mites and booklice feed on the mold. Spiders in turn dine on the hordes of crawling life. If you feel good about the drooping nets of spiderwebs hanging from your basement ceiling, think again, because the presence of spiders signals a miniature food chain that includes mold and life forms that produce allergenic fecal matter.

CONTROLLING WATER ENTRY

Minimizing moisture in your basement is an important step to controlling microscopic plant and animal life. The most obvious source is external water that finds its way in, and the most common cause of entry is improper dispersal of roof water.

When I started inspecting homes, I wanted to learn about wet basements, so I took a job with a basement waterproofing company. I looked at hundreds of homes and provided estimates for the installation of basement "dewatering" systems and sump pumps. In over 95 percent of the homes I visited, the wet basement was due to improper dispersal of roof water. I would demonstrate this by directing water from a hose onto the ground at a location near the foundation where there was (or should have been!) a downspout for roof water. Most of the time, a puddle would appear in the basement within a few minutes. I would explain to the occupants that they really needed to improve the dispersal of their roof water before investing thousands in a basement system. I had the worst sales record of anyone in the company, but as I had hoped and planned, I learned a lot and quit after six months.

When a house is built where there is a high water table, sump pumps can help control basement water. (A sump is the hole in the floor, and the pump empties the water from the sump to the exterior.)

Wherever you live, the water table is somewhere below your house. It may be 20 feet down or 20 inches, or even just 1 inch below the bottom of the concrete floor slab in the basement. If you dig a hole and the bottom fills with water, you've reached the water table. Above the water table, the spaces between the soil particles are filled with air and water vapor; below the water table, these spaces are filled with liquid water. The layer above the water table, where there is air and vapor in the soil, is called the vadose zone. People prefer to have their foundations in the vadose zone rather than below the water table, but sometimes topography disappoints us.

The sump pump keeps a high water table beneath the bottom of the floor slab. A pump should be kept low enough to prevent water from overflowing the sump. It should not be placed too low, though, for if there is a high water table, the pump will run continuously, creating a water-dispersal headache and using too much electrical power. The motor may also burn out more frequently with constant use.

One woman who lived near a lake had this problem with her pump, which was at the bottom of the sump under approximately two feet of water. The pump ran almost continuously, discharging water through a long hose that ran over the lawn to the curb. Where the water flowed out, the curb and asphalt were wet, and the pavement was green with algae. The water table was high, so every house on that side of the street had a similar hose across its lawn. Hers was the only "green river," however, because none of her neighbors had their pumps positioned as low as she did. I explained that she should raise her pump, since the level of the water table in her basement was about equal to that of the lake surface. She was essentially trying to empty the entire lake that bordered all the backyards on her side of the street.

Some people depend too readily on sump pumps instead of taking care of an underlying problem. I inspected a home with a sump pump that was operating frequently. As soon as the pump drained the sump, water rushed back in. At first I thought the water table was high, but this wasn't the case. Even though all the fixtures were off and the water meter dial was motionless, I noticed a peculiar hissing noise in the vicinity of the water main. I recommended that the seller inform the town's water department. A representative discovered that the city water main was broken in the street and that millions of gallons of water had been lost. Coincidentally, when the city main was fixed, five neighbors were also able to disconnect their sump pumps because they no longer had water in their basements.

I've found some strange things, including frogs, in basement sumps. Some items like dead mice, moldy toilet paper, and other biodegradable debris that find their way into sumps can be a source of air quality problems. Keep your sump clean and install a nonbiodegradable cover that can be easily removed for periodic checks. If there is a high radon level in the soil, the sump can also be a source of radon gas in the basement, and you may have to install an airtight radon cover (see "Radon Gas" later in this chapter).

When the pump operates, be sure no water squirts out of the pipes or splashes out of the sump. In one home the sump pump was housed in a closet. Near the end of the discharge cycle, water squirted out of the weep hole and splashed onto the drywall. All the walls of the closet were covered with *Stachybotrys*, a potentially toxic mold.

A last caution about sump pumps. Power failures often occur during heavy storms, and you may lose your electricity precisely when you need it most. If you depend heavily on a sump pump to keep your basement dry, consider installing a battery-operated backup pump. If you are in a rural area, you may want to have a power generator on hand, because batteries have a finite lifetime. But never operate a gasoline-powered generator indoors, or you face the danger of asphyxiation while trying to keep your basement from drowning!

BASEMENT RAIN FORESTS

Surprising as it may seem, humidity and condensation rather than leaks or flooding cause most basement mold problems I see. Water that condenses on uninsulated cold-water pipes or on a pressure tank associated with well-water storage can drip onto the floor or soak into stored goods. If the pipes in your basement sweat like this, installing foam insulation tubing around them will prevent condensation. Insulation for copper and other piping comes in various diameters to fit most common pipe sizes. You can also put closed-cell foam insulation around a well-water pressure tank.

In most basements, foundation masonry (stone, brick, concrete blocks, or poured concrete) is cooler than the upstairs walls and floor. During the summer the temperature of the masonry is often below the dew point of the basement air, and moisture will condense on the masonry and even on goods stored close to or touching the masonry.

BIODEGRADABLE DUST

Whatever type of foundation you have, masonry wall and floor surfaces acquire a layer of house dust for several reasons. First, microscopic plant fibers, such as cellulose from sawdust and lint, adhere to the rough wall surface. As airflows carry other particles over the cellulose fibers, suspended biodegradable particles (such as skin scales and pollen) collide with the fibers and stick. Second, spiders are constantly traversing foundation walls, foraging for insects. They leave a trail of fine silk to which dust can stick. When I look under the microscope at surface samples I take from a foundation wall, I'm always amazed to see vast networks of spider silk.

Many foundation walls are also covered with at least a fine layer of mold or actinomycetes (soil organisms) growing on the dust. Eventually, every particle of biodegradable dust that lands on basement masonry will probably be consumed by some living organism, particularly if the relative humidity (RH) is high. (To avoid this ecological progression, see "Drying Out" later in this chapter.) Even faint airflows can disturb this dust, which aerosolizes spores and other allergens.

Foundation walls and floors that are painted and smooth are easier to keep clean. Surfaces can be vacuumed with a HEPA vacuum and disinfected with dilute bleach (one part bleach to sixteen parts water) or with a 9 percent hydrogen peroxide solution, though avoid stirring up irritating dust during cleaning. In addition, be extremely careful not to get peroxide on your skin or in your eyes, because, like bleach, hydrogen peroxide is a powerful oxidizing agent and can cause bodily harm (please refer to chap. 24).

Dirt floors, however, can never be cleaned. A significant percentage of soil consists of living organisms, and their digestive enzymes are poised to receive the nutrients we shed. With a ready food source and adequate soil moisture, mold and other microorganisms will proliferate. Moisture also evaporates from the soil, increasing the RH of the basement. If you have a dirt floor in your basement, I urge you to have a contractor install a concrete floor over a vapor barrier and crushed stone. This work should be done under containment conditions.

FIBERGLASS CANOPY

Many basements and crawl spaces have exposed fiberglass ceiling insulation between the joists for the first floor; most building codes even require insulation. Unfortunately, exposed fiberglass insulation attracts rodents. The fiberglass also acts as a filter and can accumulate significant amounts of biodegradable dust and allergens. In approximately one-half of the homes that I inspected that had exposed fiberglass insulation below grade, moisture levels (RH) had at some point been excessive, and vast populations of microfungi (often along with mold-eating mites) were growing in ceiling fiberglass insulation that looked clean (see chap. 2). If there are pets in the home, then the fiberglass sometimes contains pet dander particles, which besides being an allergen is also mold fodder. And if dusty insulation becomes damp from condensation or a pipe leak, mold will have the moisture it needs to grow, regardless of the basement's RH levels.

Once a mold spore germinates, it sends out hyphae that travel along the glass fibers and digest any adhering particulates they encounter. Mold-eating mites move in thereafter to dine on the spores and hyphae. When people walk on the floors above moldy insulation, or when work is done on basement piping or electrical wiring, the insulation may be disturbed and clouds of allergenic particles can be aerosolized. Fiberglass insulation that is contaminated in this fashion can be extremely difficult to identify as a source of indoor air quality problems.

Installing fiberglass insulation with the vapor barrier side (usually tar paper) down will prevent biodegradable dust from accumulating in the fiberglass, but it will not stop the paper in the barrier from getting moldy if moisture condenses in the material. If mice have infested the fiberglass, mouse urine stains could be visible on the vapor barrier side. I recommend installing a noncombustible covering such as drywall over fiberglass insulation in a basement ceiling. (But note that mold will still grow on drywall paper if the RH is high enough.)

In one home the owner had suffered allergy symptoms for three years, ever since moving into the house. When she was exposed to air from the basement, she developed rashes. She kept the basement scrupulously clean, but she naturally avoided entering it as much as possible, even though the walls and floor were painted and no items were stored there. The flows from the hot-air heating system also bothered her, so she placed stockings on some registers as filters and kept others closed. When the blower was operating, the stockings restricted the airflow to such an extent that air was pouring out of all the duct joints into the basement, increasing the air pressure there and disturbing the dust in the fiberglass. At the first-floor level the air pressure was reduced because the single large return was pulling air into the system, and there was an insufficient supply of corresponding air from the blocked registers.

In this home, two forces were moving air up from the basement: the excess air pressure in the basement and the reduced pressure on the first floor. When I smoke-tested the airflows, I found that air from the basement rushed through large gaps under the basement door and around pipe openings in the bathroom. The basement ceiling was insulated with fiberglass that was full of mold and mites, and airflows were carrying the allergens upstairs. The owner had a professional remove the basement insulation (under containment) and HEPA vacuum and spray-paint the ceiling structure. She removed the stockings from the heat registers, had the furnace and ducts cleaned, and added an efficient filter. Within a week, her rashes disappeared.

STORED GOODS

Possessions stored in a basement that is damp from condensation, leaks, or flooding can become contaminated, particularly if the items touch or face foundation walls or the floor. When paper goods, such as boxes or newspapers, rest directly on concrete, mold often grows at the bottom. This type of growth is helped along by floor water from leaks, but it can spread even without such leaks. Unless the mold grows up the sides, you may not be aware of its presence. When I notice rectangular black shapes on a floor—residues outlining moldy items that have been removed—I avoid stepping on them. When people do step on such spots, mold spores (possibly including *Stachybotrys* spores) and other microscopic bits of contaminated debris are disturbed and become airborne.

A physician referred one client to me after a lung biopsy revealed that the man's reduced lung capacity was due to hypersensitivity pneumonitis (HP). This pulmonary condition, characterized by immune inflammation in the lungs, is sometimes caused by chronic exposure to mold spores and other bioaerosols. The man owned a large collection of classical records that he stored in a damp, moldy basement. After he retired, his wife suggested he reorganize his collection and thin it out because it took up too much basement space. He spent several hours a day over two or three years reviewing his beloved albums, sorting them into "sell" and "keep" categories while exposing his lungs to mold spores from the microfungi growing on the album covers. The couple had to get rid of all the moldy record covers and books and have the foundation walls and ceiling structure professionally cleaned and spray-painted.

To protect items against moisture from condensation, leaks, and flooding, never place possessions up against the basement walls or directly on the floor—a common practice. Items stored in unfinished basements should be on shelves (preferably rolling metal shelving) at least two feet from the foundation walls and a few inches above the floor. You can raise things on pallets of pressure-treated wood resting on bricks or concrete blocks (untreated wood pallets can become moldy). Storing items off the floor will also keep them dry if your basement gets a few inches of water in a storm. You can also place 1.5-inch solid polyisocyanurate sheet foam insulation on the floor and up against the foundation wall, and store goods upon this backed platform.

The air that flows into and out of a home's blower system must be balanced: for every cubic foot of air distributed to all the rooms, one cubic foot of air must be drawn in by the system's return(s). When a system is not balanced, as is often the case, trouble can result.

Storing clothing and other fabric items in airtight plastic bins or bags will help protect them from excessive basement humidity. One caution, though: don't put fabric in airtight containers during humid weather. Moisture is adsorbed (bound to the surface of the fibers) before it is absorbed (trapped as liquid between the fibers). At 100 percent RH, a cotton shirt may weigh about 15 percent more than it does when the RH in air is at about 10 percent, because individual water molecules in the air are adsorbed on the surfaces of the cellulose fibers. At every level of RH except zero, adsorbed moisture will be present. When many individual water molecules (not in ice) are joined together, they behave as a liquid; when they are separated from each other and bound to a surface, they behave as if they are part of the surface they are bonded to, so a cotton shirt carrying 15 percent of its weight in adsorbed water may still not seem wet.

Cotton cloth that is dripping wet has first adsorbed and then absorbed moisture. The adsorbed water will still be present when most of the absorbed water has been squeezed out, because it takes more energy to break the bond between the water molecule and the cellulose than to wring out the liquid water. If you pack a shirt that feels dry into a plastic bag on a humid day, the adsorbed moisture will remain in the bag. As the room cools, the moisture may condense on the material or on the plastic, and if spores are present, mold may grow. If you must pack away clothing on humid days, place the articles in the dryer first. Cotton fresh from a hot dryer will have a very low moisture content, but if the material is allowed to remain in humid air, moisture will again be adsorbed onto the fibers. If possible, therefore, pack the clothing while it is still warm.

If you experience a significant basement flood, discard cushioned or upholstered items (including mattresses and sofas) that are stored in the basement if they absorbed water. Replace any cardboard boxes that have become wet, because mold spores can germinate within hours. (Also replace cardboard boxes that have been stored directly on the concrete or touching the foundation wall.) Be extremely careful about using large-volume fans to dry the basement; in a basement that is already moldy, fans can blow spores around and create significant air quality problems.

It takes far less moisture than a flood to cause trouble. One family purchased a home with a damp basement. They thought it would be safe to put all their winter clothing in a large cedar closet in the basement, but when they went to retrieve their clothing in the fall, it was covered with *Aspergillus* mold. The RH in the closet was no different from that in the rest of the basement, and though the odor of cedar may repel insects, it did not slow the mold growth down in the least.

In the end, I recommend storing as little as possible in a basement, because the chance that mold will grow on stored goods is so high.

DEADLY MOLD EXPOSURE

For those who are highly sensitized, mold exposure can even be deadly. A family who called me for help had a damp basement, and all their stored goods were covered with mold. The family's teenage daughter was experiencing anaphylaxis; she would go into shock and stop breathing, generally in the middle of the night. The cause of her illness was unknown. Her parents kept an extra mattress in her bedroom, and every night one of them kept vigil after she had fallen asleep. The cat's litter box was in the basement, and the door was left open so the animal could go up and down freely. Airflows were carrying the mold spores from the basement up into the living spaces.

I recommended the family install a pet door to the basement and hire a professional cleaning firm. Because the girl might have been sensitized to the basement dust, the workers did all they could to prevent disturbed dust from rising into the rest of the house. This extraordinary effort, similar in scope to an asbestos mitigation, entailed covering all the floors at the first level with plastic, gasketing the basement door, and sealing gaps around all the pipes that rose to the upper levels. The company also created negative pressure below grade by blowing HEPA-filtered air out through a basement window. This way, even if there were any small openings left unsealed between the basement and the first floor, air would flow into the basement rather than the other way around. To be safe, the daughter also stayed out of the house until all the rooms had been thoroughly cleaned with a HEPA vacuum. I later heard that the girl, who had been hospitalized at least three times in the months before the cleanup, needed no hospitalization afterward.

DUCT CONVEYANCE

One concerned couple called me because their young son had been experiencing chronic fevers and had been hospitalized numerous times. The child had been taking antibiotics for months to no avail. There was a hot-air heating system in the home, and the damp basement was packed full of furniture acquired from yard sales. They had biodegradable items sitting directly on the floor and up against the foundation walls. Everything was covered with *Cladosporium* mold growth.

The bottom of the furnace air return had never been secured properly, so there was a large gap. When the heating system was operating, mold spores from the basement were sucked in and blown upstairs with the hot air. With a Burkard sampler, I measured one of the largest concentrations of spores I had ever seen—about 300,000 *Cladosporium* spores per cubic meter of air—coming out of the heat register in the boy's bedroom. There were other problems in the home as well. Three of my many recommendations were to install a bottom at the return cabinet, eliminate the moldy furniture, and improve the grading around the foundation so less water would enter the basement.

Another client, referred by her pulmonologist, had been suffering from hypersensitivity pneumonitis. Because she became breathless so readily, she had been basically housebound for three years. Her house was at the bottom of a hill and also had a basement garage with a driveway that sloped sharply down from the street. The house backed up to a swamp, so the water table was high. All these factors conspired against the client, for during heavy summer rains the basement flooded, sometimes with as much as 12 inches of water. Mold growth in the basement was extensive, and the hot-air heating system was helping to circulate spores throughout the living spaces.

The woman's physician had already ordered a lab test on her blood serum for reactivity to mold (an HP screen), and it showed a mildly elevated level of IgE (immunoglobulin E) in reaction to one type of *Aspergillus* mold. I took Andersen air samples in the home and shipped the petri dishes overnight to the same lab for additional testing, which indicated the woman had elevated levels of IgE in reaction to the specific species of *Aspergillus* growing in her home.

The client had a professional thoroughly clean the basement and the heating system, and her respiratory capacity went from 50 percent of normal to 100 percent.

DRYING OUT

An unfinished basement should be kept as dry as possible to keep mold growth and microarthropod populations at a minimum. The RH should be kept at no more than 50 percent. People who realize how important it is to reduce basement moisture operate dehumidifiers, but I still find many problems in basements that are being dehumidified.

The dehumidifier coil can be full of biological growth. The coils, particularly a spiral configuration, accumulate a layer of dust that is kept constantly wet by the condensation. If you cut wood in the basement, your dehumidifier can trap lots of sawdust (and biodegradable dust can also collect in exposed fiberglass insulation and be deposited on other basement surfaces). Mold, bacteria, and other organisms grow on cellulose as well as on other biodegradable components in dust (fig. 15.1).

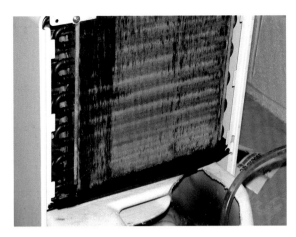

FIGURE 15.1. The filter screen has been removed from this basement dehumidifier, revealing a mold-covered cooling coil. Without adequate filtration, dust accumulates on the cooling coil as air flows across it. Water that condenses on the coil wets the dust, causing mold to grow. Most dehumidifiers are supplied with inefficient screen filters, so the coils must be cleaned regularly.

Check the cooling coils on your dehumidifier regularly, and be sure there is no biological slime clinging to them. If there is, the machine itself can disperse airborne allergens. Contaminated coils can be cleaned with a sprayer and dilute bleach or a hydrogen peroxide solution (see chap. 24) and a soft brush (do this outside), but do not bend the fins. Refer to the manufacturer's cleaning directions, and do not wet any electrical components.

I also find that many people don't empty the drain buckets of their dehumidifiers often enough. Most dehumidifiers stop running when the bucket is full, defeating their purpose. In addition, any biodegradable debris inside the bucket will fester. In humid conditions the drain bucket sometimes has to be emptied two or three times a day. One way to avoid this annoying chore is to suspend the dehumidifier above a basement sink and let the water drain through a garden hose directly into a sink. If you don't have a basement sink, you can purchase a small condensate pump (sold for use in air conditioning systems) and pump the water outside through a plastic tube. If you want to use either of these means, be sure to buy a dehumidifier with a hose fitting on the condensate tray.

A dehumidifier should be operated in a clean basement, or the air movement the machine generates can disturb and disperse allergenic dust. In addition, don't operate a dehumidifier during the winter when the air is dry or when the basement temperature is below 65°F. If the compressor is running but there is little or no water condensing (or if the coils are iced over), you are wasting your money.

Another wasteful mistake homeowners make is to keep the basement windows open when they operate dehumidifiers. This is like trying to dehumidify the air in the whole neighborhood. It's similarly wasteful to leave the door to the rest of the house open. The only way to successfully dehumidify a basement is to isolate it from the outside and from the rest of the house. If a basement consists of several areas or contains isolated areas such as storage closets, keep the connecting doors between such areas or spaces open or use more than one dehumidifier. (You can also acquire a dehumidifier with an optional duct kit.)

I recommend purchasing an expensive and efficient dehumidifier that has about three times the capacity of most less expensive models and a very efficient pleated media filter to prevent biodegradable dust from accumulating on the moist cooling coils. No matter what model you choose, the only way to know if your dehumidifier is doing its job is to measure the basement's RH separately from the machine's digital display. This means buying a thermo-hygrometer, which can be purchased in most hardware or building supply stores. Place the device in a remote corner in the basement near the floor.

THE "DO-NOTHING" DEHUMIDIFIER?

Some people install a device that has a fan to exhaust basement air to the exterior. These devices are called "dehumidifiers" because, as the fan depressurizes a basement, dryer make-up air is supposedly drawn into the basement from the rooms above. The upstairs air may not be drier, though, than the air in the basement, and if the upstairs air is cooled, the A/C system will have to run longer, negating any supposed savings that an exhaust-fan-only unit can offer as compared to a typical refrigerant-based unit. If the upstairs air isn't air conditioned, the exhaust- fan-only unit isn't effective during humid weather, when dehumidification is most needed below grade to avoid microbial growth due to elevated RH conditions.

Such exhaust-fan-only devices can also cause backdrafting of combustion products. In one home, two exhaust-fan-only–type "dehumidifiers" were installed in the basement. The homeowner's gas-fired boiler had an automatic draft damper above the standard "bell" draft hood. There was an approximately one-inch hole in the center of the damper plate to provide draft for the combustion gases from the pilot light. Unfortunately, the draft provided by such a small hole is not adequate to remove all the combustion products produced by the pilot. These gases were spilling out of the draft hood into this basement. I could smell the odor of combustion products as soon as I entered the unfinished basement mechanical room. I recommended that the homeowner either eliminate the automatic damper (which would reduce the efficiency of the boiler due to heat loss) or keep the damper and replace the gas pilot light with a spark or coil ignition. I also recommended that she try to get her money back for the two exhaust-fan-only "dehumidifiers" she had purchased and use instead a conventional refrigerant-based dehumidifier.

BASEMENT ACTIVITIES

Some people let their children play in an unfinished basement, or they exercise in the space. I don't recommend that unfinished basements be used in this way, because basement dust tends to be contaminated with mold spores and microarthropod fecal allergens. When wood is sawed in an unfinished basement, biodegradable dust collects on basement surfaces. If moisture is present, either as high RH or water, mold growth will occur (and if the wood is sawed during construction, the basement can be contaminated with mold growth before the property is even occupied).

Particularly for people who have allergies or asthma, spending extended time in contaminated spaces can lead to respiratory health issues. To make matters worse, both play and exercise raise respiration rates and disturb dust, both of which can increase the severity of exposure and symptoms. I realize it's often convenient to do laundry in basements: if the basement is kept clean of dust and is adequately dehumidified, this should not pose an excessive risk. Area rugs should never be placed on concrete, however. The rug fibers capture biodegradable dust, and the rug is cooled by its contact with the concrete. Conditions of elevated RH develop in air close to the rug and concrete, and mold growth can follow.

My own basement is the exception to my cautions of using unfinished basements as living space. We are the first owners of our current home, and rather than having fiberglass insulation installed at the basement ceiling, I asked the builder to insulate the exterior of the foundation walls with two-inch-thick sheet foam and to place the same on the crushed stone before the concrete floor was poured. I also had a hot-air heater (that operates off the boiler) installed that is hung from the framing at the basement ceiling, and I run a high-capacity dehumidifier in the humid season (which in New England where I live is between mid-April and mid-October). The heater rarely operates, yet thanks to the sheet foam insulation, the basement temperature is never under 60°F in winter and always under 70°F in summer. Our basement is therefore "conditioned" and is dry as a bone, even if it is unfinished. Still, we are careful about storage, keeping all our goods on metal shelving with wheels. And we HEPA vacuum the entire basement every few months to remove biodegradable dust.

RADON GAS

In some areas of the country, the levels of radon (a radioactive, carcinogenic gas) in the soil are high. Radon can enter a basement from a sump, particularly if a system of piping to collect sub-slab water is connected to the sump. An airtight plastic sump cover may reduce radon entry. Radon also enters a basement with other soil gases through dirt floors and cracks in masonry floors and walls. These flows occur because the pressure inside the house is usually less than that of the gases in the soil. Elevated radon levels are a particular concern if people spend time in the basement. Even if the basement isn't used much, air with radon can flow to the upper floors from the basement. In general the level of radon on the first floor is one-half to one-third of the level in the basement—proof again that we inevitably breathe basement air upstairs.

A radon mitigation system draws soil gases, including radon, out of the spaces that surround a basement foundation and floor slab. A plastic pipe is sunk into crushed stone in the soil beneath the basement floor. The pipe, sealed in concrete at the basement floor, rises through the house and into the attic, where an in-line fan secured to the pipe draws the radon-containing air from the soil behind the basement masonry and blows the radioactive gas out above the roof, where it dissipates.

Unlike most unhealthy particles and gases in air, radon gas cannot be smelled or tasted, and it causes no immediate symptoms. In fact, a liter of air with radon and one without radon are nearly identical in every way, because at the action level of four picocuries of radon per liter of air suggested by the US Environmental Protection Agency (EPA), only about one atom in 30,000,000,000,000,000,000 in a liter of air is radon! Yet radioactive atoms are so dangerous that even if inhaled at this concentration, they increase the risk of lung cancer. (If you smoke and have elevated radon in your home, the likelihood of your having lung cancer increases.)

Every home should be tested for radon as recommended by the EPA. Radon test kits are inexpensive and easy to use. If the concentration in the lowest lived-in level is above four picocuries per liter, additional testing or mitigation may be needed. Mitigation systems are worth the investment to protect your health and property.

Do not install a radon mitigation system yourself; seek a licensed contractor. I inspected a house where the seller had installed a radon exhaust fan in his basement and connected it to a dryer hose at the basement ceiling that discharged beneath the rear deck. The connection at the interior was loose, and some radon-laden air poured into the basement. In addition, the discharge beneath the deck enveloped his barbecue and his daughter's sandbox in radioactive gas.

If you have a radon mitigation system, the fan should be accessible and the pressure gauge (a tube filled with colored liquid) checked periodically to be sure that the system is operating. (If the liquid levels in the tube are equal, then the fan is not operating.)

CRAWL SPACES

Some homes or additions are built over crawl spaces—shallow spaces between the ground and floor structure—rather than over full basements. Although crawl spaces are common in some parts of the country, I would never choose to live in a home with one because I have seen them cause so many indoor air quality problems. In addition, few people who have crawl spaces think of dehumidifying them.

I discourage you from purchasing a home with a crawl space unless the space is spotless and has concrete floors and walls. Crawl spaces with dirt floors make me shudder.

A CRAWL SPACE WATERFALL

I inspected an apartment for a tenant who was paying a substantial rent for his exclusive unit but had never been able to live there because the air had a foul odor that made his allergies worse. The first-floor apartment was directly above a sandy crawl space with two sources of unwelcome water. First, the downspouts dumped water directly at the foundation wall rather than directing it away from the building. When it rained, water seeped through the foundation and formed meandering streams that ran through the crawl space. Second, the crawl space contained a pond of sewage seven feet across and six inches deep at the bottom of a concrete sump that contained the uncapped clean-out for the building sewer system. And finally, rodent burrows lined several of the sand mounds near the sump.

I vacuumed the living room carpeting in the apartment, using a special filter cassette to obtain a sample of dust so I could quantify dust mite allergens. I observed the dust in the cassette with a low-power microscope and was astonished to see a silverfish scurrying frantically through the dust. The microarthropod was preying on dust mites in the dust; six mites crawled out of the dust and were upside-down on the cassette cap trying to escape their fate. It was the food chain on a microscopic level, all sucked from an apartment carpet!

I believe this living jungle was caused by the elevated moisture conditions in the crawl space below. Moisture saturated the air in the crawl space as well as the wood framing, the flooring, and the carpeting above. Microarthropods thrived in the high humidity in the carpet. In addition, an unwelcome smell rose into the apartment from the sewage pond. The tenant used the evidence of the damp stench as well as my report to break his lease.

Another desperate homeowner asked me to inspect the crawl space under his three-year-old dining room addition. The previous day he had stood outside by the crawl space ventilation louver and heard water dripping, though he could not recall having any plumbing installed in the room above. He had not looked into the crawl space in five years.

The crawl space was above grade, and when I removed the access vent and looked inside, I could not believe my eyes. White and tan tendrils of macrofungal hyphae (mycelium) hung from every joist, and dark stains covered the wall framing. The soil was damp, and there was an odor of mold. What was the source of moisture? The architect had not wanted to put gutters on the addition, and the builder had neglected to put a vapor barrier over the soil. Moisture from the damp soil evaporated into the space.

The most extraordinary part of this scene was not the fungus but the main beam. Although it superficially appeared satisfactory, it was cracked from top to bottom at the center of its longest span. The man told me he had held a party for thirty guests the weekend before. The load of all of these people had cracked the beam, weakened by the unseen decay. Miraculously, the beam had not failed. Later that day, when I told the builder about the crack, he was so concerned the addition might collapse that he rushed over to support the beam with concrete blocks. I heard from another builder about an addition that had failed within three years owing to macrofungal growth caused by excessive moisture in a crawl space (fig. 15.2).

VENTILATION

Most building codes require that crawl spaces be ventilated to the exterior. In many climates, however, these vents allow in more moisture than they "ventilate." I prefer a dehumidified crawl space that is closed to the outside and has a concrete floor or a mesh-reinforced vapor barrier over dirt. Conditions in a crawl space should be monitored. Make a point of regularly looking in. Keep a thermo-hygrometer there, and if the RH rises above 70 percent, expect to find mold growth and to face a remediation project. Try to keep the RH at no more than 50 percent. If the crawl space is small, open to the basement, and you have a dehumidifier with adequate capacity for the two spaces (check with the manufacturer), you can operate a small fan to blow dehumidified air from the basement into the crawl space.

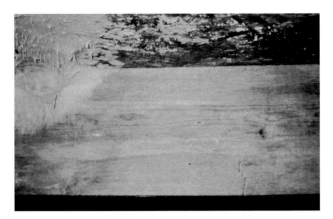

FIGURE 15.2. This is the main beam in the crawl space of a three-year-old addition to a home. The crawl space was damp, and the beam was about seven inches thick. At the upper left of the photo is the white mycelium of wood decay fungi (macrofungi) growing on the beam and on the oriented strand board covering the floor joists. The fungal growth extended invisibly throughout the beam, and after a large party took place in the room above the crawl space, the weakened beam cracked from top to bottom. The crack is visible near the right end of the beam, passing through a knot. The entire floor could have collapsed.

Still, measure the RH in the crawl space, and if necessary install a second dehumidifier there. (If you don't want to or can't enter the crawl space to check the thermo-hygrometer, have a remote-read thermo-hygrometer placed in the space and monitor conditions.)

Building codes have changed and now allow for unventilated crawl spaces, but only if they are "open" to the conditioned space above. In practice this means either supplying a small, specified amount of conditioned air from the house to the crawl space via a ducted system or including the crawl space in the furnace/air conditioning return system. I am disappointed that, after so many years of requiring ventilation that actually brought in moisture to create mold in crawl spaces, we have a new prescription to add mold spores from moldy crawl spaces directly to the interior of homes via the mechanical system. If your crawl space was built according to the code change and is part of the mechanical system, I suggest that you seal off any ducts open to the crawl space and dehumidify the space. If needed, you can install a small fan on a timer that will periodically exhaust air from the crawl space. The fan should have louvers that close when the fan is not operating.

VAPOR BARRIERS

Vapor barriers on the soil, which are also required by many building codes, are an important way to minimize crawl space moisture and biological growth. Unfortunately, vapor barriers are often torn or disrupted by careless homeowners or contractors who enter the crawl space to do work. To be effective, a vapor barrier must be airtight and be secured to the foundation wall and support columns, as well as column footings if present. "Pathways" of pressure-treated wood should be present, so people can enter and exit the crawl space without damaging the vapor barrier.

CRAWL SPACE PETS AND PESTS

I've inspected many homes that had powerful unpleasant odors that originated in crawl spaces. The odor sources are typically mold or pest infestations in fiberglass ceiling insulation or animal excrement and other biodegradable debris in the soil. In some homes the odor will be apparent upstairs even when there is no visible connection between the crawl space and the interior (fig. 15.3).

One couple thought they had a powerful mold odor coming from their basement. Although they did have significant flooding and mold growth in the basement, the odor that concerned them originated in the dirt-floored crawl space. It turned out that they had offered to take care of their daughter's cat while she was on vacation. Apparently, the cat preferred the crawl space to the litter box.

Crawl spaces also attract wild animals. Fiberglass insulation can be an attractive nesting site for bees. Even framing openings that aren't large enough to be noticed can provide access for small rodents. Some of these animals would rather nest in open fiberglass insulation than in a log or elsewhere in the wild. Mice urinate and defecate inside the fiberglass, and if they die there, the smell is even worse.

An insurance agent purchased a single-family home to use for offices. The house had not been well maintained, and after he bought the property, he had to clean the basement and crawl space thoroughly to eliminate mold. Although he had spent a great deal of money on

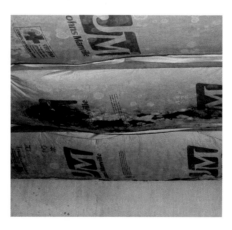

FIGURE 15.3. Rodents were nesting in the fiberglass insulation at the ceiling of a crawl space that had not been dehumidified. The rodents urinated in the insulation and wet the tarpaper insulation vapor barrier in the middle bay. Black, pink, and white mold grew on the stained paper. You can see other light-colored circular mold colonies on the paper in the other two bays. This mold was present as a result of the high relative humidity.

the remediation, an odor lingered. The crawl space ceiling insulation was covered with a plastic vapor barrier, and I could see brown stains and liquid from rodent infestations. After the insulation was eliminated and the joists were HEPA vacuumed and spray-painted, the odor disappeared.

Because crawl spaces are often damp and inaccessible, they may harbor termites (see chap. 13). In one home treated for termites, the applicator sprayed pesticide on the soil in the crawl space as well as on the floor joists. This type of "broadcast" spraying is not permitted. In this case some of the framing in the crawl space was covered with chlordane, a particularly persistent, odorous, semivolatile toxic chemical, which evaporated into the basement and moved with airflows into the upper levels of the house. One of the owners was a nurse who was chemically sensitive. She could no longer work in the hospital, where she had already been exposed to numerous chemicals and irritants. As is so often the case, her home provided no respite.

Though this is an extreme case of an overzealous and inappropriate application of a powerful pesticide, even when the chemicals are correctly and appropriately applied, they can enter the house air through a dirt floor in a crawl space. This is another reason why I feel strongly that dirt floors in crawl spaces should be sealed with crushed stone, a vapor barrier, and concrete.

SOME RECOMMENDATIONS

CLEANING AND REMEDIATION

- Keep the basement floor and walls free of dust.

- If you are sensitized to mold and dust, wear a NIOSH N95 two-strap mask when cleaning your basement.

- Painted basement surfaces are easier to keep clean.

- Professionals using asbestos-level containment should tackle remediation of a moldy basement or crawl space. Such work should include removal of mold-infested exposed fiberglass insulation. The ceiling structure (including subfloor and joists) should then be thoroughly HEPA vacuumed to eliminate all residual dust and then sealed with a light coating of spray paint to encapsulate residual allergens.

CONSTRUCTION PRACTICES

- Dirt floors in basements and crawl spaces should be covered with concrete over crushed stone and a vapor barrier. Alternatively, keep soil free of all biodegradable materials and cover the soil with a heavy-duty airtight mesh-laminated vapor barrier attached to the foundation walls. If access is needed, create "pathways" on top of the vapor barrier by laying down pressure-treated wood.

- If you have multiple spaces in your basement, use more than one dehumidifier, or acquire a dehumidifier that can be ducted.

- Follow manufacturer's directions for correct placement of the dehumidifier in your basement or crawl space.

- Use a thermo-hygrometer to measure the relative humidity (RH) separately from the dehumidifier.

- You do not have to dehumidify below-grade unfinished spaces in the heating season.

- Do not operate a dehumidifier until a moldy basement or crawl space has been remediated; otherwise, mold spores will be aerosolized by the machine's airflows.

- Check the coils on your dehumidifier and clean as needed; follow the manufacturer's directions.

- Empty the reservoir on your dehumidifier as frequently as is needed. Alternately, attach the machine to a condensate pump or position the machine so that it can drain into a sink or sump.

- Do not depend on an exhaust-fan-only "dehumidifier" to control the RH in your basement.

- Keep a sump pump low enough to prevent overflow from the sump during heavy rain, but don't keep the pump submerged below the water table.

- Keep a sump clean and cover it with a nonbiodegradable cover that fights tightly but that can also be easily removed.

LIFESTYLE CHOICES

- Avoid using your unfinished basement as if it were a living space.

- Never exercise in a musty unfinished basement.

- Don't let pets go down into a musty basement.

- Rugs and carpet remnants should not be placed directly on concrete.

- If you have a basement workshop, install some kind of ventilation system so that sawdust will be exhausted out of the space when you saw wood.

MOISTURE AND HUMIDITY

- Insulate cold-water pipes in humid areas to prevent sweating.

- Repair any pipe leaks.

- Maintain the RH in your unfinished basement and crawl space at no more than 50 percent.

ODORS

- If you notice a strong chemical or musty odor in a basement or crawl space, have the space professionally inspected.

- Research the history of the property to see if the house was ever treated for termites.

PESTS AND PETS

- Keep them out of unfinished basements and crawl spaces.

RADON

- Test your below-grade spaces for radon; follow US Environmental Protection Agency guidelines for testing.

- A licensed contractor should install a radon mitigation system.

STORED GOODS

- Store goods on non-wood pallets placed on concrete blocks. I always recommend using rolling metal shelves, however. Whatever option you choose, goods should be stored at least 18 inches to 2 feet away from foundation walls and up off the basement floor.

- As long as goods are dry, you can store smaller items in tightly lidded plastic boxes.

- Minimize the amount of goods you store in your basement.

- Seal clothing in plastic to protect it from mold growth, but only when the clothing is dry or when the RH is under 30 percent.

- Do not use a crawl space for storage.

WATER ENTRY

- Run a hose outside the foundation area where you suspect a water entry problem.

- Immediately discard cushioned or upholstered items such as sofas and mattresses that have been soaked.

- Use caution when drying out a flooded basement. If mold growth is present, fans can aerosolize spores.

- If you've had a major flood in your basement, confer with a remediation specialist about your options.

16. FINISHED BASEMENTS

In my indoor air quality investigations I have found that people with respiratory problems are much more likely to be living in houses with finished, carpeted rooms below grade. I hate to see people using such rooms because, as you will see from the stories that follow, most basements and other spaces below grade are not suited for use as playrooms, family rooms, exercise rooms, and bedrooms unless extraordinary steps are taken during construction and unless such spaces are scrupulously maintained while in use.

In this chapter I concentrate on the IAQ problems caused by finished, below-grade rooms. Even if your basement is finished, be sure to read chapter 15, because it contains information and suggestions relevant to all below-grade spaces.

LEAKS AND FLOODS

I have inspected numerous basement rooms in which water had penetrated walls and leaked under floors. In one potentially unhealthy situation, a physician called me after reading newspaper accounts of infant deaths in Cleveland, possibly caused by exposure to *Stachybotrys* mold. He and his wife had just brought their first baby home from the hospital, and he was worried about mold growth in his basement. They were renting, and when they first saw the home, they had inquired about stains on the finished basement walls. The landlord claimed the basement had flooded only once.

When I looked carefully around the finished basement, I could see signs that flooding had occurred several times, most likely from sewer backups. I also wondered if mold was growing inside the walls. Using an adapter that fit over an electrical outlet, I took a Burkard air sample directly from an outlet. The wall consisted of paneling over drywall, and by pushing on the panel, I forced air out from between the two layers. A cloud of white smoke appeared, which I assumed was drywall dust. But when I looked at that sample under the microscope, it consisted of tens of thousands of *Penicillium* mold spores. Though I did not find *Stachybotrys* mold, I still encouraged the family to move.

CARPETING

One young couple purchased a three-year-old house. After living there a few months, they decided to finish the basement. They installed walls, shelves, and carpeting and transformed the space into a family room, exercise room, and laundry area. That fall, during a heavy rain, a small amount of water leaked onto the floor from the bulkhead and soaked into a corner of the carpet under the treadmill. The wife, who was pregnant, went on maternity leave from her job in December. To keep fit, she set out on an exercise program in the basement. She subsequently experienced shortness of breath and was hospitalized; her doctors assumed that the pregnancy was causing her respiratory distress. She stopped exercising in the basement and started to feel better, but after the child was born, the woman renewed her basement exercise regimen. When she once more developed severe breathing difficulties as well as a dry cough, she was hospitalized again, and her doctors determined that her respiratory capacity was less than 70 percent of normal.

It became clear that her pregnancy had not been the cause of the condition. After she was diagnosed with hypersensitivity pneumonitis (HP), she called me. With a Burkard sampler, I found that the concentration of Pen/Asp (*Penicillium* and/or *Aspergillus*) spores was about 50,000 per cubic meter of air (I consider a concentration of 1,000 spores per cubic meter to be high). It was no surprise that I also found extensive mold growth in the basement carpet dust. I suggested the woman stay out of the basement until it could be thoroughly cleaned by a professional working under containment conditions (see chap. 23). I also recommended vinyl flooring. Within months, her respiratory capacity returned to 100 percent.

LEAKAGE UNDERNEATH

Another woman became an independent consultant and worked from her home. The family expanded office space on the first floor and moved the living room down into a lavishly renovated space in the basement. Three years later, after living and working in her home

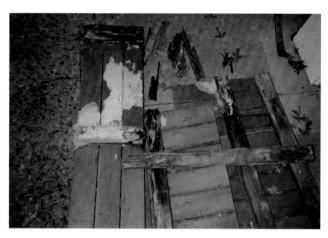

FIGURE 16.1. This decayed basement subfloor was only three years old. The back was covered with fungal growth. The white material is a mass of hyphae called the mycelium, which is the macrofungal "root structure" digesting the wood. Some of the wood sleepers were so rotted that they crumbled.
PHOTO BY STEVE GOSELIN OF ENVIROTECH (ENVIROVANTAGE SUBSIDIARY); USED WITH PERMISSION.

nearly twenty-four hours a day, seven days a week, the woman developed terrible, itchy rashes that were driving her crazy.

When I arrived, the first thing she did was point out some stains in the basement carpet. I did not expect to see stains, because she had described how the carpet was laid on a plank subfloor raised above the concrete. I checked the stains with my moisture meter, and indeed they were wet. At first I was suspicious of the family dog, but the regularity of the pattern suggested the moisture had another cause.

I recommended that she have a contractor lift some of the carpet and subfloor to determine the moisture source. After creating asbestos-level dust containment conditions in the basement, the contractor found water on the concrete and extensive macrofungal growth on the back of the plank subfloor. Apparently, rainwater had been leaking through cracks in the foundation and pooling on the masonry floor. Wood-decaying fungi (macrofungi; see chap. 2) had grown on the wood and between the planks, and moisture from the decaying wood had created the damp stain pattern (fig. 16.1).

The family ended up tearing out the entire floor because the bottom of the subfloor was completely rotten beneath the carpeting. After the flooring was up, workers noticed decay in the wall structure and began to remove that. In the end the entire finished basement was demolished only three years after it had been created and at a cost more than three times the expense of the original construction.

The extent of this particular problem might have been discovered sooner had there been access behind the walls and under the floor.

One couple I worked with bought a house with a long history of basement water problems. The seller had installed a sump pump and a drainage system under the floor to prevent basement flooding, but mold had already gotten a foothold. After living in their home for about three years, the new owners decided to spruce up the finished basement. They both worked many hours on the project, removing old carpeting and installing new vinyl flooring. They also moved their bedroom to a first-floor room adjacent to the basement stairway. They kept the door to the basement open because their children watched TV and played with their dog in the refurbished lower-level family room.

The wife began getting rashes on her face soon after the renovation was complete. At times her tongue swelled and her throat constricted. When I visited the home, I was impressed by the glistening new floor in the basement room. It was clear they had worked hard on the project. I was less impressed, however, by the film of mold on the lower two feet of all the paneled walls and the *Aspergillus* mold flourishing on many of the cellulose ceiling tiles.

The husband arrived after I had finished inspecting the basement and taking samples, and I felt it was important to explain to him all the problems I had observed. As he and I walked through the basement, he was quiet at first and avoided looking at me directly. The paneling was dark and the mold layer was not readily visible, so as I went around, I shone a bright flashlight obliquely across the surfaces, whereupon the colonies became quite obvious. I also pointed out white tufts of macrofungal growth (mycelium) protruding from the decorative ceiling beams. Little by little, he recognized the extent of the contamination.

Although I did not suggest removing the beautiful new flooring, which was preferable to wall-to-wall carpeting, my extensive list of recommendations included removing all the ceiling and wall materials, even the partitions and nonstructural wood. I suggested that they expose the ceiling structure and HEPA vacuum the exposed surfaces (including foundation walls, joists, and subfloor) to remove allergenic dust and then spray-paint the wood surfaces. The wires and pipes also had to be cleaned. The foundation walls could then be washed to eliminate loose material and coated with Thoroseal or painted. The tile as well as the masonry floor in the mechanical room could also then be cleaned. I was clear that this cleaning should be undertaken with asbestos-level containment measures to avoid contaminating habitable spaces with moldy dust. Until the remediation work was finished, I encouraged the family to stay out of the basement (and keep the dog out, too, for it could carry mold spores upstairs on its fur) and to keep the basement door tightly closed. After the basement was cleaned, I recommended eliminating all dust from the rest of the house with a HEPA vacuum and dehumidifying the basement to control the relative humidity (RH).

DROWNING AT HOME

Why do basements flood? Over the lifetime of every house, a flood will probably occur once or twice. External causes include a high water table, improper grading at the exterior, and natural disasters such as torrential rains or river flooding. Some of the more common internal sources of basement flooding are broken water heaters, frozen pipes that burst, and broken washing machine hoses. If your finished basement floods, immediately remove the wet carpeting and padding as well as any damp upholstered furniture, because it is almost impossible to dry these items in place before mold and bacteria start to grow. You may be able to save the carpeting by having it professionally cleaned, but cushioned furniture and carpet padding, once soaked, should go on the trash heap.

After you have cleaned up the obvious basement water, don't forget about the most important potential source of home contamination: the bottom of your forced hot-air furnace or basement air conditioning system. I cannot tell you how many blower cabinets I have looked into that were full of mold from water on the basement floor. In one such home, a young boy who had almost died from a bee sting was found in subsequent skin-prick testing to be sensitized to over 30 allergens, probably including some of the fungi growing in the bottom of his family's neglected furnace blower cabinet.

In another home with a finished basement that had floor water and dampness owing to poor drainage, my footsteps squished on the carpet, leaving shoe-shaped puddles as I walked. Fiberglass insulation in the walls was still wet weeks after the last heavy rain. To a height of about three feet, the back of the basement drywall was black with *Stachybotrys* mold that was crawling with mites. I even found *Stachybotrys* spores blowing out of the hot-air register on the first floor. Stains on the paper frame of the fiberglass furnace filter suggested that it too had been partially under water.

Sadly, the return air for the heating system came from the moldy basement family room. Both the parents and the children suffered from asthma as well as chronic sinus and respiratory problems. The mother was so ill and frustrated that she was prepared to tear the house down; they were even concerned about using the same foundation. They had the basement professionally remediated (see chap. 23), but they also moved to a new house. During catastrophic floods, government agencies, the Red Cross, and other trained professionals step in to help the displaced. But such organizations and professionals won't help you when you are the victim of a basement flood in your own home, even though the health consequences can be dire.

DON'T DO IT YOURSELF

I've worked with many people who took it upon themselves to remove sodden carpeting and moldy drywall and done so without wearing personal protection or isolating the area from the rest of their homes. As a consequence, they spread allergenic dust and exposed themselves to mold spores. Even if the basement flood was minor, be cautious about creating airflows that could aerosolize spores that are in another area of your basement. In one finished basement laundry room, the washing machine hose leaked. The homeowner mopped up the water and set some fans in place to circulate air so that any wall surfaces that were dampened could dry faster. Unfortunately, the airflow from the fans aerosolized spores from nearly invisible mold growth on the ceiling—growth that had been present before the washing machine hose leaked. In trying to solve a minor problem, the man created a major exposure to mold spores.

Don't wait too long to figure out what needs to be done. Mold can take root within twenty-four to forty-eight hours if conditions are conducive to its growth. And bacteria concentrations can increase dramatically within hours. Have an IAQ professional or a remediation/ restoration professional assess the situation as soon as possible.

CONDENSATION

Even in the absence of leaks and floods, it's still risky to lay carpet directly on concrete, whether in a basement or on the first floor of a home built on a slab, since moisture condenses on the slab whenever the surface temperature is below the dew point. I prefer to see resilient or ceramic tile on the floors of finished basement rooms. If homeowners insist on basement carpeting, I generally recommend covering the concrete with at least one-inch-thick XPS (extruded polystyrene) sheet foam insulation with a wood-sleeper grid on top of the insulation. The plywood would be nailed to the grid, and pad and carpeting installed on top of the plywood. (I do not recommend installing a raised subfloor because mold, moisture, and pest problems can develop in the space between the finished floor and the concrete.)

Moisture can also condense on masonry walls as well as on floors, because these are always cooler than room air. One broker felt lucky to list a lovely garden-level studio apartment. The unit had more light than one would expect from a basement unit. In one end wall, sliding glass doors opened to an inviting private patio. The apartment floors were flagstone, and the owner had plants hung everywhere, inside and out. The ambience was very appealing.

When the broker walked around the unit, she noticed that the edges of the floor along the walls were damp. She looked closely at the walls, which had been left in their original "fieldstone" condition, and she saw a sheen of moisture all along the surfaces. The only way to prevent this situation was either to dehumidify or air condition the unit to minimize moisture buildup. In both cases the windows would have to be kept closed.

One of my clients neglected to take these precautions. To surprise his wife, he built a basement studio for her craft business. The room had shelves for storage and counters for work space, and she spent many productive hours there. Unfortunately, the room was not adequately dehumidified or heated, and mold grew on all the walls. She probably developed her sinus condition from exposure to the many mold spores in the air (one study found that over 90 percent of sinus infections involve the immune system's response to fungi).[1] I recommended that the couple eliminate the room.

The likelihood of condensation is high in a small, cool space, particularly if at least one wall is masonry. One woman had a chronic cough, and when I inspected her home, I found wall-to-wall closets in a finished basement room. The back wall of every closet was the masonry foundation. Moisture was condensing on the wall, and mold was spreading to the goods stored in the closets. I suspected that the woman coughed whenever she wore contaminated clothing.

Another condensation problem led to legal action. I was asked to help defend a siding installer being sued by a customer who claimed the vinyl siding was responsible for the health problems that he and his daughter were experiencing. According to the owner, the contractor had removed all the wood siding on the house, exposing the wood plank sheathing to the weather. Before new vinyl siding could be installed, heavy rains soaked the sheathing. The customer claimed the insulation in the wall cavities had also gotten wet. He believed the contractor had covered the walls with vinyl siding before they'd had a chance to dry out. Within a month of the installation, the man's daughter had to move out of her basement bedroom because of asthma symptoms, and he himself began to experience more asthma symptoms and hoarseness. Within a few months he was barely able to speak and was fired from his job, which required a clear, audible voice. In addition to his health complaints, he stated that the contractor had done a poor job installing the siding.

When I read the man's deposition, I felt sympathetic, and I wondered if I would be able to support the contractor's position. When we arrived at the house, though, I thought perhaps it was the wrong property, because I could see none of the defects in the siding installation that the owner claimed were present. As I entered, I also noticed that his housekeeping was less than ideal. Cat food had been spilled in the kitchen, all the interior walls were yellow with nicotine stains, and there were piles of clothing and other possessions on the floors. The porch had water-stained unfinished drywall on the inside. Once thick but now flattened shag carpeting covered all the floors. The basement was damp, and all the basement walls and ceilings were covered with mold. I removed the cover from the blower cabinet of the antique furnace and took samples of the dust. I later found that this too was contaminated with growing mold.

After my visit, I seriously questioned that anything the installer could have done had caused the contamination I observed. It's possible that the nailing on the walls disturbed irritants already lurking inside the wall cavities, but it's doubtful that the single exposure of the building exterior to water could have produced the wretched indoor conditions I found. Only years of elevated relative humidity, condensation, and neglect could have created the "decor" in this partially finished basement.

INSULATION

I recommend using either foil-covered sheet foam insulation or XPS sheet foam insulation on foundation walls rather than using fiberglass batts between the studs, for two reasons. First, if a basement floods, fiberglass absorbs the water and can retain the moisture for months. The wooden framing and the back of the drywall can get damp, and mold can proliferate. Solving this problem requires removing the wet insulation and replacing the lower portion of the drywall. Second, when fiberglass insulation is placed between the studs of the wood framing, a cold space is left between the backside of the finished wall and the interior side of the foundation wall. Moisture can condense in this space, encouraging fungal growth on dust and on the wood framing.

Sheet foam insulation should be flush against the foundation wall. The side of the insulation facing inward will be near the temperature of the heated, finished room (assuming no second layer of fiberglass insulation is placed up against the studs behind the finished walls), so condensation will be at a minimum. In addition, sheet foam insulation does not absorb much moisture if there is a basement flood, and the area between the finished wall and the foundation wall will dry out faster. A word of caution: the foam insulation should not rise to the top of the foundation wall. An inch or two of the concrete should be left visible for termite inspection. No debris should be left between the finished wall and the foundation wall.

Some people consider installing SPF (spray polyurethane foam) insulation in their basements. We discuss this kind of insulation in chapter 22.

RADIATIONAL COOLING

The joint where the masonry floor and wall meet is always the coolest part of a basement room, because cold air sinks and because any object near a colder surface loses heat to that surface through radiation. Similarly, if you were to stand in front of a block of ice, heat would radiate from your body and be absorbed by the ice. The opposite occurs if you stand near a fireplace. The side of your body facing the fire feels warm because your body is cooler than the flame and thus absorbs some of the heat.

If two cold surfaces meet (such as the masonry floor and wall), the heat loss from an object near those surfaces is greater than if the object were facing only one cold surface. An object in the corner where two walls meet the floor is now facing three cold surfaces so thus will lose more heat than if the object were next to two cold surfaces. For this reason, temperatures at the outside corners of the foundation wall are usually the lowest, and the RH is the highest. In a finished basement, insulated walls are cooled by heat loss from the walls' "exterior" sides to the cooler foundation (except where sheet foam insulation is placed against the foundation wall).

Think of the space in which the wall meets the floor as the "joint zone." Within that colder area there is higher RH and thus an increased chance of microbial growth. If carpet contains nutrient dust, these conditions are conducive to almost year-round mold growth and microarthropod activity. If you look around a carpeted basement room, you will usually see spider webs in the joint zone.

If you want to have carpet in a basement room (which I discourage in principle), I recommend either using area rugs or bordering a larger carpet with up to eighteen inches of resilient or ceramic tile. With a smooth surface in the joint zone, you can wipe up any moisture that may condense and eliminate settled dust more easily.

Heat sources (heat registers, baseboard convectors) are more difficult to keep clean than tiled surfaces, so heat sources placed in a joint zone can become homes for microbial growth. In two split-level

As air cools, its relative humidity (RH) rises. When the RH is above 80 percent, a number of microfungal species can flourish.

homes with carpeted, finished below-grade rooms, I removed dust samples from the bottoms of the clogged fin tubing of the baseboard heating convectors and in both cases found that the dust consisted of almost 30 percent *Aspergillus*, *Penicillium*, and *Cladosporium* micro-fungal growth. One owner had a chronic cough; the other had respiratory distress. In both cases I found elevated levels of spores in the air in the finished lower levels. In another house, where the owner was sensitized to molds and suffered from chronic fatigue syndrome, I found *Penicillium* mold growing in the dust on a hot-air register in the joint zone of a basement room. To avoid mold growth on heat sources, the heat emitters must be kept free of all dust (see chap. 24).

In general, the RH should be below 60 percent all year round in finished below-grade spaces. To control the RH, finished basement rooms must be dehumidified (or air conditioned) in the summer and heated consistently throughout the colder months. If you air condition your finished basement, add dehumidification as needed. In a finished basement, the winter temperature should be the same as the temperature in your upstairs rooms, but not less than 60°F (so air in cooler corners won't develop high RH conditions).

Too often, people heat finished basement rooms only when they use the spaces. At other times, the rooms will cool and the relative humidity will rise, leading to mold growth.

PEST ODORS

The owners of a split-level house were concerned about a mold-like odor in the carpeted family room on the lower level. Because the house was built on a slope, the front wall of the lower-level room was partially below grade, but the rear was at grade level with a door to the exterior (called "walk out to grade"). The wife was a tutor and spent hours in the room each day working with her students. Both she and her husband were worried that the odor might impair her livelihood as well as their health. They had already gone to considerable expense to replace the boiler and install a chimney liner in the mechanical room adjacent to the family room, in the mistaken notion that these steps would remove the odor.

I found that someone had installed a concrete patio at the rear exterior wall, completely covering the untreated wooden sill that supported the wall. Untreated wood should never be buried in concrete, because excess moisture from the ground will always lead to macro-fungal decay (and to insects and other pests). In this case I could see a piece of the decayed sill at the lowest edge of the siding where some wood from a shingle was missing. The sill had been gnawed, probably by a rodent nesting there. I was never able to locate the exact source of the odor, but the carpenter who repaired the sill found that a rodent had chewed through the softened wood and gotten into the contiguous interior wall (perpendicular to the exterior wall) between the bathroom and the family room. The couple practically had to abandon the house while the fiberglass insulation from the rodent's nest was removed. Once the tufts of urine-soaked, moldy fiberglass were gone and the wall was repaired, the odor disappeared.

FINISHED PLAY SPACES

When children sit on contaminated furniture or play on moldy basement carpets, they disturb the allergenic dust and not only inhale the dust but also carry it on their clothing to other parts of the house. I have looked at many homes where children had trouble breathing when they were playing on basement carpets full of mold and mites.

In one home, a friend of the owner's daughter experienced asthma symptoms as soon as she entered the house. A couch in the finished basement contained more than 200 micrograms per gram of dust mite allergens. (More than 10 micrograms per gram is considered a risk for asthma.) When the couch was used, which was frequently, particulates rose from the cushions and even went up into the rest of the house with air flowing up through the open basement door.

Other pieces of furniture can also cause problems in basement play spaces, because surfaces close to the foundation wall tend to acquire mold growth. In one finished basement room, I was surprised to see mold growing at the front of a bookshelf rather than at the back, which was facing the exterior wall. I asked the owner, who had children with asthma, whether the bookshelf had ever been stored in an unfinished basement space. She told me that in her old house she had stored the shelf empty, pushed up against the foundation wall with the open shelves facing the masonry. In a semi-finished basement in another home, I found a couch covered with *Aspergillus* mold growth. I hope that no one, including children, had ever sat on that couch! The couch was so moldy that it couldn't be adequately cleaned, so I recommended that it be discarded (fig. 16.2).

If your child has asthma or allergies, I cannot urge strongly enough that you avoid creating finished, below-grade spaces in general and below-grade play spaces in particular. And since people can become sensitized to allergens, I recommend that children not spend extended time in finished basement spaces that are musty.

ARE WE MEANT TO LIVE BELOW GRADE?

If I could, I would encourage most homeowners to have finished basement rooms professionally dismantled. I would give a resounding

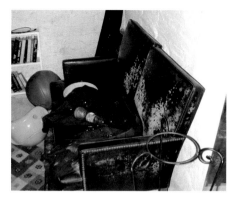

FIGURE 16.2. This moldy couch was in a basement play area. The relative humidity was not controlled, and *Aspergillus* mold grew on the couch. Mold-eating mites grazed on the mold spores, leaving allergenic fecal pellets on the leather. One child in the family had asthma symptoms and mold allergy.

"no" to adding finished rooms to a basement. I would tell occupants with allergies or asthma to move out of basement apartments.

If you have a finished basement already, I hope the suggestions in this chapter will help you minimize potential contamination. Just remember that nature is a powerful force. Life, even if it is microscopic, will prevail if nutrients and water are present.

SOME RECOMMENDATIONS

CARPETS

- Don't use carpeting in a basement space. If you insist on having carpet, lay it on a raised plywood subfloor rather than directly on the concrete, and install resilient vinyl or ceramic tile in the "joint zone."

- Area rugs are preferable to wall-to-wall carpeting, but it's best to lay them on tile or linoleum rather than directly on the concrete. Area rugs that rest on concrete must be periodically cleaned or thrown away.

CLEANING AND REMEDIATION

- If your basement has ever had a major flood, smells musty, or appears to have mold growth, don't try to clean up the area yourself. Seek advice from an indoor air quality professional. In the case of a flood, don't wait too long to figure out "next steps." Even two or three days can be too long.

- If possible, have flooded rugs and carpets professionally cleaned and dried off-site.

- Basement carpets or rugs that have gotten wet even once should be discarded if the water contained sewage, or if they smell or cannot be dried out within hours.

- If your heating or cooling equipment was in the flooded area, have the equipment checked by a professional technician. You may have to have the furnace or air handler and even some ducts cleaned.

CONDITIONING AND HEATING THE AIR

- Dehumidify finished, below-grade spaces and maintain the relative humidity (RH) at no more than 60 percent. If you depend on air conditioning, add dehumidification as needed.
- Using a thermo-hygrometer, measure the RH separately from the dehumidifier.
- Heat a finished basement consistently throughout the colder months.
- Keep registers and baseboard heating convectors free of dust.
- Baseboard heat is better than hot-air heat for all spaces, but particularly for basements.

FINISHING A BASEMENT

- If you have a raised floor in a basement room, install an access panel so that you can keep an eye on conditions beneath the subfloor.
- If you are determined to finish your basement, divide the basement into as few rooms as possible, don't add built-in benches that face the foundation, and install louvered doors on closets to facilitate the flow of heated and dehumidified air.
- Avoid using fiberglass insulation below grade.
- Refer to the resource guide for information on Building Science Corporation, which offers more advice on finished basements.

FURNITURE

- Leave at least three inches of space between furniture and finished walls.
- Use furniture with legs so that you can clean under such pieces.
- Use a leather- or vinyl-covered couch or a futon with a mattress encased with a dust mite cover.

ODORS

- If there are animal odors in the basement, you may have to remove soiled building materials.
- If a musty odor is present, even if you smell it intermittently, the basement probably contains mold growth.

- Don't let children play in moldy basements, whether the spaces are finished or unfinished. Adults should also avoid spending prolonged time there.

- If you have allergies or asthma, don't live in a below-grade space or in houses with finished basement rooms.

- Don't exercise in a musty below-grade space.

- Avoid spending long periods of time in a moldy basement.

17.

ATTICS

Your attic is part of your house. Although most of the airflow moves from habitable spaces into the attic, there are ways for allergens to reenter the house from the attic, so I encourage you to keep the attic as clean and dust-free as possible.

When you buy a new home, it's important that your home inspector go into the attic (if it's safely accessible) to inspect the insulation, ventilation, and roof sheathing and to check any attic mechanical equipment. Attics can sometimes hold deadly secrets. I recently heard about a case in which the inspector did not tell the prospective buyer there was soot on the attic rafters and sheathing, suggesting an earlier fire or puff-back in the house. The extensive damage had been concealed by repairs in the finished areas of the house. The family moved in and suffered from odors and residues of the chemicals that had been used for cleaning. The house was so toxic that ultimately it was destroyed.

SAFETY CONCERNS

I often find hazardous structural conditions in attics. While such conditions are not usually an IAQ concern, they are too important to omit from this book.

PULL-DOWN STAIRS

Pull-down attic stairs can be dangerous and, if installed improperly, can even fall out of the ceiling. Sometimes, the lever arms holding the springs are bent, so the springs can fall off and injure anyone going up the stairs. If you have a pull-down attic stairway, I recommend adding guardrails in the attic around the opening so that a misstep won't end in a tumble. Any permanent attic stairs should have a handrail.

A couple purchased an older home with wall-to-wall carpeting. The woman had asthma and was allergic to cats—far more so than she had ever realized. After she and her husband moved into the house, her asthma symptoms became so severe that she was hospitalized. While she was in the hospital, the man had the carpeting in the house removed in case the carpeting contained allergens. Before she was discharged, the woman was given an epinephrine injection pen to take home. Within twenty-four hours of returning home, the wife began struggling to breathe and went into anaphylactic shock. Her husband saved her life by carrying her outside and administering the epinephrine.

They asked me how they could make the house safe for her. When I visited, air conditioning was being installed, including an air-handling unit (AHU) in the attic, which lacked flooring and had old, loose fibrous insulation between the joists. The air conditioning technicians were carelessly storing the ducts and other components on the joists, and the equipment, including the new ducts, was dusted with loose insulation. There were even clumps of insulation inside the yet-to-be connected ducts.

I suspected that the old insulation might contain cat dander particles. In addition to recommending that the insulation be removed from between the attic floor joists (under containment conditions), I told the couple to have the floor structure HEPA vacuumed and lightly spray-painted. The new, unused air conditioning equipment and ducts also had to be cleaned. They had the attic reinsulated with fiberglass batts. After these steps were taken, that typical dusty "old house smell" disappeared entirely from the second floor. (Old insulation, filled as it often is with years of dust, dead mice, and insects, may cause the unpleasant odor characteristic of the upper levels and attics of many older homes.)

The couple also eliminated all the old house dust from the basement and living spaces, and the wife lived in the house symptom-free. Lastly, I strongly recommended that they install flooring for safer inspections of the attic in general and the mechanical equipment in particular. It's dangerous to walk on attic floor joists, because a person could trip and fall through the ceiling below. That is why I think that all attics should have some solid flooring or secured planks. At the least, there should be safe access to attic mechanical equipment.

ATTIC INVASIONS

MICE

Fiberglass insulation in attic floors is often littered with mouse droppings (see chap. 5). Although the attic may seem hot and inhospitable to us, it's relatively cooler near the ceiling of the level below, where mice burrow below the surface of the insulation and make nests. In some attics there are hundreds of finger-shaped indented burrows in the insulation. Dried mouse urine is allergenic as well as smelly, but add a mouse carcass or two, and an attic infested with mice can become really malodorous (fig. 17.1).

My in-laws lived in an old farmhouse in a rural area of New England. When Connie was growing up, there were more mice than people in the house. The house was clean, but dozens of flies were always buzzing around inside. In the winter, my father-in-law would turn the heat down in some of the unused bedrooms, and the flies would lie dormant, concealed in the window tracks. When he turned the heat on in these rooms, the insects would come alive and buzz against the glass. The fly infestation was so widespread that we sometimes found flies wedged inside the layers of folded sheets and towels in the linen closet.

I think their attic must have been the insects' breeding ground, because it was always alive with hundreds of flies. The attic was also home to generations of mice, and the flies were probably laying their eggs in mouse carcasses, which then fed the maggots. How did the mice get into the attic? The house had an attached barn, and there were openings between the upper level of the barn and the attic—openings that were rodent highways. I encouraged my in-laws to reduce the fly population by getting rid of the old insulation where the mice lived and to seal the openings between the attic and the barn.

I don't think they followed my advice, though, because they thought that mice and flies were just part of country living.

Mouse infestations can be associated with mold growth, mites, or mouse fecal material containing microbiological hazards, such as hantavirus.

"Hantavirus," Centers for Disease Control and Prevention, US Department of Health and Human Services, last updated January 31, 2019, https://www.cdc.gov/hantavirus/index.html.

SOFFIT ROACHES

Carpenter ants can nest in soffits (an overhang off the attic) where trim wood is damp from an overflowing gutter or from frequent roof-water flows. Insect pests prefer constant warmth and humidity. One entomologist I know studied cockroach nesting and feeding behavior and found that roaches live in soffits. He also discovered that when the soffits are ventilated, temperature and humidity fluctuate too much for cockroaches, so they nest elsewhere. In one experiment, soffits at both sides of a house were infested with roaches. The entomologist installed soffit vents at one side, and before long

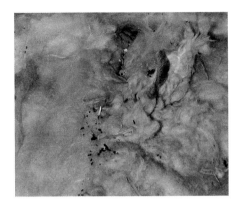

FIGURE 17.1. Mice love to nest in fiberglass insulation, whether the insulation is pink or yellow. This insulation was installed in an attic floor. There are various bits of mouse detritus in front of the slightly gray opening to the mouse burrow.

the roaches abandoned the ventilated side and moved to the more humid, unventilated side.

The presence of carpenter ants signals excessive moisture, but a cockroach infestation can cause asthma. Installing soffit vents makes the attic less hospitable to insects and is thus a step toward a healthier house.

THE FOOD CHAIN

Where there is life, there are predators. In the attic of a house in the woods, I found thousands of larval cases stuck to the rafters and sheathing. Apparently, some type of moth larvae had pupated in the attic, and numerous spiders had set up shop to take advantage of the vast food supply. Spiderwebs hung all around, and beneath each web the wood floor planks were spattered with spider droppings. Wearing a Tyvek protective suit and a respirator, I managed to scrape up about an eighth of a teaspoon of spider droppings. I sent them off to an allergist, who was going to test them against the blood serum of a few of his patients to see if their blood reacted to the proteins in the spider fecal material, suggesting allergy. Unfortunately, my precious sample was lost, but I remain convinced that these droppings cause allergy symptoms (fig. 17.2).

LARGER PREDATORS

Some of the animals that move into attics are larger. I heard about one family who purchased a home that had been abandoned for many years. They spent a great deal of money renovating the interior, but they never investigated their inaccessible attic. After all the work was done, they came home one day and found that the second-floor ceiling in the master bedroom under the attic had collapsed under the weight of raccoon droppings.

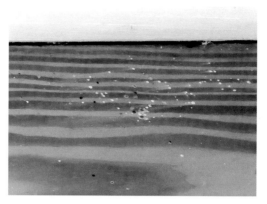

FIGURE 17.2. Some of the spider droppings on this wood floor are just white, and others are white with a dark bull's-eye at the center. This appearance is typical of spider droppings. The droppings form as a mushy liquid that quickly dries and hardens after hitting the floor, where the droppings stick tenaciously to the wood. The droppings must be scrubbed vigorously to be removed.

In an older building with a flat roof, I was inspecting a top-floor apartment for a buyer and didn't think there would be access to the "attic" crawl space. Above the kitchen table, though, was a square hatch. I stood on a ladder, opened the hatch, looked in, and faced a squirrel nest that consisted of several sections of a newspaper shredded and piled up between the ceiling joists. Running through the paper was an electric cable for the kitchen light fixture. The cable had been chewed entirely bare of insulation for about two feet. Littered around the access hole were metal pots and pans that a previous tenant had thrown into the attic for storage. Had one of those pans landed on the bare wires when current was flowing, it would have created a short circuit, igniting the newspaper, and possibly burning the house down. The only good thing that can be said of squirrels living in attics is that, unlike raccoons, they leave all their droppings outside.

Bats also live in attics. One home inspector ended up paying for a new ceiling. When inspecting the attic, he was "buzzed" by a bat. He ducked, lost his footing, slipped off the ceiling joists (the attic had no flooring), and fell through the plaster ceiling. Luckily, he caught himself on a joist before he fell into the room below.

Birds can move into attics. On one site visit to a 100-year-old home, I had inspected the entire house except for the attic eaves. I opened the eaves access door and stepped in. My client, the prospective buyer of the property, followed me, and because there was no flooring, I cautioned him to be careful where he stepped. One misstep and one of us could fall through the ceiling to the bedroom below. As we walked along the joists, our shoes made loud crunching noises. I looked down at what appeared to be white insulation and suddenly realized I was looking at feathers instead of fiberglass. My buyer, who was Spanish, exclaimed, *Caca de pajaro!* "Bird droppings!" He turned around and, stepping as fast as he could on the joists, exited through the access door and raced out of the house. The family who had lived there for decades had apparently not taken good care of the property. The attic window had fallen out, and generations of pigeons had flown in to roost.

Pigeon droppings (guano) may contain *Histoplasma capsulatum*, a parasitic fungus that can cause mild to serious respiratory infections.[1] The droppings contain spores that become airborne when the guano is disturbed. Great caution should be exercised when such spaces are cleaned, because inhaling large amounts of this dust can cause the illness called histoplasmosis.[2] If you have pigeon guano in your attic and are concerned, have a microbiology lab test for *Histoplasma capsulatum*.

A ROOF OVER MY HEAD

One of my clients had a long-term roof leak, and the water ran down two stories through a wall cavity and soaked her living room wall. She discovered the leak when she removed a picture and found the wallpaper black with mold. I subsequently found the growth to be a species of *Stachybotrys* mold, which is sometimes referred to as "toxic black mold" and which grows on wet cellulose.

We've seen over and over what moisture can do to our living spaces, and naturally the main function of a roof is to keep rainwater out. Most single- and two-family homes have gable roofs, and the top layer that faces the weather is most often covered with asphalt shingles. These shingles are fastened to wood roof sheathing that is nailed to the attic rafters. The sheathing consists of either wooden planks (typical in older homes), oriented strand board (OSB), or plywood.

As they age, roofing shingles weather, crack, and can leak. Water can also leak around chimney and pipe penetrations. This moisture can fuel macrofungal decay of the sheathing and rafters. Sometimes, water will run down a rafter and into a wall, possibly leading to macrofungal decay as well as microfungal growth (see chap. 2). To minimize the chance of such problems, a home occupant should check the attic for leaks during a heavy rain.

If you put on new roofing, keep in mind that a great deal of dust from the sheathing and rafters may be released. If the sheathing is covered with mold (and it often is in newer homes with plywood or OSB sheathing, discussed below), the dust will contain extensive amounts of spores. In normal circumstances the mold on attic sheathing does not become airborne and is generally not an IAQ problem in the rooms below, because air from the house flows into the attic and out the roof rather than vice versa. If there is an air conditioning unit or furnace in the attic, though, be sure that it is protected from the dust while the roof work is ongoing. Remove or cover any goods stored in the attic. And last, if you or anyone in your family has allergies or asthma, stay out of the house during the disturbance, since some dust may find its way into the living areas. It's a good idea to clean surfaces in rooms under the attic after the roof has been replaced.

VENTILATION

If you walk on the roof of a poorly ventilated attic that has had excessive moisture or leaks and the sheathing is decayed, you might fall through the roof.

In older homes the sheathing consists of narrow wooden planks that were installed horizontally with gaps between them. These gaps allow air to escape from the attic at the gable ends of the planks. In newer homes the roof sheathing consists of four-by-eight-foot sheets of plywood or OSB that act as barriers to the flow of air and vapors. The buildup of moisture can cause condensation on the sheathing, leading to extensive growth of mold and even delamination of plywood.

To provide attic ventilation, newer homes usually have soffit vents and a ridge vent at the top (ridge) of the roof. In theory, warmer attic air rises owing to convection and exits the ridge vent, and outdoor air is drawn into the attic through the soffit vents. Unfortunately, theory isn't always proved true in practice. First, wind direction can thwart the intended airflows. Using smoke tube testing, I have observed air exiting instead of entering soffit vents. In addition, some attics, even though they have ridge and soffit vents, are extremely hot in the summer. I believe many of the newer ridge vents just don't permit enough airflow to let the hot air out of the attic.

When ridge vents first became available, they were manufactured with baffles, a strip of metal bent upward at each side of the vent. These baffles helped reduce the air pressure when the wind blew over the vent and thus increased the flow of air out of the attic. Some people thought vents with baffles were unsightly, so the baffles were eliminated. In my view, this drastically reduced the efficiency of ridge vents. In addition, to be effective at all, ridge vents must be installed over a sheathing gap so that air can move from the attic to the outside. In older homes that have new roofing, I have often found that roofers neglected to cut away the sheathing at the roof peak beneath the ridge vent. Though the roofers had encouraged the owners to add this new feature, they might as well have left it off, for there was no gap underneath. If you pay a roofer to install a ridge vent, be sure someone cuts away enough of the sheathing beneath the vent to allow for airflow.

A similar shortcut is sometimes attempted when soffit vents are installed, as the following story illustrates. A family purchased a large home in an expensive community near Boston. They had a thorough home inspection done by a member of the American Society of Home Inspectors (ASHI) who was referred by their attorney. The ASHI inspector identified many defects, some of which the sellers refused to recognize. The broker recommended another inspector, whose role was to mollify the buyer and the seller with a second opinion. Without even entering the attic, this inspector pronounced the ventilation adequate. I was then asked to provide yet another "second opinion."

The soffit ventilation consisted of continuous strips of louvered aluminum about two inches wide. These would have been adequate except for one thing I observed when I climbed a ladder and looked closely at the soffits. No one had bothered to cut out a strip of wood behind the metal louvers. There were only a few one-inch circular holes, barely enough to provide any soffit ventilation at all.

Continuous soffit vents can provide adequate ventilation, but the wood behind them must be cut away to allow for airflow. I do not recommend installing small circular soffit vents, since they have minimal open space. In addition, more often than not, the first time that the exterior trim on a home is painted, the circular vents are painted over and become completely useless. Also, for any type of soffit vent to operate properly, the spaces above these vents should not be blocked by attic insulation.

At another property, excess attic ventilation rather than inadequate attic ventilation turned out to be an insidious culprit that nearly drove the owner mad. The first time I spoke with the man, I wondered if he was imagining things. He told me he hadn't slept for a week because vibrations in his right lung were keeping him awake at night. I was about to say I couldn't help him when I realized I was committing what I consider a professional sin: doubting the client. I decided I owed him at least a house visit, and we made an appointment.

As soon as I entered his home, the man dragged me frantically from room to room, asking questions about fiberglass and furnishings. Was the furnace too close to the wall? Could paint fumes offgassing from the walls in the newly built home be causing his problem? I kept reminding myself, "The client is right; the client is right."

Finally, he unwound a little and I was able to ask him some questions. I discovered he had been living there only a month, and for the first three weeks he had slept peacefully. What had changed in that last week? Contractors had installed a new floor in the attic just before his insomnia began. He led me to the attic, and there I saw the beautiful new tongue-and-groove flooring. As he walked about and I stood motionless near the stairway, I could feel the vibrations from each footstep. I suddenly realized that adding the flooring had stiffened the attic floor structure, making it respond to pressure the way a diving board reacts after the diver jumps up and down. The floor was behaving like a damped harmonic oscillator: the energy in each footstep bounced the floor, causing vibrations that then diminished rapidly in strength.

The large master bedroom where the man slept was directly beneath the new attic floor. Nailed to the attic floor joists at the top was the new floor, and at the bottom was the bedroom drywall ceiling. As the attic floor vibrated, so did the attached ceiling, which in consequence compressed and expanded the air in his bedroom, changing the air pressure within the room. For some strange reason the man was able to detect these pressure changes, but only in his right lung. I tested my theory by gently bouncing up and down in the attic while the man lay on his bed beneath. About 70 percent of the time he could feel the vibrations as I moved. I decided he wasn't crazy after all.

What was making the floor vibrate? The attic was so well ventilated that when the wind blew outside, it changed the interior pressure in the attic. When the attic air pressure was greater than the air pressure in the bedroom below, the floor was pushed down. When the attic air pressure was less, the floor was pushed up. In both cases the floor movement caused vibrations that were transmitted to the air in the bedroom. Before the new flooring was added, the attic structure had not been stiff enough to vibrate in this way.

I told the man he could hire an acoustical engineer, but I recommended that he first see if putting weight in the middle of the attic floor would diminish the oscillations. Since he had just moved in, all his books were still in boxes. He carried these to the attic and piled them right above his bedroom. After that he slept like a baby.

MOLD ON SHEATHING

One family called me because of chronic moisture in the attic. The sheathing on the north-facing side of the gable roof was covered with black mold, and in the middle of the winter, icicles were hanging and water was dripping from the exposed roofing-nail ends. Why was this happening? I found a large opening in the return duct in the basement, which meant much of the supply air for the hot-air furnace came from the basement rather than from the first-floor return. This reduced the pressure in the basement and drew in cold exterior air through a leaky basement door leading to the outside. The upstairs of the home was being excessively pressurized, since more air was being supplied to the spaces than was being removed by the first-floor return. A humidifier on the furnace evaporated almost a half a gallon of water into the supply air for every hour the furnace operated. Warm, moist air was being forced into the cold attic from the pressurized house through openings at the pull-down stairs, ceiling fixtures, and probably other obscure framing gaps, and the moisture was condensing on the cooler surfaces. This was the cause of the attic rain.

PREVENT ATTIC MOISTURE

Mold growth can occur if moist house air migrates up into an attic, even if the attic is well ventilated. In hot weather this moisture evaporates; in cool weather the moisture condenses on cold sheathing, leading to mold growth. In New England where I live, the mold growth is usually heaviest on the north- or northeast-facing side, as well as in locations where bathroom exhausts are vented into the attic or soffit.

Let's examine some of the ways that moist house air can flow up into an attic.

THE BATHROOM EXHAUST

On one cold day I used a nontoxic smoke pencil to track airflows from a bathroom exhaust vented directly into the attic near the soffit. While I was in the attic, the homeowner directed the smoke into the ceiling exhaust grille while the fan was off. Since the house air was warmer than the attic air, smoke was drawn into the grille by convection. The smoke flowed into the attic rafter bay directly above the exhaust. The sun was shining on the roof, so there was convection in the rafter bay that moved the air and smoke up toward the ridge vent at the peak of the gable roof. Because there was very little airflow out of the ridge vent, the roiling cloud of smoke struck the ridge pole and dropped down toward the attic floor, proving that the moist house air was entering the attic and not being vented properly. As a consequence, the sheathing was covered with mold.

OPENINGS AND GAPS

Seal openings around the chimney and pipes with tightly packed fiberglass, and construct or purchase a sheet foam box large enough to fight tightly over the attic pull-down stairs.

WHOLE-HOUSE FANS

Hot air can rise from the house into the attic through the louvers of a whole-house fan. This type of fan is normally installed in the second-floor ceiling of a two-story home, with louvers that open with the airflow only when the fan is turned on. A whole-house fan removes 5,000 to 10,000 cubic feet of air per minute from the habitable part of a house and blows it into the attic. From there, the air moves outside through the attic vents (gable-end louvers, soffit vents, or ridge vents). When a whole-house fan is working properly, all the air in a typical-sized house is replaced every three to six minutes. But a whole-house fan can be effective only if air can flow out of the attic and fresh replacement air can flow into the house. That is why it is important to keep windows open when operating a whole-house fan.

One man told me about an experience he had one winter evening when he came home from work. As he approached his home, he noticed black smoke pouring out of his attic gable-end louver vents. A fire truck was ahead of him on its way to the house. All the rooms were full of black smoke. One of his children had accidentally turned on the whole-house fan when all the windows in the house were closed. This reduced the air pressure in the house, causing backdrafting at the oil-fired boiler. As a result, the family faced a costly soot cleanup. Backdrafting can also pull carbon monoxide (CO) into a home from a chimney flue. If you have a whole-house fan, I recommend installing a kill switch in the attic so the fan can't be turned on during the winter. In the summer, always be sure enough windows are open when you operate the fan.

In another home the husband was experiencing allergies related to mold. The finished basement had repeatedly been wet, and the carpeting was contaminated with mold. The owners were planning to eliminate the carpeting and were keeping the basement door closed until they could do so. In the meantime they used their whole-house fan all summer. I was in the house during the fall and the fan was not on, so I asked the woman to set up the house as she normally did in the summer, then turn on the fan. At the second floor they kept one window in every bedroom open, but they did not keep any windows open on the first floor. As soon as the whole-house fan turned on, the entire first floor smelled of mold. I did a smoke test at the one-inch gap beneath the basement door, and it was obvious that air was billowing from the moldy basement to the first floor when the fan was running.

These two examples illustrate why there must be a sufficient supply of fresh air in the habitable part of the house when a whole-house fan is operating. This next example shows why there must be enough ventilation in the attic to allow the fan to do its job. I looked at a house where the entire family suffered from allergies. The attic contained both a whole-house fan and an air conditioning unit. The family used the A/C only during the hottest summer days; the rest of the time they used the whole-house attic fan.

When it was working, the fan greatly increased the air pressure in the attic, which contained a leaky air-handling unit (AHU) for the air conditioning. Because the attic had inadequate ventilation, air was forced by the high air pressure into the leaky AHU and blew back into the living spaces through the duct system instead of blowing out of the house through the attic vents. The attic was full of allergenic dust that was aerosolized by the air agitation and then moved with airflows back into the rooms below. If you have a whole-house fan, check with the manufacturer of the fan to ensure you have adequate attic ventilation. Keep in mind that the unobstructed (free) area of a vent is always less than the area you see, because the opening area may be reduced by louvers and screens.

ICE DAMMING

In addition to supplying moisture for mold growth, an accumulation of warm air in the attic in the winter can lead to ice damming by melting the bottom layer of the snow piled on a gable roof. The melt-water runs (invisibly) down the roofing beneath the snowpack until it reaches the soffit, which is cold because it overhangs the exterior of the house. There the water freezes on top of the shingles near the edge of the roof and creates a dam of ice, allowing water to build up behind it. Roof shingles are designed to shed water from the surfaces but are not meant to be waterproof. Water building up behind an ice dam gets under the shingles and from there leaks onto the roof sheathing and rafters. (In winter, a thick layer of ice in a soffit can sometimes be seen from the attic.) In extreme cases, water from the soffit flows down behind the siding and icicles stick out of the exterior walls. You know you have an ice-damming problem if you see long icicles hanging from the edge of your roof or gutters (fig. 17.3).

All this ice eventually melts and can cause paint to peel. One ice dam can cause all the paint to peel off that side of the house. If water

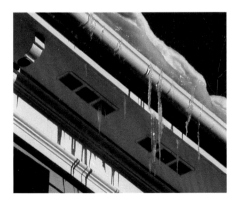

FIGURE 17.3. The roof in this photo was covered with snow. The edge of a thick layer of ice is just below the snow and above the wooden gutter. Water from the ice dam leaked under the roof shingles and into the soffit. Water from the soffit leaked from a soffit vent (the metal grille), where a slightly brown icicle formed.

If the space affected by ice damming contains visible mold growth or smells musty, you could aerosolize spores if you operate a fan to dry surfaces. Confer with an indoor air quality professional as soon as possible after ice damming has occurred.

enters insulated wall cavities and remains there long enough, micro-fungi can grow; if the dampness remains during warmer weather, the wood may even decay due to macrofungal growth. When an ice dam causes indoor leaks, be sure to dry out carpets, walls, or furniture to avoid more serious exposure to mold spores. (You may never have seen or have to worry about ice damming if you don't live in a cold climate.)

ATTIC MECHANICAL EQUIPMENT

Many newly constructed homes have AHUs in the attic or in attic eaves. Many of the problems with furnaces in basements will also occur when they are in the attic. Dust, attic air, or loose insulation fibers can enter the heating system through leaky return ducts. One arrangement that I have seen only twice but that seems particularly unsafe is a furnace humidifier in an attic system. If the attic is cold enough, the water supply pipe could freeze and break, flooding the entire house. Even if the pipe only leaks, the water can wet uncovered insulation, creating conditions conducive to mold growth. Never install a furnace humidifier in an attic.

Another problem common to both attic air conditioning and heating equipment is inaccessibility. It is difficult to service and repair equipment when the attic has no flooring. Sometimes the door to an attic is so small that the service company may not be able to use its best technician because the person is too large. If you have attic mechanical equipment, be certain there is ready access to the attic, that there is safe flooring all around any equipment that needs to be serviced, and that lighting is adequate. For families with allergies or asthma, attic equipment should preferably be isolated from the general attic space inside an insulated, ventilated, well-lit mechanical closet. This also makes it easier to maintain the equipment properly.

If you have air conditioning equipment in the attic, be sure there is an overflow tray with a float switch cutoff under the AHU. A secondary drain from the overflow tray isn't a bad idea, either, because if the condensate tray leaks, water will go into the overflow rather than onto the ceiling below. If you do have an overflow tray in your attic, check it during the air conditioning season to be sure the drain line is functioning and that no water is accumulating in the tray. On more than one inspection I have found attic overflow trays full of water and moldy debris.

One more caution: if the AHU for your air conditioner is in your attic, be sure there is adequate ventilation to keep the attic as cool as possible. The warmer the attic, the more energy it takes to cool the air within the duct system. It is more cost effective to ventilate an attic than to cool down heated air. An attic exhaust fan can be installed to increase ventilation. You wouldn't want to install such a fan in a humid climate, however, because you wouldn't want to bring in moist outdoor air into the attic. In addition, make sure that the attic floor is airtight so that cooled house air isn't exhausted.

A man with young children became concerned when the family's nanny began to feel respiratory distress a few weeks after moving into their air conditioned home. He found it curious that she was suddenly suffering from the same symptoms everyone in his family had been experiencing, and he called me to investigate. I found that the return system for the attic air conditioner's AHU consisted of a duct attached to the blower cabinet at one end and to the fabricated metal box at the other. The metal box sat on the attic floor, was partially buried in loose fibrous insulation, and was located directly above the return grille that held the filter. The grille was flush with the second-floor ceiling. I stood on a ladder on the second floor, opened the return grille, and removed the filter. Then I saw a one-inch gap between the metal box and the top of the filter holder. The seal between the box and holder should have been airtight, but because it was not, the air conditioning return was sucking attic air full of allergens and loose insulation fibers into the system, which was circulating the contaminated air throughout the house. After the family made the return airtight, installed a media filter, cleaned the ducts and AHU, and HEPA vacuumed all the rugs and carpeting, their symptoms decreased.

I investigated a similar case in which a retired couple had installed air conditioning three years before. The husband's allergies had seriously increased ever since. The AHU was in the attic. In this case the installer had never even bothered to put in a duct to the filter holder, which again was in the second-floor ceiling below. Instead, he just cut a large hole in the wood floor of the attic and secured the return duct to it, assuming that air would flow between the joists from the filter at one end of the attic to the return duct at the other end (the space between the joists was supposed to act as a "panned bay" return; see chap. 18). Unfortunately, a one-inch gap between the ceiling plaster and the bottoms of the joists allowed unconditioned and unfiltered air from the entire attic floor structure to enter the system.

We discuss heating and cooling equipment in greater detail in part IV.

ATTIC STORAGE

An attic provides a dry place to store family albums, clothing, seasonal decorations, old dishes, extra bedding, and furniture. Keep in mind, though, that attic dust can be allergenic and irritating. In older homes with balloon framing this situation can be even worse, because dust from inside wall cavities finds its way to the attic. In balloon framing, the stud bays are open from the basement to the attic, so an airflow system driven by convection can occur inside the wall cavities. If the basement is moldy, spores can flow up the wall cavities and into the attic, settling into the attic dust. (Balloon framing can be a serious hazard because it allows fires to spread in wall cavities from the basement to the attic; this type of framing is no longer allowed by building codes.)

If you plan to store possessions in an attic, be sure to minimize airflows from the house into the attic. Lastly, an attic used for storage should have a securely attached plywood or plank floor, not only to make cleaning easier and prevent someone from tripping or even falling through the ceiling below, but also because if there is fibrous insulation and no floor, stored goods can become contaminated with dust containing fibers.

LIVING IN ATTICS

While renovating their house, friends of ours turned the third-floor attic into a spacious master bedroom and bath. The bathroom ceiling sloped because it was under the roof gable. The plumber foolishly installed water pipes on top of the insulation close to the roof sheathing. After the renovation was complete, the couple went out of state for a long weekend. Before they left, the husband tried to take a shower in his new bathroom. It was a cold winter day. The master bathroom had no water, so the man assumed something minor might be wrong with the new plumbing. He showered in the old second-floor bathroom, and the couple left for the weekend.

While they were away, the frozen pipes in the new bathroom burst, and water cascaded down to all the rooms below. Fortunately, they had asked a neighbor to check the house, and the flood was discovered before the interior was completely destroyed. When I saw the house, most of the floors had buckled, the walls were sodden, and a few of the plaster ceilings had collapsed. Their insurance paid for the damage, but all the hard work and planning that had gone into the renovation was lost.

If you have pipes in your attic (or on the top floor of your house), be certain they are not on the cold side of the insulation. If you turn on a faucet in the winter and no water comes out, be warned! This means water has frozen in the pipes, and they might burst. (You can minimize the chance of bursting by allowing faucets to trickle, but first be sure that the drains aren't clogged.) And if you have any type of piping containing water in the attic and then decide to increase your attic ventilation, it's extremely important that you install insulation in a way that allows heat from the house to keep the pipes warm. It's not enough to insulate the pipes themselves, because insulation doesn't create heat—it only slows down heat loss.

If you own an older home with finished rooms under a sloped roof, there may be insulation under the floor in that top level. If large gaps exist between the floorboards, air will flow over the insulation to enter the room. This air can contain irritants that affect people with allergies or asthma. If this is the case in your home, you can either seal the cracks with caulk or install a new layer of solid wood or vinyl flooring or wall-to-wall carpeting over an air barrier. Allergens can also come from closets or bureaus built in under the eaves because they may be open to dusty construction cavities. If you have a built-in dresser under the eaves, pull out the top drawer and look inside. The space should be enclosed, and you should not be able to see rafters or attic insulation. If you can see rafters or attic insulation, create an enclosure at the back of the bureau to isolate it from the attic eaves. The interiors and exterior of the drawers, beneath the bottom drawer, and the entire enclosure should be cleaned.

Sometimes people put a carpet down on the floor in an unfinished attic and let the children play there. This is a poor idea because of the irritants that can collect in attic dust. In one home the attic dust was potentially lethal. I had almost finished the inspection when I went up into the attic. As we ascended the attic stairs, I could see a rug on the floor and toys scattered about. The attic had a sloped plaster ceiling, and the children had poked holes in the plaster as they played. I could see the wood lath and rafter insulation through gaps in the plaster ceiling.

I thought the insulation looked odd, and bits of it seemed to be ground into the rug. I feared the worst, because in some older homes, loose fibrous asbestos insulation was installed between the ceiling joists in attics. I opened the eaves closet and looked up at the rafter cavity with a mirror and a flashlight. I was astonished to find the cavity completely stuffed with asbestos pipe insulation. A former occupant had been a plumber, and he must have used the rafter bays to "store" the insulation he had removed from old heat pipes.

Another type of insulation, called vermiculite, also contains asbestos, though less than 1 percent. This insulation, sold in bags, all came from the same mine in Libby, Montana. Fortunately, it is rare to find vermiculite in homes. See chapter 22 for a discussion of asbestos testing and removal.

SOME RECOMMENDATIONS

AIRFLOWS AND HEAT LOSS

- Minimize ice damming by preventing heat loss from the house into the attic, but do not cover recessed fixtures with insulation unless the fixture manufacturer allows it.

- Install a tightly fitting insulated cover over the top of the pull-down stairs or access hatch leading to the attic.

- If your attic is accessed via a permanent staircase, install an insulated door at the bottom of the stairs.

- Install an insulated cover over the top of a whole-house fan to prevent heat loss to the attic in the winter.

- Have a kill switch for a whole-house fan installed in the attic to prevent accidental winter operation.

- Operate your whole-house fans only when the windows are open.

- Make sure the connections in an attic duct system are airtight.

- Bathroom exhausts should vent to the exterior and not into the attic or a soffit. If the exhaust hose is long, consider installing a fan near the discharge to increase airflow in the hose.

- Seal openings around the chimney or pipes to prevent moist house air from flowing up into the attic.

- When a ridge vent or soffit vents are installed, be sure adequate openings are cut below the ridge vent or above the soffit vents.

DUST AND ALLERGENS

- Don't use your attic for storage unless it has a securely attached plywood or plank floor.

- Keep in mind that gaps between attic floorboards, as well as closets and drawers built into the eaves, can be sources of allergens.

- If you have allergies or asthma, always wear a NIOSH N95 two-strap mask when you go into your attic, and avoid using your attic for storage.

- Change your clothes after spending time in a dusty attic.

- Keep attics as clean and dust-free as possible.

- Remove or cover goods stored in the attic while a new roof is being installed.

MECHANICAL EQUIPMENT

- Be sure the attic has adequate flooring and lighting for safe access to mechanical equipment.

- Don't install a furnace humidifier in an attic.

- Install an overflow tray with a float switch beneath an attic air conditioning unit.

- Periodically monitor your attic for leaks, pest infestation, moisture condensation, and other problems.

- Whenever possible, avoid placing water-carrying pipes in unheated attic spaces.

- Replace old attic insulation if it smells.

- If there was evidence of mouse infestation in the old insulation, HEPA vacuum the attic floor and spray-paint it to encapsulate residual dust before installing new insulation.

- If your attic is full of guano, consult a certified industrial hygienist, and consider sending some of the droppings to a lab to find out whether they contain *Histoplasma capsulatum*.

- Make sure gable-end louver vents have insect screens and are covered with hardware cloth at the interior.

PART IV.

HEATING AND COOLING

HEATING AND COOLING WITH DUCTS

18.

Most newer houses are heated and/or cooled by ducted systems, which include furnaces and heat pumps. A furnace is a piece of mechanical equipment in which air is heated; if the furnace contains a cooling coil, the equipment can also cool air. Furnaces can be powered by electricity, oil, or gas. Heat pumps are air conditioning units that can also produce heat and are powered by electricity, not fuel. A furnace and the indoor component of a heat pump are both air-handling units (AHUs) because they circulate air. Furnaces and most heat pumps move air through ducts, while heat pump mini-splits typically move air into and out of a space directly, without the use of ducts, although some newer installations are ducted (fig. 18.1).

Newer homes, particularly in climates milder than the Northeast, have heat pumps. Some older homes have hot-air heat without central air conditioning. Other older homes may have heat supplied by a hot-water or steam system connected to a boiler, and cooling supplied by a separate system. (Note that a furnace heats air, and a boiler heats water.)

In this chapter we discuss systems that supply heating and cooling through ducts. In chapter 19 we discuss heating and cooling systems that operate without ducts. We could write at least one book on each of the different kinds of heating and cooling equipment, but our purpose in this section of the book is to focus on some of the more common types of equipment found in homes as well as conditions of this equipment that can lead to indoor air quality problems.

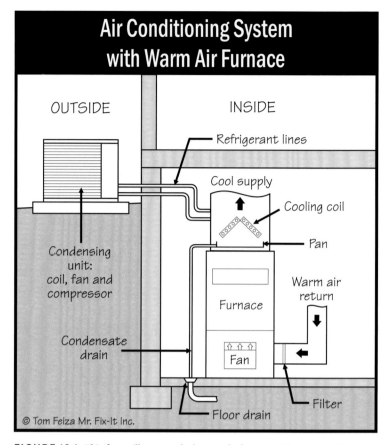

FIGURE 18.1. This figure illustrates the basics of a furnace with an air conditioning coil. The furnace is typically in a basement, and the condensing unit is usually outdoors at grade. In the winter and summer the air takes the same path, indicated by the wide arrows. Air passes through the cooling coil in the winter, but the coil is not cold because the condensing unit is not operating. In the summer, condensed water drains from the pan, either into a floor drain or a condensate pump that collects the water and pumps it into a sink, sump, washing machine drain, or to the outdoors. COURTESY OF TOM FEIZA'S *HOW TO OPERATE YOUR HOME*, WWW.HTOYH.COM. USED WITH PERMISSION.

SOME HISTORY

Today, most new homes in America are built with central hot-air heating systems. Such a system uses a network of ducts to distribute air from a heat source. Years ago, before the advent of central heat, separate rooms were heated by fireplaces or stoves. When people began to think about how a single heat source might warm the entire house, two questions no doubt arose: where to put the "fire," and how to distribute the heat from the fire to the other rooms.

The first central hot-air systems consisted of a cast-iron stove (a furnace) that usually burned coal and was mostly surrounded by a sheet metal case into which the ducts were inserted. The front doors of the stove were not encased in the sheet metal, so that coal could be shoveled in and ashes removed, and air could flow into the stove to fuel combustion. Combustion gases were eliminated through a metal vent pipe that ran from the stove into a chimney. There was a large opening at the bottom of the sheet metal case to let basement air into the space between the stove and the case. The cast-iron walls of the coal stove transferred heat to this air that then rose by convection through the ducts to warm the house. The stove walls were thus the first "heat exchangers" in hot-air systems. (The walls also prevented toxic combustion gases produced by the burning coal from mixing with the warm air between the heat exchanger and the sheet metal case.) These early furnaces were called gravity hot-air systems, because gravity (as well as convection) is what caused colder, denser house air to sink and warmer, less dense air to rise.

To carry warm air only by convection, the ducts in a gravity system had to be large—at least eight to ten inches in diameter. If you have ever seen these older systems, you know that large ducts take up quite a bit of room in the basement. Because these early furnace units were so big and had many ducts extending outward at the top, some people called them octopuses.

These octopuses depended on pathways for air infiltration (flow in) into the basement and on leaky windows, doors, and attics above grade for exfiltration (flow out). Think of the heating pattern as a convective cycle of air. Hot air rises, so as a furnace of this type heated the basement air that then rose into the ducts, air pressure in the basement dropped. Outside air was then pushed into the basement through leaks in foundations and basement windows and doors to replace the air flowing upward in the ducts (though some systems had ducts connected to openings in the foundation wall through which exterior air was brought in directly). The heated air rising by convection leaked out of the house through openings in upstairs walls and in the attic.

Gravity hot-air heating systems were inefficient for three reasons. First, the systems only heated cold basement or outside air, so they required a lot of fuel (coal was cheap back then). Second, the warmed air was leaking out of the house, so heated air was only circulated once within a home. Third, the systems had to be designed carefully, for all the ducts had to have the proper slope to maintain the convection cycle. Warm air would not flow into a duct with a downward turn, so any room fed by an incorrectly pitched duct would remain cold.

A blower and return duct were added later to increase the efficiency and comfort of a central hot-air heating system. Instead of depending on convection to move the air, a forced hot-air system uses a mechanical fan or blower to circulate the air at a rate of between 800 and 1,500 cubic feet per minute (feet³/minute). Much larger volumes of warm air could now be moved through smaller ducts. In addition, the slope of the duct was no longer relevant, because the air was being forced through the system. This means that ducts could go up, over, and around obstacles. (Today, flexible plastic ducts are used in most forced hot-air systems.) The return duct offers an avenue for air to enter the system from inside rather than outside the house. Air that has already been heated thus returns to the furnace and is recirculated, so less energy is required to maintain a consistent interior temperature.

When blowers were first introduced, furnace designers feared the increased airflow would pull debris such as paper and dust into the system, where some debris might be ignited by the coal-heated heat exchanger. To prevent this from happening, a coarse filter was added to the air intake. Other improvements included designing furnaces that could burn oil or gas rather than just coal, allowing for smaller heat exchangers that could still produce intense heat. Electric furnaces, which burn no fuel, were also introduced. In an electric furnace, air is blown over red-hot wire coils similar to those in a toaster.

A further development was the heat pump, which consists of a split system: an indoor unit and an outdoor unit. We discuss heat pumps later in this chapter.

A CLOSED SYSTEM?

Air leaks in and out (mostly at gaps around windows and doors) in all homes owing to pressure differences between the air inside and outside the house. The rate at which air is replaced in a building is called the air exchange or ventilation rate, and it is measured in air changes per hour (ACH). In a typical poorly insulated, leaky Victorian-era house, all the interior air may be replaced by outdoor air each hour (one ACH). Heat bills are high in many older uninsulated homes because nearly every hour, a volume of air equal to that of the entire interior space of the house has to be heated from outside temperature to indoor temperature.

In a modern, more "tightly" constructed and better-insulated home, the air exchange rate is reduced to about 0.25 ACH or less. Because newer homes have lower air exchanges, the heating systems recirculate the inside air. This may save money, but it also increases occupants' exposures to all kinds of pollutants, including combustion gases, radon, chemicals, and by-products of biological growth. If there is mold growth in the furnace blower cabinet or air conditioning plenum, less fresh outdoor air is available to dilute the mold spores and odors. The effects on occupants can range from occasional sneezing, coughing, and headaches to year-round allergy symptoms, respiratory distress, or other serious health effects.

RETURN AND SUPPLY DUCTS

There are two sides to the forced hot-air cycle: the return side and the supply side. Usually, there is a supply duct to every room in a home. Many years ago, when hot-air heat was first installed, there was also a return duct in every room. This balanced the airflow. Today, only one or two returns are usually installed, commonly in central areas such as in the floor or ceiling of a common hallway.

Because return ducts draw house air in, they tend to have the largest accumulations of dust and debris. (I have found toys, combs, leaves, candies, and in one case a half-eaten sandwich inside return ducts.) If a return duct is close to the basement floor, which is generally cooler because of heat loss to the concrete, the high relative humidity (RH) there can lead to mold growth in the duct dust. Sometimes, a return duct is installed within a concrete floor. This is not a good idea, since such a return in a slab or a basement floor may draw in radon gas as well as moisture. Most return ducts, however, are either in the basement ceiling or just below the ceiling joists and are connected to the furnace by a vertical section of duct and connected to return grilles on the floors above the basement.

Occasionally, I inspect a home in which the return grille on the first floor has been covered with a rug. This starves the furnace of air and limits the supply of warmer air into the rooms. In addition, the reduced air pressure created in the air-starved ducts can bend duct metal inward when the blower turns on. Then, when the blower shuts off, the metal can make a popping noise as the ducts return to their original shape. If you hear a noise like this when your blower turns on or off, be sure a rug is not covering a return grille. If your grille isn't blocked, hire a professional to investigate the cause, because the popping means that your return airflow is somehow restricted or inadequate.

Whether the system is starved for air or not, there will always be reduced air pressure in the return duct. If there are gaps or leaks anywhere in the return duct system, unwanted air from wall cavities or the basement can enter, carrying contaminants and allergens with it. If a leaky return duct passes through a moldy crawl space, odors, spores, and moisture from the crawl space are circulated through the house.

A particularly leaky type of return uses a panned bay: a duct created by covering the space between two wood floor joists with sheet metal. The top of this duct consists of the subfloor, the sides consist of the two adjacent floor joists, and the bottom is the sheet metal. Contractors use panned bays so that they don't have to reduce the ceiling height in the basement with an additional duct. I often see big openings in panned bays to accommodate wires and pipes, and more often than not these ducts are inadequately sealed at the top and the ends. Panned bays can contain allergenic dust. I've even seen moldy joists being part of panned bays. Panned bays should be clean and airtight to the basement.

CARBON MONOXIDE

Sometimes the return is not even ducted but is on the furnace itself and consists only of an opening in the blower cabinet wall. In many jurisdictions this is not allowed because it is such a dangerous practice. For example, with a gas-fired furnace, the pressure reduction in the basement induced by the blower can cause downdrafting at the furnace chimney flue. This can introduce combustion gases into the supply air, and if carbon monoxide (CO) is present, it can cause illness or death.

A return can be created accidentally at the furnace if the blower cabinet door is not fastened shut. I was asked to investigate just such a situation in which an entire family of four was hospitalized. In the middle of the night the door to the blower cabinet of the furnace had fallen off, and the next time the furnace turned on, it drew more than 1,000 cubic feet of air per minute from the basement, lowering the air pressure. Air flowed from the chimney flue back into the basement, carrying combustion products that included CO. The furnace then circulated CO throughout the house.

I always recommend installing CO detectors at or near the basement ceiling, because combustion gases are hot and therefore rise. Combustion gases can also enter your living spaces through a damaged chimney or a cracked or rusted heat exchanger, so it's sensible to have CO detectors on every level of your home, but at least outside the bedrooms (since 2008 in my home state, new homes with combustion appliances have been required to contain CO detectors). In addition, always check that the blower cabinet access panel is securely in place. (New furnaces have an interlock switch at the blower cabinet access panel. If the panel is not properly secured, the furnace will not operate.)

SPACES WHERE THERE SHOULDN'T BE ANY

Even when return ducts are properly installed, the cabinet holding the blower is part of the return system because air is being drawn into that space. Now and then in homes with ducted returns I find blower

I do not like to see returns that are not ducted. But it is not unsafe to have a direct-fired furnace with its own piped combustion air intake located in a mechanical closet with a louvered closet door as a return.

The National Conference of State Legislatures stated that, as of March 2018, "a majority of states have enacted statutes regarding carbon monoxide (CO) detectors, and another 11 have promulgated regulations on CO detectors. . . . 27 states and the District of Columbia require carbon monoxide detectors in private dwellings via state statute."

"Carbon Monoxide Detector Requirements, Laws and Regulations," National Conference of State Legislatures, March 27, 2018, http://www.ncsl.org/research/environment-and-natural-resources/carbon-monoxide-detectors-state-statutes.aspx.

cabinets without bottoms. Depending on the size of the floor gap at the bottom of the blower cabinet, this improper installation may negate the purpose of the return duct and allow unfiltered air from the level of the basement floor to be drawn into the system. In several homes that had been flooded, owners didn't realize water had soaked into the open bottom of the blower cabinet and moistened thick mats of dust that had accumulated over the years. Mold and bacteria grew there and released allergens into the airflow. If your basement floods, don't forget to clean and disinfect the entire interior of the blower cabinet, including the bottom, whether there is a sheet metal bottom or not, because water could have seeped in. And be sure to replace the furnace filter.

Another common practice is to leave out the return duct when the furnace is in a mechanical closet on a level other than the basement. I often find such arrangements in condominiums and townhouses. In this situation there is usually a louvered door to let air into the closet. In some installations, though, I have seen mechanical closets with openings left in the ceiling to furnish the return air. This air is often sucked through building cavities to the furnace. This is particularly foolish in very old homes, because dust from the cavities supplying the makeup air may contain years of accumulated allergens.

MOLDY ODOR

A woman with asthma called me because she suspected the mold odor in her kitchen was causing her headaches. A hot-air supply register and a return grille (a register has dampers for airflow adjustment; a grille does not) were located in the kitchen floor. The grille sucked kitchen air into the hot-air heating system, and the duct passed through a damp, cold crawl space under the kitchen. The woman had already had her ducts cleaned, but the company had forgotten to include the kitchen return duct, which was clogged with hair and a variety of materials such as crumbs and skin scales that were ripe for biological growth. I tested the airflow at the duct with a nontoxic smoke pencil and found that when the heating system was turned off, air moved into the room by convection from the duct. Before I left the house, I used a mirror and a flashlight to show her the festering mat that had been accumulating within the duct beneath her return grille.

Back at the office I looked with a microscope at a sample of the dust from the return duct and found it consisted of about 30 percent mold growth that was flourishing on the food and other biodegradable materials in the return duct. Numerous mites and other microarthropods were enjoying the moldy banquet. When the dust was disturbed, allergens became airborne.

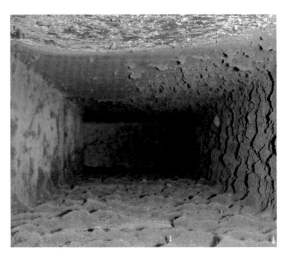

FIGURE 18.2. The interior of this return duct is unusually dirty. Mold often grows in dust like this, and mites occasionally forage in the nutrients. Allergens from outdoors and from every pet and microarthropod that ever lived in the home are stored in the dust, so ducts should be professionally cleaned before new occupants move in.

The owner was so horrified at the appearance of the leftover dust in the return that as soon as I left, she had the duct-cleaning company come back to remove the debris. The cleaners did not exercise the careful containment efforts required around a person who has asthma, so even more allergens were released into the air. It's not surprising that the woman's breathing got much worse. Utmost care must be exercised in removing allergens from an air conveyance system where a person who is sensitized lives or works. In fact, sensitized individuals should insist that a duct-cleaning company do a site evaluation before undertaking the job, to determine the scope of the work and to explain services and fees in detail (fig. 18.2).

In another home, a woman and her son were both miserable owing to mold odors and allergens coming out of contaminated ductwork that passed through a cold, damp crawl space. The problem was so severe that, though she had purchased her home only three months before, the woman was looking for another place to live. I was amazed to learn that she had paid for a home inspection before she bought the house and that the inspector had never even mentioned the crawl space or the moldy debris sitting in the ducts beneath the registers. Had the home inspector discussed the problems associated with heat ducts running through crawl spaces, the woman might not have purchased the home, since both she and her son had serious allergies.

The owner had chosen this inspector from a short list given to her by the real estate agent. Rather than just following a real estate agent's recommendation for a home inspector (even if the real estate agent is a buyer's agent), you might also obtain a referral from a friend or an attorney. I always recommend that buyers use an inspector who is a member of the American Society of Home Inspectors (ASHI), which provides a code of ethics and standards of practice and requires testing and education for membership.

SICKENING DUCTS

Dirty ducts can impair health. In one case I investigated, a woman had been experiencing debilitating symptoms, including migraines, muscle pains, swelling in the backs of her knees and calves, and tenderness in her wrists. She left her house for the first time in several years to go on a week's vacation. While she was away, all her symptoms gradually disappeared, and she was elated. She was able to move without pain for the first time in three years. Her symptoms returned within hours after she came home. Her doctor recommended she call me, because he suspected that an environmental trigger in her house was responsible for her symptoms.

I generally take Burkard air samples to determine the level of mold spores and try to identify the mold genus. When my clients are experiencing severe symptoms, however, I sometimes take Andersen air samples and send the petri dishes to a mycologist to determine what species of mold are present. In this case the laboratory found elevated levels of several kinds of mold, including *Aspergillus ochraceus*, a species that produces a mycotoxin called ochratoxin A. This dangerous mycotoxin can suppress the immune system and disrupt kidney function. Some studies have even found it to be carcinogenic.

Aspergillus ochraceus mold often grows on grains, and because ochratoxin A is so poisonous, animal feeds are routinely tested for it. Such testing is rarely undertaken in indoor air quality investigations, however. My client wanted to take this extra step, so more duct dust samples were gathered by a duct-cleaning company and sent to a specialized laboratory. In one sample[1] the lab found a concentration of over 1,500 parts per billion (ppb) of ochratoxin A (typically, grains are considered contaminated if they have even a few ppb of ochratoxin A). A lab scientist told me this was the highest level he had ever seen in any sample of any type, and he recommended the woman immediately move out. It is not clear what constituents of the mold spores caused her symptoms, but what is clear is that those symptoms disappeared as soon as she stopped living in the house.

There is more to this story. The woman had lived there for over twenty years. Why had she developed these problems only in the past three years? Three events had occurred that might have contributed to the extraordinary mold growth and its distribution. First, a water heater on the first floor had burst, possibly sending water into the ducts. Second, she had insulation installed around the ducts, and the installation had disturbed the dust in the ducts. And third, she had added a furnace humidifier that was elevating the moisture levels in the system. In addition, two other conditions had existed for a long time. First, she had never had the ducts or furnace cleaned since moving into the house. And second, the ducts passed through an unconditioned crawl space with less than two feet of clearance between the floor structure and the soil. At some locations the rusted-out ducts were resting in the dirt.

I did not recommend that the house be razed, but I did recommend it be raised to create headroom for a proper basement (eliminating the crawl space). I did not recommend cleaning the furnace and the ducts, since they were so deteriorated and contaminated. Instead, I encouraged the owner to eliminate the furnace and ducts (with asbestos-level mitigation procedures) and replace them with a hot-water heating system.

DUCTS IN A SLAB

Mold readily grows in damp cavities, particularly if the spaces are close to masonry. A duct in a concrete slab is just such a place. In the home of a family with allergies, no ducts should pass through a slab, since the accumulated dust in the ducts will almost certainly become contaminated. In addition, if the soil beneath your home has been treated for termites and your ducts pass through or beneath a concrete slab, pesticide may evaporate through gaps in metal ducts or through the walls of semi-porous (Transite-cement asbestos) ducts and contaminate the air that flows through them. (Some older homes have Transite-cement asbestos ducts installed in concrete slabs; see chap. 22.)

SHOULD PEOPLE CLEAN THEIR DUCTS?

Studies do not generally support duct cleaners' claim that the process will reduce dust and allergens in the house[2] or increase the efficiency of the system, but I believe this is because, more often than not, duct cleaning is done improperly and inadequately. If you have an air conveyance system, it's extremely important to keep the interior of the ducts, the blower cabinet, and the air conditioning coil (if present) free of dust and debris.

With proper filtration (discussed later in this chapter), ducts should not have to be cleaned more than once every five to ten years. Do not clean ducts on your own. (If you use a leaky vacuum cleaner, for example, you could spread mold spores into the house air.) Hire a company that uses brushes and HEPA vacuums to clean. Using a truck-mounted vacuum and an air "whip" in place of a brush to loosen dust just isn't adequate. To reach the ends of ducts, every floor, wall, and ceiling register must be removed during cleaning. Whenever possible, duct surfaces should be HEPA vacuumed by physical contact with the vacuum tool. A hole may be cut into a basement duct where access through existing openings is limited. Making holes in the duct does not damage the system as long as the hole is properly sealed after the job is completed.

Ducts in general can either be insulated at the outside or the inside. Internal fibrous lining material in ducts captures biodegradable dust that can lead to microbial growth deep within the fibers. Such ducts cannot be adequately cleaned. (In general, I don't like to see exposed fibrous lining material anywhere in an air conveyance system. Closed-cell foam or foil-covered fiberglass insulation is preferable.)

If anyone in your family is sensitized to dust, great caution should be used during cleaning. The ducts should be under negative pressure so that any dust made airborne within the system is not released into the house air. People with allergies or asthma should vacate the house while the ducts are being cleaned, and the house should be aired out after the job is done.

Most people think it is adequate to clean only the ducts, but there is far more to an air conveyance system than just the ducts. It's essential that the blower and blower cabinet as well as the air conditioning coil (if present) be cleaned at the same time and with the same caution. Whenever possible, the blower should be removed for cleaning. After a system is cleaned, there should be little or no dust visible in the entire system. (Tell the service provider you plan to check with a mirror and a flashlight.) This is particularly important for an allergy-prone family.

One woman from out of state called me because her father, who had asthma, was hospitalized with a collapsed lung after his ducts had been inadequately and sloppily cleaned.

I feel strongly that people with allergies and asthma should not live in homes with forced hot-air heat with air conditioning, because there is too great a chance for year-round circulation of allergens. (If you have hot-water or steam heat and a separate air conditioning system, you will only be exposed to allergens from the duct system during the air conditioning season.) I have been contacted by many families suffering from allergies even after they had their ducts cleaned. In one case, an ultraviolet "disinfectant system" had been installed, and in other cases, electronic filters had been added to the furnaces. None of these costly "solutions" worked, because the blowers and blower cabinets were untouched and thus were left contaminated with mold growth.

Some cleaning companies advertise various duct treatments such as spray coatings and biocides. I do not believe these are needed except during cleaning of the air conditioning coil and condensate tray.

Spray coatings will glue the residual dust in place and only make it harder to clean the ducts in the future. Biocides may kill some percentage of the organisms present in the ducts, but just because mold and bacteria are killed doesn't mean they won't still be allergenic if by-products of this microbial growth become aerosolized. In addition, as soon as the solution dries out and a new layer of dust containing new spores and bacteria accumulates, biological growth can recommence when moisture conditions are suitable. Finally, some biocides may become airborne on coated dust particles and cause air quality problems of their own.

There are two types of nonmetallic ducts that in my opinion cannot be cleaned adequately. One type, made from rigid fiberglass board coated on the outside with aluminum foil (called duct board), can be rectangular or round. In residential installations when the interior fiberglass surface of such ducts becomes soiled and contaminated with microbial growth, the ducts cannot be cleaned because the material is porous. Mold-contaminated, rigid fiberglass ducts must be replaced by metal ducts.

The other type of duct is flexible and consists of a thin layer of plastic on the inside and outside, with fiberglass in between and a thin metal spring-like spiral to stiffen the inner plastic and maintain the duct opening. The interior plastic surface is smooth, but the metal spiral creates ridges, making the duct difficult to clean thoroughly. In addition, the duct is often compressed during installation because it is so flexible, and this makes it hard to reach all interior surfaces. Compared with most solid metal ducts, flexible ducts are inexpensive, and it is cheaper to replace them than to clean them if they are in an accessible space such as the attic or unfinished basement. Unfortunately, flexible ductwork is sometimes installed in ceilings, where it cannot be replaced without great expense. This is why I recommend that installers use metal ducts.

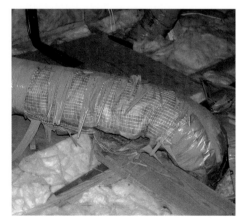

FIGURE 18.3. This section of flexible duct consists of a (shredded) gray vinyl outer wrap, a white fiberglass mesh enclosing a layer of pink fiberglass duct insulation, and a spiral metal wire embedded in a layer of thin plastic. This inner plastic layer (through which the duct air passes) is not visible in the photograph. Without the outer wrap, the insulation is peeling away from the inner duct.

Flexible ducts are covered in about an inch of fiberglass insulation held in place by a very thin vinyl wrap. The wrap on some flexible ducts spontaneously deteriorates (a condition I have seen primarily in attics), allowing the insulation to fall off. Once this occurs on attic ducts, you are heating or cooling your attic rather than your living spaces, and in the cooling season outside moisture will condense on the exterior of the exposed uninsulated surface of the cold ducts. Periodically check the exterior of your flexible attic ducts; if the outer thin plastic layer has fallen off, replace these damaged ducts (fig 18.3).

TOO MUCH MOISTURE: CENTRAL HUMIDIFIERS

Many people think that forced hot-air heat is dry, so they install humidifiers on their furnaces. After you read this section, I hope you'll think twice about doing this.

A retired couple purchased a condominium in a three-year-old complex. They were the first family to occupy the unit. During the sell-out phase the unit had been used for storage, and it was the last condominium to be sold. As soon as the couple moved in, they had a contractor install a furnace humidifier. In addition, since the unit was air conditioned, they never opened their windows. Shortly thereafter, the wife started having chronic upper respiratory infections. Her husband sneezed frequently, and both had trouble sleeping.

I entered the scene six months later. I measured the moisture content of the inside air and found it was four times that of the outside air. I went to the mechanical closet and saw a drum-type humidifier consisting of a cylinder-shaped sponge pad that rotated within a tray of water. When I removed the cover and the pan, I was overwhelmed by the putrid odor. Numerous large colonies of mold were floating on the surface of the tray. The water in the entire tray was colored amber and brown by filamentous growths beneath the surface, and there was also a thick layer of crystallized minerals present. I looked at a sample of the water with a microscope and saw bacteria and several genera of microfungi, including *Alternaria* and *Epicoccum*. Exposure to spores from both of these molds is associated with allergies and respiratory symptoms.

I also took Burkard air samples in the condominium. Considering the extraordinary extent of contamination in the humidifier tray, I was surprised to find there were not many mold spores in the air. But even when I don't find high levels of mold spores in the air, people may still experience increased asthma and allergy symptoms due to contaminated humidifiers in their homes. In such situations the humidifier tray may contain crystallized minerals along with biological growth and its by-products—the chemicals that mold and bacteria contain and excrete. When the water films break on the humidifier sponge and the water drips from the rotating drum, allergens may become airborne within small water droplets. When the water droplets evaporate, even smaller particles remain suspended. If they become airborne, any dust particles from the tray water will also be covered with allergens. The particles then become surrogate allergens and can be inhaled (we discuss surrogate allergens in detail in chap. 3). Such particles settle on furniture and carpets and can be re-aerosolized when the surfaces are disturbed.

Though I didn't find many mold spores in the air in this case, I did find *Epicoccum* spores in dust from the carpet. In the sample I took from the blower cabinet, I found a dried-out amber flake of minerals full of *Alternaria* spores. This flake was a clear indication that particles were being ejected from the humidifier and entering airflows in the system.

Why was there such prolific mold growth in the humidifier tray? I hadn't a clue until I looked at the dust samples from the hall floor. These contained typical settled air particles (skin scales, cellulose), but what was most unusual was that almost half of the dust consisted of biodegradable starch granules. I asked the owner if she used body powder containing starch or whether she did a lot of baking. She said no but she also told me that during construction, her condo had been used by contractors who might have mixed starch-containing wallpaper paste in the unit for their work elsewhere. The starch granules from the dry powder must have become airborne and accumulated in the ducts. When the heating system was operating, granules found their way into the humidifier water, where they became nutrients for mold and bacteria. Ironically, another of the woman's complaints was that she had to constantly clean dust from the floor and other surfaces.

Because the mold spores found in the carpeting most likely had originated in the humidifier, I recommended removing the carpeting. I also recommended removing the humidifier and having the ducts and furnace professionally cleaned. A few years later the woman called me. She was so congested that her voice was barely audible. She reported that they had had the heating system cleaned and the humidifier removed, but they had kept the contaminated carpeting. I told her I thought the carpeting was releasing airborne allergens every time someone walked across the fleecy surface.

One study of central humidifiers undertaken by Pennsylvania State University scientists for ARI (American Refrigerant Institute, called the Air Conditioning and Refrigeration Institute at the time of the

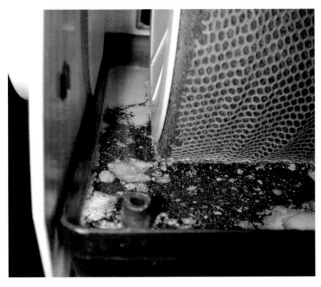

FIGURE 18.4. This portion of a contaminated furnace humidifier sickened occupants. In the lower portion of the photo is the water-filled tray with actinomycetes floating on the surface (actinomycetes are allergenic bacteria that grow like fungi with spores and hyphae). The honeycomb material at the right covers the sponge that rotates in the water to humidify the air. As the sponge rotates, it picks up allergens from the tray. Humidifiers like this should be removed.

study) concluded that humidifiers were not a source of microorganisms.[3] Other studies of both portable humidifiers and central humidification systems concluded otherwise.[4,5] My experience leads me to agree that humidifiers can be a source of microbial growth, because in my inspections I often find a correlation between contaminated humidifiers and occupants with symptoms (fig. 18.4).

As you might guess, I would discourage anyone from using a furnace humidifier, except possibly a trickle or steam type. These have no water reservoirs to support biological growth. Any system with a humidifier should be inspected at least monthly to ensure there are no leaks and that no water is soaking into any fiberglass material that may be lining the furnace or ducts. In addition to creating a growth environment for contaminants, a leaking furnace humidifier can corrode a heat exchanger or a furnace vent pipe, allowing potentially lethal combustion gases to escape.

I often tell clients that central humidifiers have two operating conditions: broken in the off position, and broken in the on position. During one of my indoor air quality lectures, I asked a group of 70 experienced home inspectors if any of them had ever seen a furnace humidifier that was operating properly. This group represented over

100,000 completed home inspections. I didn't see a single hand go up, but I did hear a lot of laughter. We discuss portable humidifiers in chapter 11.

AIR CONDITIONING: A MAJOR SOURCE OF BIOLOGICAL CONTAMINATION

In my opinion, central air conditioning represents one of the greatest potential sources of biological contamination indoors. In a central air conditioning system, air is blown across a cooling coil. In apartments or condominiums in many larger buildings (see chap. 14), cold water may be circulated to the coils from central chillers. A chiller could be either on a roof or in any space adjacent to the building. In single-family homes and smaller multi-unit buildings, compressors may supply refrigerant. Regardless of the cooling source, in all but the driest climates, as the air cools, moisture condenses on the coil and water drops into a pan called a condensate tray. Dust and moisture meet in the tray and on the coil (fig. 18.5).

The insulating fiberglass lining in the AHU can also become wet if water splashes onto it from the coil or drips from a leaking condensate tray or from a condensate tray with an improperly installed drain line. These conditions are ideal for biological growth. Even if parts of the moldy soup dry out, particles can still become aerosolized by airflows.

Rather than be concerned about indoor air quality, most heating, ventilation, and air conditioning (HVAC) technicians focus on keeping the equipment maintained so it will be efficient and will provide a comfortable level of cooling. Building occupants should therefore understand how their HVAC systems work and be sure that they are properly maintained. If you or anyone living in your house or apartment has allergies or asthma, be especially vigilant about checking the cleanliness of the indoor components of your air conditioning system.

One young woman rented a townhouse in which previous tenants and the landlord were not careful about keeping the central air conditioning system clean. She moved in during the summer and within two weeks began to feel short of breath. A physician found that her blood oxygen was low. Several months later, she was diagnosed with a peculiar pulmonary condition, eosinophilia granuloma. At the same time, she found out she was pregnant. Her doctors were greatly concerned that the fetus might have been affected by the oxygen deprivation she had experienced early in her pregnancy. She vacated the townhouse, and her symptoms decreased but resumed whenever she returned to the unit to pick up possessions.

I found that the condensate tray for the air conditioning coil was leaking into the fiberglass lining below. The insulation was dirty and

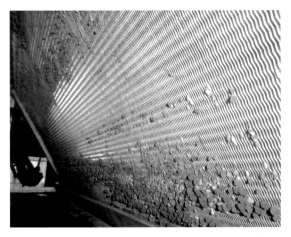

FIGURE 18.5. The strange blobs of dust on this air conditioning coil caught my eye. I sampled the blobs, and they consisted almost entirely of *Cladosporium* mold growth (along with another unidentified mold). The home occupant suffered from chronic pneumonia.

full of mold. Airflows passed over the contaminated insulation, disturbing the irritants and carrying them into the air. Luckily for this young woman, her baby was born healthy.

As this story illustrates, the biggest danger in central air conditioning systems is water leaking onto surfaces that contain nutrients. This is why NAIMA (North American Insulation Manufacturers Association) recommends that if fiberglass lining in ducts and air-handling units becomes moldy, it should be replaced.

Chin Yang, a microbiologist, did a study of fibrous lining material from A/C systems and found that about 50 percent of the 1,200 dust samples he looked at were contaminated with mold growth.[6] The reason that more people aren't sickened by these conditions is that about only 10 percent of people are allergic to mold.

A sweat-sock odor (or any musty odor, for that matter) coming from the air conditioning system is an indication of biological growth. You may notice that this smell is particularly strong when the air conditioning first starts up. This is because air that has been sitting around the contaminated materials near the coil becomes saturated with the smell of mold, bacteria, or yeast and thus contains a higher concentration of the odor. I have sampled the dust in hundreds of air conditioning units and almost always find biological growth because two basic elements to support life are present: water and nutrients. Get rid of one or the other and the chances of microbiological growth are greatly reduced.

I cannot state this strongly enough or often enough: if you have central air conditioning, it is essential that you keep the interior of the AHU completely dust-free (ducts should also be cleaned as needed).

Water should flow only through the condensate drain line; it should never leak or overflow from a central air conditioning unit. In my opinion, fiberglass lining should never be exposed close to a cooling coil, because if the material contains dust nutrients, it is a perfect environment for the growth of microorganisms.

If you want to know whether
the dust inside a return contains allergens, you can send a
dust sample to a laboratory for
analysis. If you are sensitized,
wear a NIOSH N95 two-strap
mask when handling the dust.

Vacuuming contaminated insulation, as I have often seen attempted, is not a solution because the organisms causing the trouble are deep within the insulation. In addition, vacuuming such insulation with a non-HEPA vacuum can aerosolize other allergenic particles. If you have a dirty return duct, have it professionally cleaned, because you can't really tell by looking whether the dust is contaminated. Adequate filtration is also essential in keeping an air handler free of biodegradable dust.

FILTRATION

Proper filtration prevents dust buildup but is especially important for air conditioning. As noted earlier in this chapter (and before the advent of air conditioning), air filters were initially used to prevent fires from starting on heat exchangers. What is the primary purpose of filtration today?

I've often heard it said that "a filter in a heating or air conditioning system helps keep the indoor air clean." In my opinion, this is not the purpose of filtration in a mechanical system; rather, the primary purpose is to keep the equipment clean. Without efficient filtration in place, dust can build up in an air handler, and microbial growth may ensue. Then the mechanical system can circulate by-products of this growth within a building.

For decades, coarse filters (that you could see through) were used in hot-air systems, and many homes still use similarly coarse filters. These filters do not prevent biodegradable materials from accumulating within an air handler and in my opinion are responsible for a significant percentage of IAQ problems.

A testing methodology has been developed that compares the filtration efficiency of all types of filters. Filters today are classified according to their MERV (minimum-efficiency reporting value) rating. For air conditioning, ASHRAE (American Society of Heating, Refrigerating and Air Conditioning Engineers) recommends a minimum of MERV 8 filtration. For families with allergies and asthma, I recommend using MERV 11 or MERV 14 pleated-media filters. The higher the MERV rating, the more efficient the filter, but also the more difficult it is to push air through the filter. A HEPA filter has a MERV 16 rating, and few standard blowers in air handlers have the capacity to push air through a HEPA filter.

Expensive HEPA bypass
filter systems are available
as add-ons to air handlers.
These units pass only a small
amount of the return air over
the HEPA filter; the bulk of
the air passing over the coil is
not filtered by the HEPA filter.
That is why I recommend that
the best pleated-media filter
that the system can handle be
placed before the blower, so
that all the air passes through
the filter.

To prevent the accumulation of dust and skin scales on the air conditioning coil and air handler's interior surfaces, including the fiberglass lining, use a pleated-media filter with a minimum rating of MERV 8 and change the filter at least twice a season. (If you run the AHU most of the year, you may want to change the filter more often.)

We discuss the importance of filtration in mini-splits in chapter 19.

ULTRAVIOLET LAMPS

A growing number of HVAC technicians are recommending the installation of ultraviolet (UV) lamps in residential HVAC systems. UV light has been divided into three categories. Typical black lights produce UV-A radiation, which is not particularly harmful. UV-B radiation is more energetic, causes tanning, and is associated with skin cancer. UV-C radiation is more energetic still and is referred to as "germicidal" because it can destroy the chemical bonds in molecules. The UV lamps installed in HVAC systems produce UV-C radiation.

Are UV-C lamps useful in disinfecting the air moving through a residential HVAC system? My answer is "no." Air moves through such a system too quickly, sometimes as quickly as 10 feet per second, too fast for a UV-C lamp to have much of a germicidal effect. Can such lamps disinfect surfaces in a residential HVAC system? Again, my answer is "no," for several reasons. Most contamination occurs at the front (incoming) side of the coil. Proper UV-C lamp installations in larger commercial HVAC systems contain several long lamps, placed so that the entire front side of the coil is irradiated to destroy microorganisms. In residential installations the UV-C lamps are usually too small to be effective in disinfecting surfaces, and sometimes the lamps are placed at the back (exit side) of the coil. (I saw one UV-C lamp improperly installed perpendicular to the airflow, preventing surface irradiation altogether.) UV-C lamps also produce ozone gas, which may smell like fresh air but which is irritating to inhale and is one of the chief components in smog.

Installing UV-C lamps in residential HVAC equipment can be expensive. I once inspected seven air handlers that supplied heating and cooling to a large house. Each of the air handlers contained a UV-C lamp. The filter in each air handler was inadequate. All the return plenums were full of moldy exposed fibrous lining material, and there was visible mold growth in all the blower cabinets. Mold spores were being circulated on airflows throughout the ducts. The air handlers were about ten years old, or halfway through their useful life. The air handlers would have had to be dismantled to be properly cleaned. My client decided instead to replace all seven air handlers. If he had spent money in the first place on upgrading the filters rather than installing UV-C lamps in the air handlers, he would have made a better investment and protected himself and members of his family from exposure to mold spores.

UV-C lamps can cause burns, blindness, and cancer, so UV-C lamps should never be looked at directly. If you have a UV-C lamp in your air handler, turn the lamp off before you or anyone else opens up the air handler. But in the end, you would be better off removing the lamp and upgrading the filtration in your HVAC system.

One of the paradoxes of air conditioning is that the system blows cold air that may be saturated with moisture. Ideally, we would like an air conditioning system to produce cool, dry air. This is difficult to achieve, however, because the RH rises as the air temperature drops. Moisture condenses as humid air passes over a cooling coil, but the air remains cold and close to its dew point. Although air conditioning clearly reduces the moisture content of air, operation of the equipment is controlled by a thermostat, a device that responds only to temperature. (In hot, dry climates, condensation may not be a problem because the moisture content of the air may be very low.)

In hot, humid climates, air conditioning set at between 75°F and 78°F can control the RH. In homes that are intermittently occupied or vacant during the summer, however, cooling the indoors is somewhat of an energy waste, as it is not necessary to keep the interior cool when no one is home. It is still necessary, though, to prevent the RH from rising above 80 percent, or mold growth may occur. When a house will be empty for an extended period of time during hot, humid weather, it makes sense to have a separate dehumidifier to keep the RH no higher than 65 percent. Then the air conditioning thermostat can be set in the 80s. The dehumidifier should drain by gravity into a sink or bathtub rather than be connected to a condensate pump, which could break down while the property is empty.

HEAT PUMPS

A heat pump's blower and heat exchange coil (together called an air-handling unit) are indoors, and the compressor is outdoors. Through heat exchange with the outside air, a heat pump system can both heat and cool inside air. Most heat pumps also have electric heating coils that act as backup if the compressor breaks down.

One allergic condominium owner had serious problems because her heat pump was installed in a mechanical closet without a ducted return. A hole was left in the wall so that air could come from the unit's laundry room, but the laundry room had a solid door. There was also an opening in the ceiling of the laundry and the adjacent hallway. I suppose the designer thought air would flow from the ceiling grille in the hallway into the laundry room and from there into the mechanical closet.

This wasn't what happened, unfortunately. The mechanical closet on the owner's floor was wedged between those of the condominiums above and below. There were large openings—larger than needed—for pipes in the floors and ceilings, interconnecting the three closets. One of my client's complaints was that she could smell coffee in the morning before she wanted to get up, because the owner of the condominium below hers was an early riser. In the evening she was choked by cigarette smoke that got drawn into her mechanical closet from the unit above.

Perhaps she wouldn't have minded these smells so much if she hadn't also been experiencing year-round bronchitis, sore throat, and allergies. She was late meeting me at her home for my site visit because she was returning from the emergency room after a severe episode of breathing difficulty. Before moving into the condominium, she had been an avid jogger, but she hadn't been able to run for months.

I found that the filter in the mechanical closet had fallen to the floor and the air conditioning coil was covered with mold; because of the shared airflow among the three units, any contamination in the other units was distributed throughout her unit too. I recommended that she stop using the heat pump, put in electric baseboard heat instead, and depend on window air conditioners for cooling. Because the wall-to-wall carpets contained dust from the moldy heat pump, I encouraged her to install hardwood flooring. I also told her to get rid of her down comforter and pillow.

She was able to jog again within days of turning off the heat pump. Once she installed wood flooring, all her symptoms decreased until one day when she returned home from errands and once again had so much trouble breathing that she was hospitalized. She subsequently found out that the filters on heat pumps throughout the buildings had been changed that day. Those heat pumps were also contaminated, and dust had become airborne in the hallways. In the end, because she could not control the air quality in the common areas of the building, she was forced to sell her condominium and move.

In another heat pump horror story, a man with a history of sinusitis moved into his new home and shortly thereafter developed nosebleeds, swollen and teary eyes, and dizziness. I removed the cover that concealed the heat pump coil and was startled to see a light-colored circle over 12 inches in diameter in the black fiberglass lining close to the coil. I took a sample of this material and with my microscope discovered that the entire mass of the circle was *Penicillium* mold. This mold growth probably occurred because air flowing through the fins released moisture droplets that were then deposited on the dirty fiberglass lining.

AIR-TO-AIR HEAT EXCHANGERS

Since the air exchange rate of buildings has been so drastically reduced owing to airtight construction practices, the concentration of indoor pollutants has increased. Just bringing fresh outdoor air into a house comes with an energy penalty. Outdoor air in the winter is cold and has to be heated if brought indoors; outdoor air in the summer can be hot and humid and has to be cooled and dehumidified before being brought indoors.

Air-to-air heat exchangers, also known as HRVs and ERVs, were created to get around the energy penalty associated with bringing fresh air into buildings. These are relatively small units that typically have four ducts (two to the exterior and two to the interior) and two blowers, one to bring fresh air into a house and one to exhaust stale air out of a house. Air-to-air heat exchangers have a "core" that allows heat to be transferred in the winter from warm indoor air to the incoming cold exterior air, and in the summer, if air conditioning is present in the house, the core uses the cool indoor air to cool the incoming outdoor air. In this way, about 80 percent less energy is used to heat or cool unconditioned outdoor air that is brought into the home.

There are differences between an HRV and an ERV. An HRV (heat recovery ventilator) is an air-to-air heat exchanger that only allows for the transfer of heat energy. An ERV (energy recovery ventilator) has a slightly different core and allows moisture (but not air) to pass between the incoming and outgoing airstreams. This helps reduce indoor moisture levels in hot and humid climates. HRV and ERV technologies are recent innovations, and given the airtightness of new homes, installation of these technologies would appear to be necessary. In the province of Ontario, Canada, this technology is required for all new construction. To decide which type of ventilation system is best for your home, discuss your options with an HVAC professional.

Bringing some fresh air into a home via an HRV or ERV is important but not without problems. I have looked at many of these devices. Some of them run continuously, so a great deal of outdoor and indoor air is being processed. In the spring, summer, and fall, outdoor air can be full of pollen and mold spores. Indoor air is always full of skin scales that occupants shed and also contains lint from clothing and furnishings. Skin scales, lint, and pollen grains are biodegradable, so all HRVs and ERVs are equipped with filters to eliminate aerosolized dust. In most of the units I've inspected, though, the interiors were filled with dust and mold growth because of inadequate filtration as well as poor maintenance.

There should never be any visible dust inside an HRV or ERV unit. I always recommend that the filters supplied by the manufacturer be eliminated and that supplemental, in-line filter units be used. An in-line filter unit is nothing more than a box (about the size of a countertop microwave) containing a filter inside lying at an angle and one round opening at each end of the unit for attachment to a duct. (One brand of in-line filter comes with a MERV 12 filter that is too restrictive, so this filter should be replaced with a properly sized MERV 8 filter.) HRVs, ERVs, and in-line filters should be located in readily accessible areas because they must be inspected on a regular basis, perhaps even monthly, and cleaned as needed. I only recommend using disposable pleated-media filters, because washable filters can never be cleaned adequately. Disposable filters may have to be replaced several times a year, depending on the dustiness of the indoor and outdoor air.

Building occupants' health can depend on the condition of HRVs and ERVs. In two homes that I inspected in which occupants were experiencing allergy symptoms, the air-to-air heat exchangers were moldy. The occupants' symptoms abated as soon as these units were turned off. If you have one or more of these devices in your home, always follow the manufacturer's recommendations for maintenance and cleaning. It is also extremely important that the units have adequate filtration.

SOME RECOMMENDATIONS

AIR CONDITIONING (INCLUDING HEAT PUMPS)

- A cooling coil should always be safely accessible for cleaning and inspection.

- If there is any debris on an air conditioning coil, have the coil professionally cleaned and disinfected.

- Be sure the condensate pan is not leaking, and have it cleaned regularly by a technician.

- Check that the condensate line has a trap and that it is not clogged.

- Lining that is near the coil and blower should be made of non-fibrous material such as closed-cell foam made for the purpose. Fiberglass is acceptable if covered with foil for easier cleaning.

CARBON MONOXIDE

- Install carbon monoxide (CO) detectors in your home. Follow the manufacturer's instructions for installation and maintenance.

DUCTS

- Ducts should not run through concrete.

- Hire professionals to clean your ducts, and make sure they take great care not to spread allergens into the air.

- When the ducts are cleaned, have the blower cabinet and blower (as well as the air conditioning coil, if there is one) cleaned of all dust.

- If the fiberglass insulation lining your air-handling unit (heat pump, furnace, or air conditioner) or ducts has gotten wet or is moldy, have it replaced with closed-cell foam. Be careful that contaminants are not spread into the air while the work is being done.

- Inspect the ducts by removing a register and looking in with a mirror and flashlight.

- If you have fiberglass ducts in your home that have become contaminated, replace them with metal ducts wherever possible.

- If flexible ducts have become contaminated, consider replacing those that are accessible.

- Don't use biocides or adhesive sprays in ducts.

- Be sure your return is properly ducted and airtight.

- A panned-bay return should be clean and airtight to the basement.

FILTRATION

- Use an efficient pleated-media filter (such as a MERV 8 or MERV 11 filter) to prevent dust accumulation.

- A filter should not be installed directly beneath a cooling coil because when the blower is off, water can drip from the coil onto the filter and mold growth can ensue.

- Do not use washable filters, because they can never be adequately cleaned.

- I don't recommend electronic filters because they have to be cleaned at least monthly.

- I also do not recommend electrostatic filters because they cannot be adequately cleaned.

- The filter holder should be airtight at the perimeter to prevent air bypass.

HUMIDIFIER

- Get rid of any furnace humidifier that contains a tray full of water.

- If you must have a central humidifier, use a steam or trickle type.

- A furnace humidifier should be inspected regularly and cleaned as needed.

- In cold weather, the relative humidity should be controlled to minimize condensation on windows (see chap. 11).

- Add supplemental in-line filtration to an energy recovery ventilator (ERV) or heat recovery ventilator (HRV); remove the original filters from the ERV or HRV unit.

- Clean an ERV and HRV as needed to remove biodegradable dust.

- An air-to-air heat exchanger should discharge moisture from condensation into a drain line.

- A fresh-air intake should be located away from mulch and other sources of contamination.

19.

HEATING AND COOLING WITHOUT DUCTS

The kind of horror stories you'll read in this chapter can almost always be avoided by engaging qualified professionals to maintain your heating and cooling system(s) and by using common sense in monitoring the equipment.

HEATING

ELECTRIC BASEBOARD HEATING CONVECTORS

A baseboard electric heating convector works rather like a toaster. Neither one has a motor, but both have metal filaments that heat up when electricity passes through them. Both also require little maintenance, but the high temperatures they generate can cause fires.

Curtains can be scorched if they touch electric baseboard heaters. In one basement apartment, I found an extension cord resting on the heater. All the cord's insulation had melted at one spot, and the cord was stuck to the heater's metal cover. A short-circuit could have started a fire if the metal hadn't been painted, which supplied a thin layer of insulation. Electric baseboard heaters can be a particular worry in children's rooms, where plastic toys and other combustibles may end up near or inside the heating unit. On one inspection, I found the child's pillow on top of the heater.

At another property, I saw an open door that was completely flush with the front of a baseboard heater. Apparently, the door was always kept open. As I started to close the door, smoke rose from a blackened band of charcoal at the bottom where the wood was smoldering. Why hadn't the owners noticed the problem? To answer this question, I have to describe the burning process. "Burning" is the chemical combination of oxygen with carbon-containing materials. The more oxygen there is, the faster are the chemical changes that take place. With an increased rate of chemical change, more heat is produced, and therefore higher temperatures are reached. Earlier in the book we looked at the thermal decomposition of wood, which produces combustible vapors. When wood burns with a flame, it is these vapors that are burning and that supply the energy to decompose more wood. Three ingredients are required for wood to burn with a flame: an ignition source, sufficient heat, and enough oxygen.

But wood can decompose without a flame when enough heat energy is supplied. Think about a fireplace. You arrange the wood and light the logs, but sometimes the "fire" smolders rather than burns. Smoke is produced (more smoke than when the fire is burning, but there is no flame). If you pick up a bellows and blow air onto glowing embers, a flame appears because the increased flow of oxygen speeds up the chemical change and thus increases the temperature. If you try to burn wet wood, the fire may also smolder because some of the heat is being spent on evaporating the moisture within the cellulose structure rather than fueling thermal decomposition.

When I started to close the door in this basement, I moved the wood at the bottom of the door away from the baseboard heater, introducing more oxygen to the heated wood surface. The rate of chemical change in the wood increased, producing smoke. If you have baseboard electric heat or supplementary electric heat in any room in your house, be sure that nothing combustible ever comes in contact with the heaters.

HOT-WATER BASEBOARD HEATING CONVECTORS

Baseboard heating convectors can also be part of a hot-water heating system. Connie and I like this kind of heat because the convectors aren't so hot that they can cause fires when combustible materials come in contact with convector surfaces. Hot-water heat also doesn't produce strong airflows that can stir up dust the way a ducted system does.

RADIATORS

Radiators can be filled with either steam or hot water, depending on the kind of heating system present in the building. Radiator surfaces can be hot to the touch, so care must be taken to avoid body contact.

Some families with small children install radiator covers to prevent little fingers from touching hot radiator surfaces directly; still, the covers can themselves be quite hot. That said, you should have little concern about combustibles (such as curtains or furniture) coming in contact with radiator surfaces. Later in this chapter, we discuss some of the problems that can develop when radiators are heated by steam. We talk about cleaning radiators and baseboard heating convectors in chapter 24.

RADIANT FLOOR HEAT

In this kind of hot-water heating system, pipes are installed beneath the floor. The heat is transferred to surfaces in contact with the pipes, and these surfaces in turn warm the room. This is a wonderful, even kind of heat. When the pipes leak, however, the floor may have to be ripped up to get to the pipes if they are inaccessible. I've inspected homes in which the radiant heat pipes were installed in the concrete slab (the floor of a basement or the concrete upon which a house with no basement is constructed). If those pipes leak, some of the concrete must be removed, resulting in a mess. Sometimes, such pipes are just abandoned and a hot-water baseboard heating system is installed in the house.

If you have radiant heating in which the piping is looped within the flooring, be sure you know where to find the shutoffs for the boiler and loops. Since the loops are not visible, if you have a basement and the radiant floor piping is above the subfloor at the basement ceiling, be sure to check periodically under the basement ceiling for leaks.

BOILERS

A furnace heats air, whereas a boiler heats water. Both a furnace and boiler can run on electricity or, depending on the type of burner, can use either gas or oil for fuel. Inside a gas-fired boiler or furnace, the burners produce a gas flame, not much different from the flame on a gas stove. With an oil-fired boiler or furnace, a burner pumps a fine mist of oil into a stream of air moving from a blower into the combustion chamber. An electric spark from a transformer ignites the mixture of fuel and air.

The mist, an aerosol of microscopic oil droplets, forms as the liquid is sprayed through a small hole in a nozzle. So long as the opening is smooth and clean, the shape of the oil spray is straight and symmetrical. If the nozzle is dirty or clogged, the mist may point to the side rather than to the middle of the combustion chamber. The flame may then touch the sides of the chamber, resulting in incomplete combustion, which produces soot and possibly carbon monoxide (CO).

When oil burners are serviced annually, often the nozzle is replaced.

There are two kinds of boilers. The most common type is a forced hot-water boiler, in which water is heated and then circulated through radiators or baseboard convectors or, in the case of radiant floor heat, through tubing in the floor. The less common type, a steam boiler, boils the water and turns it to water vapor ("steam") that then travels through pipes into radiators or, in older homes, convectors.

BOILER NEGLECT

When rooms were heated with their own stoves or fireplaces, people knew they were dealing with fire. With the advent of central heat, however, the flame moved into the basement, out of sight and out of mind. Rather than shovel coal into the stove or wood into a fireplace, all people had to do was turn up the thermostat. Heating equipment is now generally hidden away (and we don't have to remove the ashes), so the equipment can be neglected.

One man who was selling his house had called the gas company several times because he smelled something in the finished basement where his children often played. I inspected the house as part of a real estate transaction. I noticed the odor of combustion gases the moment I went down into the basement. I was concerned because combustion gases may contain CO. As I inspected the boiler, I made a point of kneeling to avoid breathing hazardous gases that I suspected were hanging in an invisible cloud below the basement ceiling.

I looked with a mirror and a flashlight to see if combustion gases were leaking out of the boiler. Combustion gases from a gas flame contain over 50 percent water vapor, and when the hot gases hit a cold mirror, the moisture condenses just as it does when your glasses fog up on coming inside on a cold winter day or when you leave an air conditioned room and walk out into hot, humid air. In all these cases, moisture from the air condenses onto cooler surfaces because they are below the dew point.

The mirror fogged when I held it near the combustion chamber, so I decided to measure the CO concentration in the basement with my Bacharach Monoxor II. The concentration was elevated at the ceiling, about 20 parts of CO per million parts of air (20 ppm). In a house, the CO concentration should normally be zero but should not exceed 9 ppm—the "acceptable level." Even at 9 ppm, though, people who are sensitive to combustion products may feel sick. And it isn't just the CO that is unhealthy; combustion gases even without CO present can also cause symptoms because they too are toxic. As soon as I completed my measurement, the real estate agent, who was tall and had been standing next to me, left the basement for some fresh outdoor air.

You might think the seller would have been upset by my findings, but in fact he was elated because at last he knew his worry about the odor in the basement was justified. It didn't cost a lot to fix this serious problem. The gas pressure had to be adjusted at the gas control, and accumulated rust chips that had fallen from the heat exchanger had to be removed from the gas burners. The excessive gas pressure and the rust chips had distorted the flame, resulting in incomplete combustion and the production of CO.

DELAYED IGNITION

Most people who burn oil have a service contract with their oil delivery companies for annual maintenance of the boiler. Unfortunately, the annual "cleaning" usually entails only replacing the oil filter and the burner nozzle. The heat exchanger passageways may get cleaned only when the homeowner complains about soot or odors. If you have oil combustion equipment, be sure the interior of the heat exchanger is inspected annually and is brush-cleaned at least every other year.

In one apartment building the oil-fired boiler had not been adequately serviced. My client, a young mother, was living on the second floor. The large boiler was confined in a small mechanical room in the basement. Soot and a strange odor were entering the woman's apartment, and ever since quitting her job to stay home with a new baby, she had had a strange taste in her mouth, a dry throat, and frequent headaches—all of which seemed worse in the winter. The management company had attempted to solve the problem by lining the chimney—an expensive procedure. They were also planning to rebuild both the walls abutting the chimney in the woman's apartment and the walls in the apartment below, where another occupant had similar complaints.

When I inspected the boiler, I could see that there was delayed ignition (the oil burner was firing too long before the spark ignited the fuel). This allowed the oil mist to build up in the combustion chamber so that when the flame hit it, a small explosion ensued, characterized by a thumping *whoosh!* In the confined space of a combustion chamber, an explosion creates excessive pressure, driving combustion products and unburned fuel droplets outward.

When this type of explosion produces black clouds (owing to incomplete combustion of the fuel), it is referred to as a puff-back, which can blow the observation door off a boiler or fill an entire building with soot. The cleanup from puff-backs can be costly but is usually covered by homeowners' insurance.

After spending about twenty minutes in the smoky mechanical room, I too got a headache and had a metallic taste in my mouth—exactly the same symptoms my client was experiencing. The management company had the burner serviced and adjusted so that the fuel ignited sooner, and that relieved the problem in both apartments.

To check for delayed combustion, it's a good idea to watch your boiler (whether fired by gas or oil) when it first ignites. Don't stand too close, though, as I learned on one inspection. When a commercial gas boiler with delayed ignition lit while I was standing nearby, my pants were engulfed in the burner flame. Fortunately, the flame rollout was brief and was not hot enough to set fire to my trousers. On another prepurchase home inspection the buyer and I were trapped in a low crawl space in front of the horizontally mounted furnace. I had pointed out the location of the emergency power shutoff switch and was explaining how to change the furnace filter when the broker raised the thermostat. As the gas-fired furnace ignited, the flame rollout was so huge that the floor joists above were engulfed in flame. I was so terrified that the buyer had to remind me where to find the shutoff switch.

RUST LEADING TO MOLD

In one home, a simple boiler leak led to mold growth and occupant allergies. I was asked to investigate the home because the owner was concerned about the lack of heat to the bedroom radiators and the moisture that condensed on the second-floor windows in the winter. I found water dripping from the boiler circulator. As water leaked out, air entered the system and found its way to the bedroom radiators. When the radiators became fully air-bound, hot water could not circulate through them, and the bedrooms stayed cold. The low bedroom temperature led to mold growth on the exterior walls. The amount of rust around the leak site confirmed that the condition had been a problem for quite a while—in this case, fifteen years. In addition, the water that dribbled out of the boiler all evaporated into a relatively small crawl space. This moist air infiltrated the home from the crawl space and condensed on the windows upstairs. Mites foraged in the mold in the closets and along the bedroom baseboards.

More often than not, rust on the outside is a sign of water leakage. Water should never be leaking from a boiler that is operating properly. If you see water, don't just put a pot there, as I have seen so many occupants do. Have the leak fixed. Know where your boiler shutoff valve is located so that if it leaks badly, you can turn off the water supply (fig. 19.1).

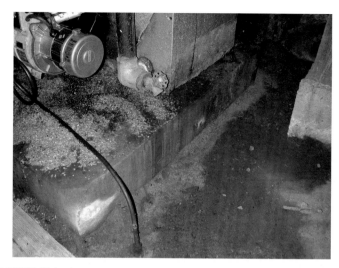

FIGURE 19.1. The extensive amount of rust staining suggests that this oil-fired boiler leaked for many years. The boiler supplied heat to evaporate the water from the leak, which led to elevated levels of humidity in the basement and in the habitable rooms above. There was a mold problem in the basement and a significant mite problem in the home, probably due to the boiler moisture. The home occupants suffered from many allergies.

SOOTIER OIL FLAME

Because an oil flame is sootier than a gas flame, oil-fired boilers always require more attention and maintenance than those that burn gas. The combustion chamber and heat exchanger inside an oil boiler need inspection and cleaning at least annually. I often find boilers that have not been serviced for several years. When such a boiler fires up, smoke and sometimes even red-hot, glowing bits of soot can blow out of the front of the case. When I shut down the burner in a boiler and look into the observation door with a mirror and a flashlight, I sometimes find that the heat exchanger "passageways" are completely blocked by rust, fuel impurities, and debris deposited from the ceramic combustion chamber liner. When the passageways are blocked like this, there is barely any chimney draft. The combustion products have to go somewhere, and they often end up in the basement.

FIRES BURN

One last observation that may seem ridiculous: Boilers have fires inside, and the metal vent pipe from the boiler to the chimney can be extremely hot, in some cases over 400°F. I often find the instruction booklet lying on top of the boiler case, in direct contact with the vent pipe. Such booklets are often scorched (making them difficult to read). I tell everyone who has a boiler to make sure there is nothing combustible within three feet of the equipment.

DIRECT-VENTED BOILERS

In traditional boilers and furnaces, hot combustion gases are vented through metal pipes into the chimney flue, where natural draft draws the gases to the exterior. In most new high-efficiency combustion equipment, gases are vented directly to the exterior through plastic piping. This type of equipment does not depend on natural draft to draw out the combustion gases; instead, a blower pulls the gases out of the combustion chamber and pushes them through the vent piping to the exterior. Direct-vented boilers are common in new construction in New England, where I live. Because the equipment is so much more efficient than traditional equipment, additional heat is extracted from the combustion gases, so the gases are cool enough to be vented through plastic rather than metal vent piping.

I have found two problems with this kind of equipment. In many homes the vent pipe joints are not airtight, and because the gases are under pressure, they stream into the house air. Even when the pipe joints are airtight, combustion gases can leak back into the house (infiltrate) through leaky windows and openings in the foundation or around the vent pipe itself. (When combustion gases exit through a chimney rather than being direct vented, the gases enter the air above the roof and from there rise into the atmosphere.)

I feel strongly that oil-fired equipment should not be direct vented through the side of the house, because the combustion products have a powerful odor that usually finds its way back inside. I have had a number of clients who became ill when combustion gases spilled from direct-vented equipment. One family I worked with had a direct-vented, gas-fired boiler in the basement, and the chimney was no longer being used. I found that large amounts of combustion gases, which contain moisture, were leaking into the house from the vent piping as well as from outside through the wall gap around the vent pipe itself. I recommended they vent the boiler back into the chimney flue, if allowed by the manufacturer. When I called several weeks later to see if they had noticed an improvement in the air quality, they said the only difference was that the air was so dry their daughter's hair became charged with static electricity when she brushed it. The family may have been missing the moisture from the combustion gases, but I knew their indoor environment was a lot healthier.

If the equipment is direct vented, the vent pipe should never be located beneath a window or near a dryer exhaust pipe, for in such cases combustion products can flow back into the house, depending on the wind direction at the exterior.

STEAM DISTRIBUTION

When the boiler in a steam heating system is not running, the radiators and pipes are full of air. When the boiler has been running for some time and the radiators are hot, all the pipes and radiators are full of water vapor. Thus there must be some mechanism to allow for airflow in and out of the system as the boiler cycles on and off.

Most steam radiators have a metal air vent (often shiny) at the side, allowing air to bleed out of the system as the water vapor is arriving and into the system as the vapor condenses when the radiator cools. The air vents are small but essential components of a steam heating system. If an air vent isn't working properly, it's either stuck open or stuck shut. If the vent is stuck open, steam pours into the house in a steady stream, condenses on nearby surfaces, and may cause wood floors to decay, paint or wallpaper to peel, and mold to grow near the radiator. In some homes, many of the vents leak so badly that the paint on the outside of the house is peeling because moisture from the house has migrated through the sheathing and condensed behind the paint film. Conversely, if the vent is stuck shut, water vapor will not be able to enter that radiator because the radiator is full of trapped air, and the room will lose its heat source.

When all radiators are working, a large volume of vapor is circulating throughout the system, and air in every heated room is warmed. In a house in which only two of ten radiators are working because the air vents on the others are stuck shut, much less vapor circulates. If the thermostat is in a room in which the radiator is not working, it takes much longer for the two working radiators to warm the house air enough to reach the thermostat's temperature set point. During this time the burner in the boiler is firing and burning fuel. Much of the heat being generated is going up the chimney instead of making steam for the radiators, and the resulting combustion gases are that much hotter.

Although a thermostat has temperature gradations, the burner on any boiler can only be either on or off. When you turn the thermostat up, the burner ignites. When the air near the thermostat reaches the temperature you have set, the burner turns off.

AIR VENT PHANTOMS

Even properly operating air vents can be sources of irritants. I was once asked by a housing agency to determine why a new boiler was making an elderly occupant feel ill. She complained of a sickening odor. Even though CO is odorless, the fire department had tested for it and hadn't found any of this gas. The situation had become serious: the woman's family was demanding that the new boiler be replaced. The housing authority, which had subsidized the boiler's installation, obviously hoped to avoid this expense.

When I arrived, a crowd was waiting for me: the woman, two of her grown children, their attorney, the plumber who had installed the boiler, and representatives from the housing authority and the boiler manufacturer. It was tough for the whole group to crowd into the basement, but we managed. I sensed a lot of hostility. The woman's children were upset because neither the installer nor the manufacturer believed anything was wrong, and the installer and the manufacturer suspected that the woman was imagining the smell.

I found nothing unusual about the boiler or its installation. Next, I went to look at the distribution system—the radiators. I went upstairs, and as the water vapor was about to arrive, I held a clean glass upside down over the air vent of the dining room radiator while air was exiting. I quickly inverted the glass and took a sniff. There was a fleeting odor of heated rubber. I repeated the test and asked the woman to take a sniff. She immediately recognized the smell that had been making her sick. The manufacturer's representative said there was a rubber gasket in the boiler, and I think it must have been off-gassing when it was heated.

I recommended that the housing authority attach small plastic tubes to each of the air vents and lead them outside through holes in the walls. In this arrangement, whenever the water vapor entered the radiators, it would push the smelly air outside the home rather than into the rooms. Those little plastic tubes saved the housing authority a lot of money, and I suspect that once the gasket stopped smelling, they were able to remove them. In the meantime, I heard from the housing authority representative that the house looked and sounded like a teakettle as vapor briefly puffing from the tubes condensed to steam in the cold exterior air.

In this case, only the woman herself was bothered by the smell. Other emissions from steam air vents can affect more people. In one apartment building, a chemical had been added to the boiler water to minimize corrosion. This chemical, called an amine, can cause skin irritation. A small amount of it evaporated into the air within the heating system, and when the water started to boil and steam moved through the pipes, this air was pushed out the vents. Some people in the building found the air irritating.

Earlier in the chapter I referred to water vapor in heating pipes as steam or water in its gaseous state. Unfortunately, "steam" has two meanings in common usage: water vapor (the gaseous state) and tiny water droplets (the liquid state) suspended in air. When liquid water is boiled inside a steam boiler, the water becomes vapor inside the heating pipes. When the vapor is released through the radiator air vent, it condenses into droplets in the cooler room air. Water vapor is not visible, but suspended droplets of water are because they reflect light.

PIPE POLTERGEISTS

A steam heating system sometimes makes banging and hissing noises that sound as if a ghost is trapped inside. The hissing is caused by the air vents as they cool periodically and let steam out. The banging is produced when hot-water vapor (the gas in the pipe) encounters cooler condensed water in radiators or pipe elbows. As it cools from the contact, the vapor condenses from a gas to a liquid, which takes up less space. The water implodes as it rushes in to fill the space that had been taken up by the vapor. In the process, the water hits itself and the interior walls of the pipes. The energy from the impact causes vibrations that are transmitted along the pipes or radiator and that we perceive as sound.

A properly constructed steam distribution system is designed so that all the condensate water from the radiators and pipes will flow back to the boiler without leaving behind any pools of water. If a radiator is not pitched properly toward the valve for the steam pipe, a puddle accumulates inside the bottom of the radiator, creating conditions that lead to the banging noise. Banging can be produced anywhere within the system where water accumulates, but the noise is most likely to occur in two places: at an elbow somewhere in the pipe system where the angle is less than 90 degrees, or at the valve at the bottom of the radiator.

People tell me that banging radiators have kept them awake at night through most of the winter. If you have noisy radiators, you may only need to place two small wooden shims under the radiator legs to alter the slope. Another hint: be sure the valve at the bottom of the radiator is opened all the way, to give lots of room for the vapor to enter and the condensate water to drain back into the pipe.

HEATING AND COOLING

HYDRO-AIR SYSTEMS

A hydro-air system has a boiler that heats water that is pumped to air-handling units (AHUs) that produce heat. The AHUs also contain air conditioning coils that cool the air. This kind of system seems increasingly common in newly constructed, large houses. If you have this kind of system in your home, the information and advice about air conveyance systems in chapter 18 will also be relevant.

HEAT PUMP MINI-SPLITS

A heat pump mini-split can supply both heating and cooling and consists of one or more indoor units mounted on walls, usually near ceilings, with tubing to the exterior for coolant lines and separate tubing to drain condensate water. A single mini-split compressor (located outdoors) can serve two or three indoor mini-splits.

A heat pump mini-split is not nearly as deep as a through-wall air conditioner, which contains a built-in compressor. The wall-mounted indoor unit of a mini-split system contains a finned coil for heating or cooling, a blower to move the air, and a practically useless filter. Nearly every mini-split that I have inspected had mold problems. I put part of the blame for such problems on government efficiency requirements to reduce energy consumption at the expense of air quality.

ASHRAE (American Society of Heating, Refrigerating and Air Conditioning Engineers) recommends that air conditioners have nothing less than a MERV 8 filter. In order to meet government-mandated SEER (seasonal energy efficiency ratio) equipment, mini-split manufacturers reduced the power of the blowers to the point that they could not pull air through such an efficient filter, so most mini-split units are equipped with a filter that is hardly better than an insect screen. As a result, dust builds up in the mini-split unit, especially on the blower blades and plastic supply vanes. When you look at one of these units that has been operating for a while, you will most likely see spots of black mold on the supply vanes and on the gray dust coating the blower blades. The fins of the cooling coil may also be covered with dust and mold growth. By-products of this microbial growth can then be carried on airflows into habitable spaces (fig. 19.2).

Initially, there was no easy way to clean these units, but now there are kits for consumers as well as for heating, ventilation, and air conditioning (HVAC) professionals that consist of bag enclosures with a drain at the bottom to collect the cleaning agents that are sprayed onto the mini-split components. Regular cleaning of a mini-split is essential, particularly for people with allergies or asthma. A mini-split must also have an internal drain for condensate water.

Some people who already have baseboard or radiator heat install mini-splits to provide cooling. Other people install a separate, ducted air conditioning system.

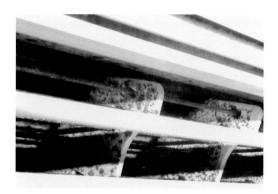

FIGURE 19.2. The dark staining on the plastic vanes for the mini-split supply is mold growth. There was also mold growth on the blower blades. All mini-splits have inadequate filtration, so dust builds up on the coil, blower blades, and supply fins. High humidity in the supply air leads to mold growth in the dust. The only way to avoid mold growth is to regularly remove all dust from visible components.

SEPARATE HEATING AND COOLING SYSTEMS

Some homes I have inspected have hot-water or steam heating systems and separate air conditioning systems.

One winter, I inspected a house in a six-year-old development of 11 houses. As I drove down the street, I noticed that each roof held a thick layer of snow. As I approached the house I was to inspect, I could see that on this particular roof the snow layer was uneven and shallower than the layer on other roofs, and enormous icicles were hanging from the roof edge (refer to "ice damming" in chap. 13). I asked the owner what made his house different from the other 10 houses. He said that his heating system was the same as the systems in the other houses, but his house was the only one with a separate air conditioning system.

His air conditioning unit was in the attic and was not airtight. When the A/C system was not running, warm air from the house rose up by convection through the open ceiling diffusers (vents) into the air conditioning ducts in the ceiling of the second floor and flowed via openings in the A/C system into the attic space. The warmth from that interior air was melting the snow on the roof.

If you live in a house with hot-water, steam, or electric heat and a separate A/C system in the attic, it is extremely important to close the A/C supplies (most have dampers) and cover the returns in the heating season. The easiest way to do this is to wrap aluminum foil or plastic wrap around a new filter and place it inside the grille. If you do not close off the supplies and returns, moist house air can migrate into the ducts and fuel mold growth. This is particularly true of a return grille in a ceiling outside a bathroom (all those hot showers).

Just be sure to open the supplies and uncover the returns before you turn on the air conditioning system.

If you have a hot-water or steam heating system and are planning to install air conditioning with the AHU in the attic, don't place the return near a bathroom. Remember, too, that if any duct runs through an unheated attic, the duct will be cooled in winter, which can lead to condensation inside the duct. Make certain that the ducts are free of all dust when installed. (I have seen installers dragging new ducts through loose attic insulation, so the ducts were contaminated before they were even installed.) The attic should also have safe access so the equipment can be inspected and cleaned as needed.

One HVAC contractor in Minnesota described an odor problem in a home with an attic AHU and flexible ducts. The supply ducts for the AHU rested on the attic floor joists in a wavelike pattern. At the top of the joists the ducts were supported, but in the space between them the ducts drooped. The contractor told me he had removed gallons of water from these ducts. Apparently, warm, moist air from the house rose by convection into the ducts, and water condensed and accumulated at the bottoms of the loops. Mold grew in the puddles.

VERTICAL STACK FAN COILS AND UNIVENTS

Vertical stack fan coils are common in multi-unit buildings, and univents are typically installed in school buildings. We discuss these ductless systems in chapter 14.

DOMESTIC HOT WATER

THE BOILER HEATS THE WATER

There are two ways to use a boiler to heat water for domestic use. Both systems use hot water from a boiler to heat cold water, but in one case, cold water is heated inside the boiler (a tankless system), and in the other case, water is heated in a storage tank that is separate from the boiler (an indirect-fired system).

In a tankless system, cold water passes through a piping coil immersed within the hot boiler water. Heat is then transferred from the boiler water to the coil, and from there to the cold water passing through the coils. In an indirect-fired system, the piping coil is located inside the separate water storage tank. Hot water from the boiler flows into the coil, and heat is transferred from the coil into the water surrounding it.

In a tankless system, mineral deposits can accumulate on the inside of the tubing walls, restricting the water flow. In an indirect-fired

In a number of houses I inspected, the dust inside return ducts located in hallways outside bathrooms contained mold growth, including *Alternaria* and *Cladosporium* mold. Children with significant allergy and asthma symptoms were living in at least two of these homes.

system, minerals can build up in the water tank but on the outside of the coils in the tank, which will not restrict the water flow.

If your hot water is supplied in any way by your boiler, then the boiler is running all year round and there is some heat loss from the boiler to the basement, even if the boiler is insulated. In basements of homes with tankless coils or indirect-fired heaters, I usually find significantly less mold growth because the basements are warmer and the relative humidity (RH) is thus lower during the summer.

HOT-WATER HEATER THAT DOESN'T DEPEND ON THE BOILER

In many homes the hot-water heater for domestic hot water is not connected to a boiler and is either powered by electricity or uses gas or oil for fuel to heat the water. You may have this kind of more traditional hot-water heater in your home. We discuss such hot-water heaters in chapter 20.

A HEAT PUMP HEATS THE WATER

The newest innovation for domestic water heating is the heat pump water heater. These water heaters use electricity to operate a heat pump and are designed to take heat from the air in its surrounding space (such as a basement or garage) and use it to heat water. If you live in a warm climate, such an arrangement makes sense because you can remove heat from warm air. If you live in a colder climate, however, taking heat from any interior space in winter means that you will have to use other fuel-burning equipment to replace the heat removed by the heat pump, so I would not recommend using a heat pump water heater in cold climates.

SOME RECOMMENDATIONS

BOILER

- Whether your boiler burns gas or oil, the interior of the combustion chamber should be inspected on a regular basis (at least annually) and cleaned as needed.

- If there is rust on the burners or on the exterior case of your boiler, the boiler may need maintenance.

CARBON MONOXIDE

- Have your heating company check your equipment for carbon monoxide (CO) in the basement and in the combustion products.

- Install CO detectors; follow manufacturer's instructions.

DUCTS

- If you have separate heating and cooling systems and an air handler in your attic for cooling, seal all duct openings (return grilles and supply registers) during the colder months when the air conditioning is not running. Don't place a return grille in a hallway outside a bathroom.

- If you are installing a ducted air conditioning system that is separate from your heating system, be sure that the ducts are clean before they are put in place.

LEAKS AND FLOODS

- Install floor-water alarms near your boiler and hot-water heater.

- Have someone monitor your home while you are away.

- Know where to find the water shutoffs for your boiler.

- Know where the shutoffs for the boiler and loops are for your radiant floor heating system.

MINI-SPLITS

- Keep the components of a mini-split clean, including the filter, coil, blower, and the supply louvers.

RADIATORS

- Steam radiators should be pitched toward the valve, which should be completely open when the radiator is in use.

- Be sure that radiator air vents are working properly.

- Don't paint steam radiator vents.

SAFETY

- Be sure that combustibles (including clothing, boxes, and plastic) and electrical cords are not in contact with electric baseboard heaters or metal boiler vent pipes.

- Nothing combustible should be placed within three feet of a boiler.

20. MORE ON HEATING, COOLING, AND FUEL

HEATING

PORTABLE ELECTRIC HEATERS

In our home, Connie's office is above our attached two-car garage. In very cold weather, the room is chillier than other rooms on that level of the house. On such days, she depends on an electric oil-filled radiator to warm her office. Our daughter-in-law grew up in the South and is thin-skinned when it comes to cold weather. When she and our son were first married, we would set the heat in the house at 72°F because we wanted her to be comfortable. She was toasty, but we were sweating! Now we keep the thermostat at our usual 68°F, we run another oil-filled radiator that we have in the guest room, and we lend her a cozy jacket to wear in the rest of the house.

In addition to conducting site visits, I also offer phone consultations. It's clear in many of these conversations that the heating systems are sources of contaminants. I recommend that people turn off their heat and depend on oil-filled radiators for a few days, to see if their symptoms abate. If they feel better when the heat is turned off (and they usually do), their next step is to have the system thoroughly inspected by a heating, ventilation, and air conditioning (HVAC) technician or an indoor air quality professional who knows something about mechanical systems. Home inspectors can also be helpful resources in such situations. The American Society of Home Inspectors (ASHI) has a website where you can find ASHI-qualified home inspectors in your area (see the resource guide).

I only recommend oil-filled radiators for supplemental heat, because other kinds of portable heaters can be fire hazards.

WOOD STOVES

Some people use wood-burning stoves as primary or secondary heat sources in their homes. If this is the case in your home, it's important to have your chimney inspected on an annual basis to be sure there is no buildup of creosote that could ignite, resulting in a serious fire threat. This caution is also applicable for stoves and burners that burn wood pellets for fuel.

One couple told me about a near-death experience in their vacation cabin in the mountains. There was a steep hillside behind the cabin, which was heated by a woodstove. The uninsulated metal chimney pipe exited the living room wall at the first floor, rose above the second floor at the outside of the cabin, and ended well below the peak of the roof.

Before the couple and their two young children went to sleep, the husband partially closed the stove's damper so the fire would last as long as possible into the night. The wind outside was sweeping down the hill, moving over the top of the chimney pipe, and hitting the peak of the roof. The cold outside air was forced down into the chimney, pushing the combustion products from the glowing embers back into the room through the combustion air hole at the front of the stove. Burning embers produce large amounts of carbon monoxide (CO), and the cabin was filling with this deadly gas. The husband woke up nauseated and dizzy. Suspecting what was wrong, he opened all the windows to air out the cabin.

To remain in the cabin safely while the stove was burning wood, the family had to increase the draft going up the chimney. They kept the living room window on the uphill side slightly open, and this did the trick. Why? Because the force of the wind coming down the hill and into the window increased the air pressure in the cabin, pushing air back up the chimney and carrying the combustion products with it. In other words, it reversed the downdraft.

HOT-WATER HEATERS

The most common kind of water heater is a separate tank fired by oil, gas, or electricity (the most expensive energy source). (See chap. 19 for a discussion of other kinds of hot-water heaters.) The biggest drawback I find with fuel-burning water heaters is spillage of combustion gases caused by inadequate chimney draft. In some newer homes with high-efficiency heating systems, blowers are installed to eliminate the combustion products. If the heating system and the water heater share a common vent pipe and the chimney draft is inadequate, combustion gases from the furnace or boiler can be blown out the water heater vent pipe into the basement air.

This problem is more likely to occur with a gas-fired water heater than in an oil-fired one, because there is an opening at the top of a gas water heater. The opening, called a draft diverter, is there to prevent downdrafts from blowing out the pilot light. Combustion gases from a boiler or furnace can exit through this opening. (This problem does not occur with an electric water heater because it doesn't burn anything and therefore doesn't need to be vented.) The combustion chamber in a gas-fired water heater is at the bottom, where there is an access cover. I have seen many gas-fired water heaters that malfunctioned because of blockages in the vent system, allowing hot combustion gases to exit at the access. The temperature of the gases was so high that it melted the plastic knobs on nearby valves. The same caution thus applies to vented water heaters as to boilers and furnaces: don't place combustibles nearby.

One problem common to all types of water heaters is leakage, both slow and catastrophic. Slow leaks can cause all kinds of mold growth, depending on where the leak is and how long it has been occurring. I recommend that homeowners check their tanks for leaks at least weekly. When a water heater breaks, cold water flows uncontrolled into the basement, mechanical closet, or wherever the water heater is. Make sure you know where the shutoff valve for your water heater is and use it if the heater breaks (for safety's sake, turn off the fuel or power supply first). When water heaters are in living spaces such as finished basements or in mechanical closets in apartments, I recommend adding an overflow pan with a floor-water alarm. Some hardware stores carry these alarms; you can also find distributors of these devices on the Internet.

Water heaters come with either a five- or a ten-year warranty. The difference between the two warranties has nothing to do with the quality or construction of the tank. A water tank contains either one or two magnesium rods, which protect the tank from corrosion in the same way that a zinc coating protects a galvanized nail from rusting. Over time, the magnesium rod dissolves. If a heater has one rod, the lifetime under typical water conditions is five years; with two rods, it's ten years. Be sure to check your warranty, and consider replacing your water heater if it's well beyond its warranty life (or you may come home one day and find your basement full of water!).

If you are going to be away from home for a time, ask a friend or neighbor to keep an eye on your boiler and water heater. Make sure this person is reliable. One of my clients made the mistake of asking the wrong person to watch her house while she was away for the winter. Something went wrong with the boiler, and the heat went off. Pipes burst and flooded the house. When the woman returned,

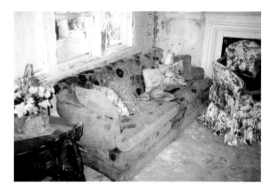

FIGURE 20.1. This moldy couch was in the living room of an unoccupied home that flooded from a heat pipe leak inside the kitchen ceiling. The leak continued for months during the winter. *Stachybotrys* mold grew on the kitchen ceiling drywall, which eventually collapsed, spreading *Stachybotrys* spores throughout the home. Many large, black *Stachybotrys* colonies developed from individual spores on the damp couch.

the entire house was wet, and a soggy bill for 30,000 gallons of water was waiting for her. Mold was growing on the living room couch, the bedroom lamps, and all the interior walls. The kitchen ceilings had collapsed, and the recently refinished wood floors were so buckled and warped from swelling that they looked like frozen waves. The house was "totaled" and scheduled to be gutted and completely renovated. Fortunately, the damage was covered by an insurance policy (fig. 20.1).

COOLING

SWAMP COOLERS

We live in New England, where most of my investigations occur, so I have never seen a swamp cooler. Some people living where it is hot and dry in the summer use swamp coolers for cooling the air. This system consists of a water reservoir with an evaporative pad and a blower. The same principles apply: wherever there are nutrients, water, and air, microbial growth can ensue. The airflow into a swamp cooler must be completely free of dust if microbiological growth is to be avoided, so efficient filtration is needed as well as regular maintenance to keep wet surfaces free of biodegradable dust. Some people add antimicrobial compounds to the water reservoir.

WINDOW AND THROUGH-WALL AIR CONDITIONERS

Many older homes don't have central air conditioning, so people depend on window or through-wall air conditioners for cooling. Most of the window air conditioners that I have looked at were full of mold

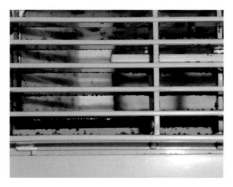

FIGURE 20.2. I have never seen a window air conditioner that had adequate filtration. As a result, dust builds up on the cooling coil, blower blades, and supply vanes. Condensed water on the cooling coil leads to mold growth on the coil, and high humidity of the discharge air from the cooling coil leads to mold growth on the blower blades and the vanes of the supply louver (pictured here).

growth owing to inadequate filtration and lack of maintenance (see chap. 24). Keeping all dust out of the air conditioner reduces the likelihood of mold growth within the unit. Attaching supplemental, electrostatic filtration material to cover the entire air intake grille can help prevent the collection of dust on the cooling coil, blower, the interior of the unit, and the supply louvers. (And replace the filter at the beginning of every air conditioning season.)

In cold climates, most people remove window air conditioners and store them in a closet, attic, or basement. Then, when spring moves into summer, those air conditioning units are reinstalled. Rarely are they cleaned first.

I can't tell you how many window air conditioners I've seen sitting on the concrete in moldy basements or stored in attic eaves that were full of ancient, allergenic dust and even mouse droppings. During use in humid climates, window air conditioners acquire mold growth and should be cleaned before being turned on each year. Sometimes, a wall or window air conditioner has to be cleaned in place. It is far less effective to clean such units in place, however. If you own a moldy unit and it cannot be removed for cleaning, consider replacing it, especially if you or anyone in your household has allergies or asthma (fig. 20.2).

PORTABLE AIR CONDITIONERS

A portable air conditioner is one that sits inside the room being cooled rather than being installed in a window or wall. Typically, a portable unit has wheels to facilitate movement. These air conditioners have one or two hoses that must be connected to a panel inserted tightly into a window. When air in a room is cooled, heat must be removed, so one hose exhausts hot air to the exterior. If you have a portable unit with two hoses, the second hose brings in outdoor air to cool the unit's compressor. Portable air conditioners suffer from the same risk that all devices with cooling coils face: water condenses on the cooling coil, and if there is dust on the coil, microbial growth will ensue.

Unfortunately, none of the portable air conditioning units that I have seen come equipped with adequate filtration; typically, the filter consists of nothing more than a screen. This means that keeping the coil clean is of the utmost importance. Connie and I own one of these air conditioning units and attach supplemental electrostatic filtration material (which we replace annually) to cover the entire air intake grille.

Some of the older, portable air conditioning units have a reservoir to collect condensed water. Such a machine will shut off if the reservoir isn't emptied. Newer units use heat from the compressor to evaporate the condensed water, and the moisture is then exhausted through the hose to the exterior. Most portable air conditioners can also be operated on the dehumidification mode, but again the same precautions apply regarding filtration and the cleanliness of the coil.

FUEL PROBLEMS

All fuels are sources of energy, and energy can be dangerous. Electricity is not technically a fuel, but it is certainly a source of energy and is not without risks. For example, many fires start in buildings with faulty wiring. Electricity is delivered continuously, as is natural gas. If you have gas supplied to your home, a constant supply of gas has to flow through the pipes from a remote source. If your fuel source is oil or propane, you must have a storage tank somewhere on the premises.

All sorts of problems can occur with the use of fuel in homes, and these problems can affect the indoor air quality as well as occupants' health; in fact, some of the problems can be life-threatening.

OIL SPILLS AND LEAKS

Oil spills and larger leaks are pungent and injurious to health. One young woman made an offer on a split-level home with a finished basement. On her first visit to the house she noticed a solvent smell, but she ignored it because the property seemed so perfect for her. The house had just been painted, so she assumed the paint might be causing the smell. Six months after she moved in, the solvent smell lingered, and the woman began having respiratory trouble. In the middle of her first winter in the house, the heating system ran out of oil. The oil company came and filled the tank with about 250 gallons of oil, but a few days later the tank was empty again. She then made the connection between the solvent smell and the bottomless oil tank.

Apparently, there was a pinhole leak in the oil line that had been installed beneath the concrete slab in the basement. Oil had been leaking for years under the basement floor, and the rate of the leak had clearly increased. Oil had even spread into the well water. Many steps were taken to try to eradicate this nightmare. The basement was excavated about eight feet down, and hundreds of gallons of oil and barrels of saturated soil were removed. The contamination was so widespread, however, that a complete cleanup was impossible. To minimize the chance that the oil remaining in the soil under the house would cause fumes to spread into occupied spaces, a radon mitigation system was installed in the basement.

Many of the numerous mitigation steps were necessary, but many mistakes were also made. First, not enough of the contaminated soil was removed. Second, open drums of oil and soil were left in the basement, where they off-gassed fumes into the air. Third, the fan in the radon mitigation system had a leak, and the fittings for the pipe to the outside were loose. Instead of blowing the air through the pipe to the roof and the exterior, the system was sucking air laden with oil fumes out of the soil, and some entered the house, making the situation even worse.

What happened to the house was sad, but what happened to the owner was a tragedy. She had originally bought the house in part because it had a basement office. She wanted to work where she lived, not only for the convenience but also to avoid paying rent for a separate office space. To minimize her mortgage payments, she had put all her savings into the down payment when she bought the house. She originally called me because her home made her feel sick, but she grew so ill from inhaling the oil fumes that she became chemically sensitive and had difficulty working.

The insurance company initially refused to pay for a proper oil cleanup, and because she was afraid of losing the house, she continued to pay her mortgage even though her income was drastically reduced and she could no longer spend time there. She decided to sue the insurance company, and her attorney asked me to return and investigate the conditions. By this time, two years had passed. To track the levels of contamination in the soil beneath the slab, the mitigation company had installed in the basement a "monitoring well": a vertical plastic pipe placed in a hole dug down to the water table. I unscrewed the cap to this well and dropped in a small glass vial attached to a six-foot string. When I raised the vial, I saw a layer of oil floating on top of the water. In the end the owner and the insurance company reached a settlement so that she was able to buy another house. I hope her new house has gas heat.

STRIKING OIL

Another homeowner looked out her kitchen window and to her dismay saw an oil geyser so high she couldn't see the top. She rushed outside to where the oil-delivery truck was parked and screamed at the driver. The hose from the truck had sprung a leak right in the middle of her yard. Oil was raining down onto her property, saturating the soil and laying in a film on top of her kiddie pool. This was a serious cleanup problem, but at least the oil was not inside the building (yet), as it is in so many other cases.

The mitigation company came to clean up the sandy soil but unfortunately never warned the owner about some precautions she should take during the removal of the contamination. On cleanup day the smell of oil in her house was so strong she opened all the windows and inserted fans to blow "fresh" air into the house. She sucked in the contaminated dust and sand instead.

The dust and sand were coated with oil and covered the interior of her house, including furniture, floors, and rugs. I took samples of sand from the basement floor, and even these reeked of fuel oil. The last time I spoke with the family, they were living in a trailer on the edge of their property. I never found out what ultimately happened to the house and its occupants.

In another home built into a hill, the basement was at grade level, and sliding doors opened to the front and side yards. The oil fill pipe was in the rear to the left of the house. The homeowner noticed that the fuel in his tank was low and called for a delivery. The tank was filled, but unfortunately someone in the oil company's office sent another tanker. The second deliveryman climbed the hill, put the hose nozzle in the fill pipe, and returned to his truck to eat his lunch. The man must have looked up from his sandwich, noticed oil pouring down the hill, and rushed out to turn off the pump. A neighbor saw him frantically trying to climb back up the oily slope to retrieve the hose, but he kept slipping down at each attempt.

No one told the owner about the afternoon's event, and when he entered his basement that evening, he noticed a strong odor of fuel oil. He looked on the floor, and there were puddles of oil everywhere. Apparently, his lawn was not the only oil-soaked victim: the excessive pressure had caused the oil tank in the basement to burst.

The company cleaned up the oil spill, but the family called me two years afterward because they had all become chemically sensitive. The owner had a home business in the basement but could no longer work there because he was so bothered by the lingering smell of oil. I noticed a strong odor of oil in the basement when I entered. There was a one-inch gap between the foundation wall and the floor. Somehow, no one realized that oil from the spill had run beneath the slab, and now fumes were entering the basement from the soil through that gap.

If your basement smells of oil, determine the cause and eliminate the source. If oil has leaked into the concrete and the smell remains after the concrete has been washed, don't hesitate to replace the contaminated portion of the slab. If you use oil for fuel, here are a few more suggestions to improve safety and reduce the likelihood of problems.

First, check the bottom of your oil tank. If it's difficult to see, use a bright flashlight and a mirror. If you see hanging oil drops and rust stalactites or signs of repair, insist that the oil company evaluate the condition of the tank. A new tank costs a lot less than cleaning up a basement full of oil. Second, if your oil line is buried in concrete, install a new line in a leak-tight liner. In addition, install an oil safety valve. This allows oil to flow out of the tank only when the burner is calling for fuel. Third, if you have an older tank that is not in use, have it pumped out and removed. It's not a good idea to save an old oil tank thinking you may switch back to oil in the future. Old tanks may have concealed interior rust that is not visible, particularly if they have been sitting for several years with condensed moisture inside. When a tank is removed, be sure the oil fill and vent pipes are taken out at the same time, or your neighbor's oil may accidentally be delivered into your basement.

BURIED OIL TANKS

A student from one of my home-buying courses called to tell me about her experience with a buried oil tank. She was moving to Oregon and had used a non-ASHI (American Society of Home Inspectors) home inspector the broker had recommended to inspect the house she was considering buying. During the inspection, she expressed concern about the asbestos boiler insulation. The inspector stuck a screwdriver into the insulation and flicked off a piece, exclaiming, "You people from out East are too worried about environmental issues." Then she asked him about the buried oil tank in the backyard. "Nothing to worry about," he replied.

She purchased the home while she was still living in Massachusetts and hired a local company to remove the oil tank. On the day of the excavation, she received a long-distance call at work from the excavator saying that the removal would probably cost four times the original estimate. Later the same day, she got a second call with a revised fee ten times the original estimate. In the end, the cleanup cost her many thousands of dollars. Had a more vigilant home inspector done the inspection, he or she might have recommended that the buyer have the seller remove the tank before the closing.

Removing buried oil tanks can be very expensive if oil has leaked out of the tank into the surrounding soil. I know of removal/remediation jobs that cost well over $60,000. Fortunately, the odds of having a leaking tank are about 1 in 200. Nevertheless, it's not worth the risk of continuing to use an old buried oil tank or even to have one on your property.

GAS EXPOSURES AND EXPLOSIONS

In this chapter and others, we have cited examples of problems related to exposure to low levels of gas and gas-combustion products, particularly for people who are chemically sensitive. If you use gas as a fuel, be insistent about having small leaks repaired. If you smell gas, don't think you are imagining the odor, even if the gas company thinks you are. If necessary, purchase your own TIF8800 combustible gas detector and test for gas leaks yourself (but don't try to make any repairs!).

All combustion products can be unhealthy, and all fuels are potentially dangerous. Gas explosions are probably less common than oil leaks, but the effects can be far more devastating. One chemically sensitive woman asked me to look at her new house because she thought it was making her ill. She told me she had become chemically sensitive after her many surgeries and hospital stays. She had originally been injured because she was blown out of her home in a gas explosion that demolished the house, leaving her disabled and in a coma for over a year. What had caused this disaster? She had lit a cigarette—her last, in fact—after a gas repairman left the cap on a basement gas pipe open.

On September 13, 2018, utility workers for Columbia Gas were replacing some low-pressure piping for the system when high-pressure gas was accidentally sent through the system to homes, schools, and businesses in several Massachusetts communities. The high gas pressure resulted in fires and explosions in almost 80 homes. One teenager died in a car when an explosion knocked the chimney off the roof and onto the car in the driveway. Many homes went without heat for weeks.

We heard about a propane explosion in the Vermont town near where Connie grew up. The house was heated by propane, and officials believe that there was a propane leak in the basement. The house blew up in the middle of the night. Fortunately, no one was hurt, but the house burned to the ground (fig. 20.3).

Several other homes in Vermont either burned to the ground or blew up due to propane leaks. Many homes in rural areas have

In some states, including Massachusetts, the law requires removal of an abandoned, buried oil tank. So long as there is no contaminated soil present, removal costs should not be exorbitant.

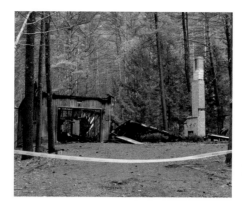

FIGURE 20.3. Propane gas leaked in the basement of this burned-out home. The gas was ignited and exploded, sending one occupant and the couch he was sleeping on into the air. The occupants escaped, but the house burned to the ground.
PHOTO BY MICHAEL DUDLEY; USED WITH PERMISSION.

Utility-supplied (natural) gas is less dense than air, but propane is denser than air and collects near the floor. Natural gas floats up and dilutes itself in air, but propane gas remains concentrated in air. In either case, if the concentration of propane gas in air is high enough, an explosion is possible.

propane heat or appliances fed by propane. If your home is heated by propane or your appliances are fed by propane, be sure that the equipment is checked periodically. Propane itself is odorless, but a chemical is added to the gas to give it a rotten egg odor so people can detect a propane leak (but the odor indoors may be stronger near the floor). If you suspect you have a propane leak, the gas should be shut off, the building vacated, and the supplier or even 911 should be called immediately.

SOME RECOMMENDATIONS

WINDOW, WALL, AND PORTABLE AIR CONDITIONERS

- Install the best filtering material that is compatible with your unit.

- The filter should be installed so no unfiltered air gets onto the cooling coil and so it is not in contact with the coil.

- If you cannot upgrade the filter, install supplemental, electrostatic filtration material over the air intake.

- Filters should be changed each season or more frequently if dusty.

- If you live in a multi-unit building and have a through-wall air conditioner in your unit, ask the building's maintenance personnel to clean the unit and upgrade the filtration.

- At the end of the cooling season, store a window air conditioner in a clean, dry space. You can also wrap it in plastic so long as the surfaces are dry. (See chap. 24 for a discussion of cleaning window air conditioners.)

- Be sure no water from the window air conditioner (or wall heat pump) drips to the inside.

HOT-WATER HEATERS

- Know where the water shutoff valve and gas or electric switch are located.

- A hot-water tank with a ten-year warranty is preferable to one with a five-year warranty.

- Do not place anything combustible within two feet of a gas-fired hot-water heater.

- Install a floor-water alarm near a hot-water heater. If you have a central alarm system, see if the floor-water alarm can be connected to that system.

- Ask a neighbor or friend to check your water heater for leaks if you will be away from home for an extended period of time.

OIL

- Have an oil safety valve installed and make sure that the oil line is in a leak-tight liner above, not under, the concrete floor.

- If there is an oil smell in your basement, determine the cause and eliminate the odor source.

- Repair all oil line leaks as soon as possible.

- If you have a significant oil leak, hire professionals to do the cleanup. Be sure the odor of oil is gone when told that the cleanup has been completed.

- If you have an abandoned oil tank on your property, check the law in your state regarding requirements for removal.

- If the tank must be removed, the work should be done by professionals.

- If you are still using an older underground oil tank, have it tested for leaks or removed.

- Check the bottom of your basement oil tank for rust and leaks. The tank may have to be replaced.

- If your basement oil tank has been removed, be sure the fill pipe and vent pipe have also been eliminated.

PROPANE

- If you suspect you have a propane leak, turn off the gas, vacate the premises, and call 911.

WOOD STOVES

- Be sure the damper is closed when the stove is not in use, particularly if you have an exterior chimney.

- Don't close a damper when there are still warm embers in the stove.

- If the boiler and wood stove (or fireplace) flues are within the same chimney, look into installing a damper that fits onto the top of the solid-fuel flue.

- Have your chimney inspected on an annual basis to be sure there is no buildup of creosote that could ignite, resulting in a serious fire threat.

- See chapter 7 for more recommendations on burning wood.

PART V.
CLEAN IT UP— INSIDE AND OUT

RENOVATION AND NEW CONSTRUCTION

21.

Your family grows, you decide to work from home, you need more space for your art—any number of life changes can mean that your current home is no longer large enough or arranged in a way that meets your needs. In these circumstances, should you renovate or move?

There are many details to remember and deadlines to meet when buying a house. For people who want to live in a healthy indoor environment, the search for a new home is particularly complicated. And that's just the buying side. When people sell a home, they have to clean it up, prepare it for the market, and try to get used to strangers marching through and making comments about the furniture and the decor.

Even though real estate transactions can be traumatic, particularly when air quality is an issue, people continue to buy, sell, and move. Whether you stay in your current home or move to a new one, renovation will probably enter your life along the way. The intent of this chapter is not to offer general construction advice but to provide some guidance for families with allergies, asthma, and chemical sensitivities, as well as for people who want to minimize their exposures to indoor contaminants, irritants, and allergens.

Although some people seem to pick up and move at the drop of a hat, most choose moving as a last resort. Moving can be fun and exciting, but it can also be a nightmare.

OUR OWN STORY

When I'm not investigating indoor air quality problems, I'm just another homeowner—a prospective buyer and seller. In the more than forty years we've been married, Connie and I have moved five times. I really dreaded our next-to-last move. We were living in a small house we had thoroughly restored, and everything was to our liking. We had even designed the kitchen with the counters and cabinets higher than usual, since we are a tall family.

There were only two serious problems with the house. First, we were running out of room. Our children were getting older and bigger, and they were beginning to have their own social lives. One night my wife and I were sitting at the kitchen table, moaning about feeling more and more squeezed in our own home. At first, our two children had their bedrooms and we had the rest of the house. Now we felt as if we had our bedroom and they had the rest of the house. We lived in a city, and unfortunately there was no space on the lot for an addition. The second problem was that the house had a forced hot-air heating system, which was beginning to bother me as well as our son, who has asthma. It was time to move again.

We found a large Victorian that was "de-habilitated." The floors were covered with old wall-to-wall carpeting and glued-on cork tiles. Some of the original architectural details had been plastered over. The kitchen and bathrooms were old, and the pink walls in some of the rooms made me see red. I was dreading what faced us, but the house had forced hot-water heat and the space we needed, and it was in our price range. We made an offer and were rebuffed. We tried one last time, making an offer that was to expire at 11:00 p.m. At 10:00 the broker called to let us know the sellers were probably not going to agree to our terms. We were so relieved that we would be looking forward to yet another lovely (though crowded) winter in our little jewel of a house that we decided to celebrate with a glass of champagne. The phone rang again before we even removed the cork. "Congratulations," the broker said. "We reduced our commission, and the sellers accepted your offer. You have a new home."

Before we moved in, we updated the kitchen and baths, had the carpeting removed and the floors sanded, tore down some false partition walls, and painted the rooms. After we moved in, there was still much to do on both the interior and the exterior. We took care of leaky pipes, broken sash cords, and wiring that had not been professionally installed. We graded the land around the house and landscaped the yard. We had to cut away bushes that were growing right up against the house, and we hired people to trim trees whose branches extended not only over our roof but also the neighbor's roof. We had a mason fix many of the loose and cracked flagstones on the back patio. The asphalt driveway was crumbling, so that too needed to be redone.

One of the first things we did after we moved into the house was to hire a contractor to replace the roof shingles on the turret. At the same time, the workers repaired and replaced some of the decayed soffit. As soon as the work started, I began coughing, and I continued to cough after they had finished the job, packed up, and left. Even though the work was on the exterior, the hammering must have disturbed ancient moldy dust in the soffit, wall cavities, and attic. The dust could then enter the house air through electrical outlets, openings in window jambs, and other obscure pathways like pipe chases, abandoned ducts, and gaps in the flooring. Clearly, some fine particles in the disturbed dust were irritating my lungs. Two weeks after the workers left, we HEPA vacuumed surfaces and aired out the house, and at last I stopped coughing.

RENOVATION DUST

Dust is an inevitable by-product of renovation, including painting, so people with allergies, asthma, and other environmental sensitivities need to stay away from the areas where the work is taking place. When large-scale projects such as moving walls, installing windows, laying new floors, and adding rooms are being done, I recommend that people not stay in the house at all. If that's not possible, or if the job is not extensive, the work area can be physically isolated from the rest of the house. Remove personal possessions, hang heavy plastic over the doorways, and operate a fan on exhaust in a window in the work area.

Buy your own drop cloths, because those owned by the contractor can be contaminated with all sorts of allergens and irritants (dander particles, mold spores, and dust from plaster or lead paint), either from other jobs or from a contaminated storage area. If you have a hot-air heating system or central air conditioning, be certain the supply registers and return grilles in the space are covered while dusty work is under way. If heat supplies and returns have to be functioning in the work area, install high-quality filter materials over them. Alternatively, you can operate oil-filled radiators for heat or window air conditioners for cooling.

Even if the construction area is isolated, workers should still be cautious as they come and go through the house. Dust from their clothing, shoes, or from construction materials carried in and out can easily settle into rugs and furniture. If workers must move through other rooms in the house, lay down heavy construction paper to make a path. If necessary, isolate openings to other rooms with hanging

Negative air pressure will occur when an exhaust fan makes the air pressure lower in a particular room than the air pressure in adjacent rooms. Air from adjacent rooms will then flow into the room with the fan rather than vice versa.

It is critical during renovation or construction to prevent construction dust from entering a duct system.

plastic and have soiled materials removed through a window or a basement door leading to the exterior. Walls and floors that are being dismantled can contain irritating dust and mold. Lightly spraying water on walls and floors that are to be demolished or on surfaces that are to be swept can help reduce dust aerosol.

At the end of the day, don't let the workers clean up with a shop vacuum unless it has a HEPA filter, since this may defeat all your precautions. (The filtration in most shop vacuums I have seen was inadequate, and dust was spewed into the air when the vacuum was running.) If possible, use a HEPA vacuum for all cleaning, and be sure the work area is kept sealed until the cleaning is complete. When the job is done, damp-wipe all the surfaces.

Even smaller projects such as hanging a picture, putting in a new electrical outlet, or installing a phone line can kick up irritating dust. When you drill a hole to hang a picture, for example, plaster dust is released into the air and onto carpeting. If the wall is covered with horsehair plaster and you are allergic to horses, you may cough or sneeze. Whenever I disturbed the horsehair plaster in a home that Connie and I used to own, I had someone operate a HEPA vacuum while I worked. Changing a sash cord in an old double-hung window isn't major renovation work, but you are still disturbing potentially irritating dust, so be cautious. If you are bothered by dust, wear a NIOSH N95 two-strap fine-particle mask when you or others are doing even minor renovation work in your home. Take your mask off after, not before, you change your dirty clothing.

PETS AT WORK

Sometimes I see dogs on construction sites because workers have brought their pets with them. If you are renovating your home or building a new one and are allergic to dogs, be sure none of the workers keeps a beloved pet inside for company. A few weeks of daily bombardment with dog dander particles are enough to thoroughly contaminate any hot-air system.

OIL AND LATEX PAINTS

Oil paints today are made with ingredients similar to those in lead paint, except that the pigments do not contain lead. About half of the volume of liquid in a can of oil paint consists of volatile thinner. Indoor spaces that are being painted fill with solvent fumes as the thinner evaporates. Some states have banned oil paints.

Today, most paints are water based (latex) and do not contain significant amounts of linseed oil or solvents. Latex paint does contain pigment and binder, but instead of being mixed with the water as a continuous fluid, the pigment and binder are suspended in water. The binder is dispersed as microscopic oily droplets, similar to the way butterfat is distributed throughout cream. This type of mixture is called an emulsion.

In latex paints, chemicals must be added to keep the oily droplets from coalescing and to prevent microbial decay during storage in the can. (If old latex paint smells sour, don't use it; there is microbial growth present.) Other chemicals are added to control flow (viscosity).

After latex paint is applied to a surface, the water and some of the other added volatile chemicals evaporate. Once the water is gone, all the oily droplets coalesce to form a coherent paint film. The pigment particles that were suspended in the water end up stuck in the film. Latex paint on a brush and in freshly applied films can be removed with water because the droplets are still dispersible. But once the water evaporates and the droplets coalesce, water cannot remove the paint because water and oil are immiscible (they do not mix).

The air in a room may be irritating while the water and chemicals added to latex paint are evaporating. Although the risk of exposure to VOCs (volatile organic compounds) is far less than with oil-based paint, those with chemical sensitivities should still be cautious about entering a space that has recently been painted. If off-gassing from oil or latex paint bothers you, check in your hardware store for the most environmentally safe paint.

When water-based paint first appeared on the market, it was called latex because the white binder emulsion resembled latex "milk," a natural product gathered from rubber trees much like the way that sap is collected from maple trees to make syrup. As far as I know, latex paint never really contained latex from rubber trees. Today, "latex paint" is a generic term for water-based paint, which is completely synthetic; the binder is generally acrylic or vinyl. People with latex allergies should of course check with the paint manufacturer to be certain the emulsion is latex-free, but it is unlikely that any room painted with a newer, water-based paint would present a latex risk, despite the moniker.

PAINT WITH MILDEWCIDE

Some clients want to use paint indoors that contains mildewcide. If dust collects on a surface that has been painted with this kind of product, mold can still grow in the surface dust if there is excess moisture in the space. The best way to prevent mold growth indoors is to keep painted interior surfaces clean and dry. Paint with mildewcide can be used at the exterior.

PAINT STRIPPING AND PAINTING

People with asthma probably shouldn't strip paint without checking with their physicians, and anyone doing such work should use respiratory protection. Regardless of the method, removing paint entails exposure to dust and fumes.

Connie's mother had a miscarriage after she spent the afternoon painting the sides of a deep, in-ground rectangular pool with an oil-based paint. There was little ventilation, so she was exposed to solvents. I also read a newspaper story about a man who was using a chemical stripper to remove paint at the bottom of a closed stairway. The vapors from this particular paint stripper are denser than air, and because he was in a small, enclosed space, the vapors eventually displaced the air where he was working. The fumes contained the solvent methylene chloride, which in high concentrations is a "narcotic" and makes people drowsy.[1] The man probably became confused, and according to the newspaper account, he died from asphyxiation.

What is the purpose of having a toxic solvent in paint strippers? Paint, if properly applied, sticks like glue. Paint films on wood are particularly tenacious because the surface is uneven. To get an idea of the microscopic appearance of a wood surface, imagine cutting across a bundle of straws, exposing the numerous parallel channels. Paint flows into the channels, and when it hardens, it fits like a key in a lock. The solvent methylene chloride has a unique property: it diffuses into the paint film and makes it swell, just as water makes a dry sponge swell. Once the film swells, it becomes flexible, and its bond with the wood is weakened. The paint can then be more easily scraped off the surface.

A few brave souls strip paint with heat guns, which produce toxic smoke as the paint is thermally decomposed. The film becomes less viscous and therefore softer as its temperature rises. There is thus a temptation to overheat the film and speed up removal. Unfortunately, this produces more smoke (in part owing to thermal decomposition) and increases the likelihood of fire. Many buildings, including historical ones, have burned to the ground because of impatient or careless use of heat guns.

Most people sand a surface to prepare it for repainting rather than stripping off the old paint layers. Sanding creates dust that should be contained. The area should also be sealed and ventilated during painting. Be sure to allow time for any volatile compounds to evaporate from the paint film before moving back into the space (see chap. 23).

HOME OFFICES

Many major renovations are undertaken to add office space to a home. More and more people are working from their homes, and the old "study" is evolving into a professional office with desks, swivel chairs, copiers, fax machines, computers, and the like.

I encourage people to increase the ventilation in a home office. Install exhausts for office machines or place such machines in their own well-ventilated spaces. Photocopiers may emit small amounts of ozone (a potentially irritating gas) and styrene (another irritating, volatile organic compound and a potential carcinogen). Photocopying uses a high voltage on an electric wire. If you have ever smelled a shirt hung outside to dry on a sunny day, you can recognize the odor of ozone gas. Even though the smell may remind us of stepping out in the fresh air, excess levels of ozone gas are associated with air pollution.

Another odor that comes from copiers is produced by heated plastic. An image being transferred to paper initially consists of powdered black ink that contains carbon, plastic, iron particles, and small amounts of solvents. The paper then passes through a fuser: a very hot wire in a glass tube. The ink melts when it absorbs the radiant heat from the fuser, and this causes the plastic to stick to the paper. Some of the heated plastic thermally decomposes, producing by-products that can be irritating. Plastics in computers, video monitors, and cables also off-gas irritants or can even smell like mold!

If you find that the air in your home office is bothering you or if you are chemically sensitive, I recommend you purchase metal office furniture. Remember that dust mite allergens can accumulate in the cushions of an office chair. A leather-covered chair is a good alternative.

OTHER CAUTIONS ABOUT ADDITIONS AND NEW CONSTRUCTION

Whether you are building an addition to your home, living in a newly constructed house, or planning to build a home from the ground up, I have several pieces of advice to share.

CRAWL SPACES

It's always cheaper to build an addition over a crawl space than over a full basement, but don't be seduced (see chap. 15). If you must have a crawl space, be certain the floor is poured concrete and install XPS (extruded polystyrene) insulation at the exterior of the walls and beneath the concrete floor. If you cannot install XPS at the exterior, the walls of the crawl space should be insulated with foil-faced sheet foam such as Thermax (a minimum of one inch thick or whatever is required by the building code in your locale). Check with your local building department on the requirements for use of sheet foam in basements. I don't recommend insulating between the floor joists with fiberglass because the insulation collects biodegradable dust and attracts rodents. (See chap. 22 for a discussion of spray polyurethane foam, or SPF, insulation, which is installed both below and above grade.)

Lastly, a clean crawl space should be open to a dehumidified basement. If the crawl space is large, you can dehumidify it separately. A crawl space with a dirt floor, visible mold growth, or a musty smell should not be left open to the basement. Isolate such a space both from the basement and the exterior, and dehumidify it separately. It's always best, though, to cover a dirt floor or have a musty, below-grade space professionally remediated under containment conditions.

INSULATING ABOVE GRADE

In a retrofit installation when insulation is blown into walls, the air used pressurizes the wall cavities and disturbs the dust in the cavities. This air has to come out somewhere, and most of it exits to the exterior through the holes drilled in the siding. But some air can enter the living spaces through electrical outlets, switches, and window gaps. If you are planning to have insulation blown into your home and are allergic to house dust, seal all gaps in interior walls with removable painter's tape and arrange to be out of the house during installation. When the installation is complete, you should HEPA vacuum your home and air it out well.

CARPETING

I discourage people with allergies or asthma from installing wall-to-wall carpeting in renovated or new spaces. I inspected one new house in which the installed carpeting was off-gassing so strongly it was difficult to spend time there. Most manufacturers recommend that people ventilate a house thoroughly after installing new wall-to-wall carpeting.

DUCTED SYSTEMS

In every new house I inspect, I look into the ducts with a mirror and flashlight and find all sorts of debris: sawdust, drywall dust, pieces of wood, and even tools. On one inspection I found a doughnut bag with food and a coffee cup inside, and the duct was full of sawdust and plaster dust. I told the buyers to insist that the heating system and ducts be professionally cleaned (a costly effort) before they closed on the house.

They asked me to reinspect the property shortly before the closing date, and I made a point of checking the duct where I had seen the doughnut. The duct looked cleaner, but when I removed the register and looked in with a mirror and flashlight, I could see that someone had cleaned only the end of the duct by inserting a vacuum into it. Now that old doughnut was even farther away, joined by a roll of duct tape. Even if people are just having floors sanded, I always recommend that hot-air heating systems and ductwork be sealed or protected by filters if possible, then thoroughly and professionally cleaned after the work is finished. When you purchase a new house, insist that the air conveyance system be as clean as surfaces in the rest of the house (fig 21.1).

When Connie and I downsized, we committed to a house before it was even built. We chose hot-water heat by baseboard rather than hot-air heat. The house had a separate ducted air conditioning system. I insisted that the ducts be sealed as soon as they were installed and that the air handlers not be installed until construction was complete and the house had been thoroughly cleaned. Luckily, the house was constructed during clement weather, but if need be, we were ready to supply oil-filled radiators for heat. We also chose hardwood flooring instead of carpeting. We made a lot of choices to help create a healthier indoor environment, and even though it involved great expense, it was worth it.

I corresponded by email with a woman in the Midwest who told me she developed asthma and mold allergies after her home was flooded. She tried everything she could think of to clean up the house, but her efforts seemed futile. She decided to sell the house and build a new one that would be environmentally safer for her. She hoped she would

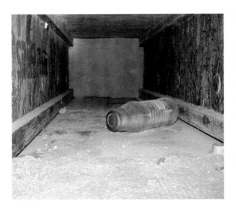

FIGURE 21.1. This photo was taken by placing a camera inside a panned-bay return duct in a newly constructed home. The walls of the return duct consist of a pair of "I" joists supporting a floor. The duct "bottom" in the foreground and the rear-end seal consist of fiberglass duct board, which is yellow when clean. The bottom of the duct is covered with sawdust from construction (and a juice bottle from a thirsty worker!).

be able to stay in the old home until the new house was ready, but the air made her feel so ill that she began to sleep in her car.

She wanted to have baseboard heat in the new house instead of hot-air heat, but the builder persuaded her to install a forced hot-air system with air conditioning. The new home was completed in the middle of the summer, and she turned on the air conditioning as soon as she moved in. Within a few days, her asthma symptoms increased. The air conditioning had been operating when the builders were working on the house, and I suspect the entire interior of the air-handling unit (AHU) became coated with construction dust that then got wet from condensation. She suffered for months and even considered moving again, but she ended up replacing the ducts and having the AHU professionally cleaned. All the internal fibrous lining material had to be replaced.

FLOODING

A home that has been flooded can be renovated, but any possible sources of concealed decay must be eliminated. One family purchased a home that had been extensively renovated after a serious flood. Many of the ceilings and walls had been replaced, and new bathrooms and a new kitchen had been installed. Unfortunately, the warped maple flooring had been left in place but covered with wall-to-wall carpeting. After the renovation, the husband, who worked on small carpentry projects in the basement, began to have trouble breathing. He was diagnosed with asthma and severe allergy to mold, and he was finding it increasingly hard to control his symptoms.

I found large clumps of fine dust hanging in strings from the basement floor joists. Each clump was directly below a gap in the plank subflooring. When I looked at the dust samples with a microscope, I found they consisted of numerous *Penicillium* mold spores, decayed cellulose, bits of carpet padding, and microarthropod fecal material. I suspect that water was trapped between the subfloor and floor after the flood, and extensive decay and mold growth followed. Whenever anyone walked on the carpet above, the loose maple floor flexed, and allergenic dust was forced out of the spaces between the subfloor and floor and into the basement air (though some of the dust stuck to the joists). Immediately after my visit, the owner decided to remove the dust from the joists. He did not wear a mask and touched the material directly. Within hours he was wheezing and had hives. He is planning to remove the carpeting and maple flooring. Before new hardwood flooring is installed, the moldy subfloor will also have to be replaced.

If you have dust allergies, handle dust that may be contaminated with the utmost care. If you are considering purchasing a home that has been renovated, be sure to find out if there has been any flooding.

IRRITATING OR ALLERGENIC CONSTRUCTION MATERIALS

Construction materials can be irritating to some people. Although suppliers of paints and other building materials may claim their products are less irritating than other products on the market, any product can be a threat to chemically sensitive individuals. Try to obtain a sample of the material before it is applied or installed to see if you find it irritating or allergenic. Surprisingly, one material you should check before it goes into your building is wood. In the basements of many new homes I have found floor joists covered with mold. The surface of even pressure-treated wood (wood treated with copper arsenate to prevent decay caused by mold and insects) can support mold growth. The preservative protects the cellulose, but the sugars in the wood sap probably leach to the surface and provide food for microorganisms. And biodegradable dust that collects on such surfaces can be more fodder for microbial growth.

In the first decade of the twenty-first century, drywall was imported from China to rebuild homes that had been damaged by hurricanes. The drywall emitted sulfurous odors that sickened occupants and blackened copper wires. The chemical emissions were stronger in warm and humid climates. The defective drywall had to be replaced in thousands of homes.

SOME RECOMMENDATIONS

HOME OFFICES

- If you are chemically sensitive, install an exhaust system for home office copiers and printers, or place these machines in their own well-ventilated spaces.

REAL ESTATE SALES

- If you are selling your house and you have allergies, ask the listing broker to alert agents that prospective buyers should not bring pets into your home.

RENOVATION AND CONSTRUCTION

- During renovations, physically isolate the work areas, cover or remove personal possessions, and create negative air pressure.

- Use clean drop cloths.

- In an air conveyance system, install filter material at supply registers and return grilles.

- Rather than operating the heating or cooling system during renovation or construction work, consider using oil-filled radiators for heat or portable air conditioners for cooling. Close and cover supplies and returns.

- Keep out of the work areas. If you must enter, wear a NIOSH N95 two-strap mask.

- Seal all gaps in exterior walls and arrange to be out of the house during installation of blown-in insulation. HEPA vacuum your home after the procedure has been completed (refer to chap. 24).

- Clean surfaces and air the house out thoroughly after renovation projects.

- If you are sensitized to volatile organic compounds (paints, varnishes, cleaning compounds, etc.), test any products before they are used to be sure they don't bother you.

- If you have mold allergies, make sure that the wood being used in the project is not covered with mold growth.

MORE ENVIRONMENTAL HAZARDS

22.

In this chapter we discuss more environmental hazards as well as a type of insulation that, if not properly installed, could result in noxious odors and potential hazards to health.

LEAD

LEAD IN PAINT

Lead paint is a particular problem in areas where the housing stock was built prior to 1978, when lead paint was banned. By now, most people know the dangers of lead paint, but I still hear stories about homeowners who are doing their own renovations. When repainting walls in an older home, people might sand old paint that has lead in it. One young couple was putting their house on the market because their second child had just been born and they needed a larger home. The listing real estate agent suggested they could increase the home's appeal by repainting the interior. They began preparing the walls and woodwork for painting while they were still living in the house. They were diligent, so they thoroughly sanded all the surfaces in the century-old house. The house was marketed before all the painting was completed, and the couple received a strong offer more quickly than they had anticipated.

The buyers hired me to do their prepurchase inspection and arranged to have a lead paint inspector at the property the same time I was there. While I was testing electrical outlets in the new baby's room, I noticed a look of great concern on the lead inspector's face.

A few minutes later, he took the buyers and me outside for a consultation. He said the levels of lead in the house were the highest he had ever seen; even the infant's blankets and teddy bear were contaminated with unsafe levels of lead dust. He told us he was going to warn the sellers to evacuate the home immediately.

Lead paint was an oil-based paint that consisted of pigment, linseed oil, and solvent. The lead was in the pigment as a finely ground white powder. The obvious purpose of pigment is to color paint, but a less obvious yet even more important function is to hide the color of the surface below. One reason lead pigment was so widely used in the past is that it has extremely high hiding power. The linseed oil formed a binder for the powdered pigment, and the solvent thinned the pigment and binder so that the mixture could be applied with a brush. After the oil paint was spread, the solvent evaporated, leaving a viscous film of pigment and binder. Oxygen from the air combined with linseed oil in the coating so that it thickened, eventually "drying" to a hard plastic film. A very small amount of a sweet-tasting chemical called lead acetate (referred to as "sugar of lead") was sometimes added to paint to speed the drying. Paint containing lead pigment does not taste sweet, but people have believed that it does because of the chemical additive's common name. (A substance can only taste sweet if it dissolves in saliva. Lead pigment cannot dissolve in saliva and therefore cannot taste sweet.)

Paint that peels from a surface usually comes off in large chips, and children can get lead poisoning by eating those chips. I believe, however, that most children are poisoned by ingesting lead paint dust. Paint that is weathered, worn, or sanded from a surface consists of either microscopic pigment particles or barely visible dust particles. Children who touch the surfaces and lick their hands can easily ingest particles that settle on surfaces or mix with other types of dust in carpeting.

If you want to do cosmetic work in an older home, don't start sanding the painted surfaces (or let anyone else do so) before you've had the paint tested for lead. Most hardware stores sell inexpensive lead paint test kits, or you can hire a lead paint inspector to do the test for you. If lead paint is found, it should be encapsulated or removed by a professional according to whatever local, state, and federal regulations apply.

A house should always be thoroughly cleaned (including the furnace and ducts of an air conveyance system) after lead paint has been removed. One woman had many environmental concerns about her new home. Because she had young children, she wanted to be sure it was as clean and safe as possible before she moved in. The house

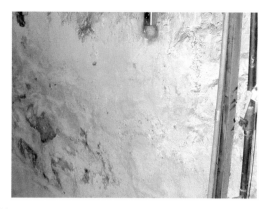

FIGURE 22.1. This stone foundation wall in the basement of a Victorian home was first coated with a yellow "white wash" containing chrome yellow pigment, a lead-containing compound. Years later, the yellow coating was covered with white paint. Dampness in the stone wall caused the paint to peel away from the white wash, allowing fine dust containing the lead pigment to fall to the floor.

had already been de-leaded, and she asked me for some suggestions for improving indoor air quality (IAQ). I removed the grille from the floor return duct. The area just inside the duct had been thoroughly vacuumed, but I could see a mat of dust more than an inch thick when I used a mirror and flashlight to look deeper into the duct. I took a dust sample and sent it to a laboratory for lead analysis. The lab found over 1,100 parts per million (ppm) of lead in the dust. I told the woman to postpone moving in until her furnace and ducts were professionally cleaned and the whole house completely HEPA vacuumed afterward. Some of the ducts might even have had to be replaced.

A young family with an asthmatic child had an accepted offer on an older home. They were concerned that the house might have a moldy basement, and their home inspector suggested that they hire me to inspect the basement. There was some typical mold growth on the ceiling, but what struck me as odd were the mounds of fine yellow powder at the base of all of the stone foundation walls. The walls had been painted white, but beneath the layer of white paint was a deteriorating yellow coating that had probably been placed on the foundation decades earlier (fig. 22.1).

As a chemist, I am familiar with the components of some yellow pigments and was concerned that the readily aerosolized, fine yellow powder might contain lead chromate: a yellow pigment used before lead was banned. I took a sample of the dust to a lab for analysis, and it indeed contained lead chromate. The dust on the basement floor was so fine that it could have been deposited in dust all over the house, so I recommended that the buyers have the dust in the entire house tested for lead before proceeding with the purchase. I don't know what happened in this transaction, but I hope they took my warning seriously.

LEAD IN SOIL

The soil around a home whose exterior has been repeatedly scraped and then repainted with lead paint can have high lead concentrations, although a great deal of the lead in soil is residue from leaded gasoline. If you live in an older home and have young children or plan to have a flower or vegetable garden, it's a good idea to have the soil around the house tested for lead. Because of the potential risks, children should not play in soil within three feet of an older house.

If children play in a lead-contaminated area, the dirt that sticks to their shoes can be carried into the house, particularly if they wear sneakers with waffle-patterned soles. The lead contamination can then be distributed into rugs or wall-to-wall carpeting, and people who sit on such rugs and carpeting will be exposed—especially children who sit and play on the floor. Lead dust that is introduced into carpeting from contaminated soil, used drop cloths, or sanded surfaces can never be completely removed, no matter how frequently the carpet is washed or vacuumed. The carpet will continue to be a hazard for years to come. (As I mentioned previously, vinyl and wood floors are preferable to carpeting because smooth surfaces capture less dust and are easier to keep dust-free.)

LEAD IN CARPETING

If you suspect that your carpeting is contaminated with lead dust, take a vacuum sample of the dust and have it tested. If the concentration of lead is high and the lab notes a health risk, get rid of the carpet as soon as possible, using the same caution as for the removal of any lead-contaminated material.

ASBESTOS

Asbestos is a mineral fiber that for years was frequently used in construction materials because of its unusual properties. For example, asbestos fibers are not combustible, so they were used for fireproofing. Pressed together and shaped into cylinders, asbestos fibers were used as pipe insulation. Asbestos fibers reinforced floor tiles, joint compound, and exterior roof and wall shingles. Asbestos (like horsehair) was added to skim plaster, both to strengthen the material and to give it texture.

Plaster containing asbestos is a composite, a mixture of two or more materials that has properties superior to those of the separate

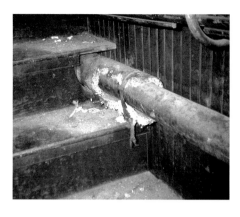

FIGURE 22.2. For years, heat pipes were wrapped with asbestos-containing insulation. Some forms of the insulation were brittle and crumbled under pressure. The treads on this basement stairway are covered with asbestos-containing dust that was aerosolized with every step.

ingredients alone. For example, paper falls apart when immersed in water, and thin layers of wax are brittle, but if you soak heavy paper in wax, the composite can be used as a container for liquid (milk, for example), and it doesn't break when bent. Particle board, another composite, is made of "sawdust" and glue. Concrete and asbestos also form a composite. Concrete that is less than an inch thick breaks easily. If enough asbestos fibers are added, the concrete is strong even when thin, and the resulting composite can be formed into roof tiles or siding shingles.

WHERE MIGHT YOU FIND VISIBLE ASBESTOS

I have seen many homes with older hot-air heating systems (the "octopuses" I referred to in chap. 18) that had the furnaces and ducts wrapped in asbestos insulation. We had asbestos pipe insulation in our own Victorian, and the day after the closing and before we moved in, I hired a professional remediation company to remove all of it. I prefer removal to encapsulation (or wrapping) because the cost of the two options is about the same and, more importantly, if any repair to the heating system or pipes is needed, asbestos-containing materials (ACMs) will still have to be disturbed even if they are encapsulated (fig. 22.2).

Asbestos can be found in areas other than in the basement. I inspected one house that had been foreclosed and then abandoned. The roof had been leaking, and the moisture had caused widespread damage to the ceilings and walls—a shame, because the hundred-year-old house had many wonderful architectural details. The oak and maple floors were littered with chips of plaster from the walls. When the house was built, a skim coat of plaster textured with asbestos had been applied to make the walls look like stone. I could see small tufts at the edges of the broken chips. The buyer sent samples of the chips to a lab for testing, and the results were positive. Before selling the foreclosed home, the bank was forced to do a costly cleanup.

One buyer asked me to inspect a recently renovated multimillion-dollar home on a large lot. She warned me that the seller had disclosed that the fifty-year-old roofing shingles were made of an asbestos-cement composite. I looked at the roof from the ground with binoculars, and the shingles seemed to be in satisfactory condition. But when I went up to the attic bedroom and looked out the dormer window onto the roof surface, I could see that the shingles had worn thin and that white tufts of asbestos were sticking up where the concrete had weathered away.

It then occurred to me that the asbestos eroding from the surface of the roof might be ending up in the gutter and then in the soil around the house. I put a ladder up at the front of the house near a porch gutter. The debris in the gutter was white. The buyer took a sample of the gutter debris and sent it to a lab for analysis; it was 25 percent asbestos! Where the gutters were overflowing at another spot, soil was splashing up against the side of the house. I took a sample of the caked-on dirt, and that too was sent for analysis. The sample contained 10 percent asbestos. Needless to say, mitigation of the roof and soil was needed, and it proved costly. If your house has or ever has had asbestos roof shingles, there could be a significant level of asbestos in the soil around the building.

Asbestos can be disturbed during renovation. One family installing new flooring in a finished basement used a floor sander to remove the old glued-on floor tiles. The tiles contained asbestos, and the collection bag for the sanding machine allowed contaminated dust to escape into the air. The house dust became so filled with asbestos fibers that family members developed skin rashes. The entire house had to be professionally remediated.

If you suspect you have asbestos-containing materials inside or outside your home, have the materials or soil tested by licensed professionals.

ASBESTOS REMOVAL

Inhaling asbestos fibers can cause a rare type of chest cancer called mesothelioma, which can appear years after someone's exposure to asbestos fibers. There are three common mineral forms of asbestos fibers: amosite, chrysotile, and crocidolite. Fortunately, chrysotile, the form of the mineral most widely used in the United States, is generally considered the least carcinogenic.

Asbestos-cement siding shingles generally are not as much of a concern because they are not subject to erosion by rain the way roof shingles are. Asbestos siding can also be painted, which helps prevent release of fibers. If you want to remove asbestos siding, the same care must be exercised as in removing roof shingles containing asbestos.

I was inspecting the outside of one house and noticed numerous light-colored chips on top of the soil. I suspected that the chips might be broken bits of asbestos-cement shingles. I asked the owner about them, and she proudly replied that it had cost her only $500 to have a neighbor remove all her siding. Unfortunately, the neighbor was not qualified to do the work.

If you know you have ACM on your roof, heat pipes, or furnace, do not remove the material yourself. Always have asbestos professionally removed, or you and your family could be breathing in the fibers for years to come.

SPRAY FOAM INSULATION

In the 1960s, building codes began to require insulation in newly constructed homes. In surfaces and cavities exposed to the exterior or unconditioned spaces, insulation reduces heat loss in cold weather and heat gain in hot weather, thus reducing the consumption of energy.

For many decades, fiberglass and cellulose insulations dominated the insulation market. More recently, spray polyurethane foam (SPF) insulation has become popular. Unlike fiberglass and cellulose, which can be purchased and installed as-is, SPF must be "manufactured" on-site. Formed by rapidly mixing two liquid chemical components pumped from 55-gallon drums and fed through a spray gun nozzle, the SPF mixture is sprayed onto a surface, typically inside a wall, ceiling, or roof cavity, but sometimes also directly on a foundation wall.

The two liquid components in SPF are referred to as A and B. Component A consists of isocyanate compounds; component B consists of a polyol compound but also contains a fire retardant and may contain a catalyst to speed the chemical reaction necessary for installation of the foam. When the A and B liquids are mixed in the spray gun, a violent chemical reaction takes place that produces bubbles and a great deal of heat. The chemical reactions continue as the foam accumulates on the targeted surfaces. The reaction subsides within seconds, and assuming that the surfaces are compatible with SPF and are clean and dry, a solid foam sticks to the surfaces onto which the SPF components have been sprayed.

There are two different kinds of SPF insulation in common use. The first type is open-cell foam (a sponge is an example of open-cell foam). Open-cell insulating foam can be applied in a single application to a final depth of up to six or more inches. The solidified foam is crumbly and porous. Since there are openings between the individual foam cells, moisture and air can flow, albeit extremely slowly, through the foam, so although open-cell SPF is an air barrier, it is not a vapor retarder.

The second type of foam is called closed-cell foam. It is denser than the open-cell foam and is very hard. There are no openings between the foam cells, so neither air nor water vapor can move through the foam. Since the foam-forming reaction produces a great deal of heat, and the dense foam does not allow for movement or heat or moisture, closed-cell foam must be applied differently than open-cell foam is applied. Most closed-cell foams cannot be applied in a layer (called a "lift") thicker than two inches (though some newer "high-lift" products allow thicker lifts). Depending on the depth of insulation needed, at least two or three lifts are typically installed. The lifts are supposed to be installed one on top of another, but only after a 20- to 30-minute interval between lifts to allow for cooling.

If closed-cell foam is installed too thickly, the heat from the chemical reactions within the foam cannot be dissipated quickly enough to prevent the interior temperature of the foam from exceeding the decomposition (chemical breakdown) of the foam and catalyst. This decomposition can produce odorous chemicals.

There are many other variables that can complicate the installation of SPF and lead to problems in the foam. For a proper installation, the surfaces onto which the foam is to be installed must be dry and should not be less than the published lower temperature limits or more than the published upper temperature limits for the particular formulation. Many manufactures have seasonal formulations that are catalyzed to work optimally with a range of ambient and substrate (surface) temperatures. The individual A and B components must be heated to about 125°F before being mixed. The drums of chemicals should never be stored at temperatures below freezing and should not be used beyond their shelf life (typically about six months). The chemicals must also be combined in an exact ratio of one part component A to one part component B at a pressure of at least 1,000 pounds per square inch (psi), though some formulations (such as those available to do-it-yourselfers) can be processed at lower pressures.

In view of all the technical variables that must be controlled and the conditions that must be present before and during SPF installations, it's no surprise that some installations result in problems. It is my understanding that about 1 in 500 (.2 percent) or 1 in 1,000 (.1 percent) SPF installations are associated with long-term odor emissions and other defects such as cracks and delamination.

We have worked with people who were so strongly affected by the odors (the chemical emissions) from SPF insulations that they had to have all the insulation removed. Some people became so sensitized to the chemical emissions that they were forced to move out of their

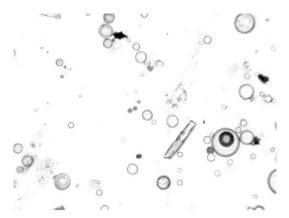

FIGURE 22.3. At the center of this micrograph of dust from the inside of a duct is a chain of three pink-stained Pen/Asp (*Penicillium* or *Aspergillus*) mold spores that measure approximately 3 microns in size. The many other round particles are spheres of spray polyurethane foam (SPF) insulation that settled from the air into the open duct during installation of SPF insulation in a home addition. The spheres could then be circulated within the duct system. The largest SPF sphere at the right contains a gas bubble; attached to the large sphere is a smaller, pink-stained SPF sphere. Eventually, all the SPF spheres will take up stain and turn pink (light micrograph).

homes. One family was having their dream house constructed and chose to have SPF insulation installed in every exterior wall cavity. The insulation was not installed properly, and the resulting odors were so irritating that the family could not live in the house. In another home in which SPF was installed only in the attic, the odor of the insulation was so strong that the homeowner sold the property. The buyer was a contractor, and he removed the entire roof to eliminate the problem.

Since the principal component in the A side is a mixture of isocyanates, a great deal of research has been done pertaining to installer exposure, because isocyanates are highly toxic and carcinogenic. Little research, however, has been done with respect to installers' exposures to B-side chemicals, and even less research has been done with respect to installers' or occupants' exposures to SPF dust.

I have taken hundreds of air samples in homes with SPF insulation. In a number of these homes I found many microscopic "droplets" of solid foam in the air. These sphere-shaped droplets form as the mixed chemicals exit the spray gun, producing a cloud of aerosol (atomized particles). The droplets contain all chemicals in the foam; some of these droplets are small enough to be inhaled deep in the lung (fig. 22.3).

There is another reason to be concerned about SPF dust. Because foams are highly combustible, they must be formulated with fire

The do-it-yourself foam kits are low-pressure kits and do not produce much atomized foam.

retardants. There has been a great deal of public concern regarding the presence of fire retardants in furnishings and clothing. One of the fire retardants of concern is TCPP, which is the principal fire retardant in most spray foams. TCPP stands for tris(1-chloro-2-propyl) phosphate. This chemical can compose up to 20 to 30 percent of the B component. It is therefore important that all dust resulting from an SPF insulation be cleaned up with a HEPA-filtered vacuum before re-occupancy.

If you are considering having SPF insulation installed, search the Internet using the terms "spray foam" and "odor" to get an idea of what has been happening with respect to SPF. Check for reviews of the installers you are considering hiring. Only use an installer who has at least five years of experience installing SPF. Make sure your installer has a rigorous air quality management plan designed to protect your home. Never enter a home while SPF is being installed, and remain away for at least a day or two after the job is done (the re-occupancy time is typically provided by the foam manufacturer in the company's literature and should be conveyed to you by the installer). Consider hiring a third-party professional to oversee the project, especially if it's a larger job.

If you have already had SPF installed in your home and there is a significant odor problem as a result, there are some steps you can take to mitigate the odor. If the insulation is in the attic, a small exhaust fan that operates in the attic 24/7 and blows air to the exterior can reduce odor infiltration into the rooms below the attic (or adjacent to the attic, if the attic consists of eaves). Chemical odors cannot penetrate aluminum foil, so you can also cover the offending SPF with a radiant barrier consisting of paper laminated with aluminum foil. The only odor that can then escape the foam is the odor that might leak through seams and around the perimeter of the barrier. (You can even cover a wall with this barrier, stapled to the studs, if the insulation has been installed in the wall cavity and the SPF is still exposed.) If a closed-cell foam installation in an attic is off-gassing a dead fish odor, you can have the foam spray-painted with a shellac-based paint. This may be effective (test a small area first), because shellac consists of an acid, and the dead-fish odor is produced by the amine catalyst, a base. The acid in the shellac film can neutralize the base causing the odor.

SPF is an outstanding insulation and when processed and installed properly can outperform any other type of insulation. Manufacturers should educate installers on safe and proper techniques for their SPF work before the insulation is banned the way urea formaldehyde foam insulation (UFFI) was banned (UFFI was a type of foam insulation used in the 1970s that made people ill).

ELECTROMAGNETIC FIELDS

A growing number of people are calling us because they are concerned about electromagnetic fields (EMFs) emanating from electric-operated equipment and devices, including household appliances, Wi-Fi networks, computers, and electrical equipment such as transformers, wiring, electric meters, and panels. Many people are also concerned about EMF from battery-operated devices such as cell phones.

One client of ours who is sensitive to chemicals and EMFs worked hard to cleanse her house of substances that could cause her to have symptoms such as headaches and fatigue. She lived in a fairly isolated area with no power stations nearby, used low-VOC (volatile organic compound) paints and unfragranced body and cleaning products, and had hard flooring throughout her house rather than carpeting, which can off-gas odors (that "new carpeting" smell). She also had a minimal number of electric devices in her home. Still, she worried about intermittent power outages that sometimes occurred in the area, so she decided to have a generator installed outside her house. She asked the installer to put as many of the electrical components for the generator as possible at the exterior of the house.

She began to experience headaches shortly after the generator was installed. I don't think she realized that the electric panel for the generator would be in her basement. She tried to live with the situation for a month or so, but in the end she decided to have the generator and all its electric components removed from her property. She lost quite a bit of money but felt better.

Among many health care professionals, the jury is still out regarding the potential deleterious effects that EMFs can have on human health. More research seems to have been done in Europe than in the United States on this issue. One review of studies[1] stated that "The major part of exposure to magnetic fields originates from household electric devices that are used commonly by the general public," but the study goes on to state, "such exposure is extremely limited."According to the study, an exception to limited exposure would be the presence of electric underfloor heating (radiant). In conclusion, the study's authors assume that more research will be done to "gain a complete picture of the exposure levels."

If you believe that you have symptoms of exposure to electromagnetic fields, the World Health Organization provides a fact sheet[2] about this condition. Some of the remediation steps taken to reduce exposure to EMF include reducing the number of Wi-Fi devices in a home and increasing the distance of a bed from exterior wiring (the service entry cable) and interior sources of EMF such as digital clocks.

In a home Connie and I lived in, the lights once started blinking; the lights intermittently got brighter upstairs and dimmer downstairs. The neutral wire for our new electrical service had not been properly connected outside the home, so the electrical connection was not adequate. Every time the lights blinked, I measured about 10 amps of power going through my water main to the street instead of going through the neutral wire of the electrical system and into the power grid. In another home where we lived across the street from a hospital, I measured 16 amps of current coming intermittently into my home from the water main. When electric current flows through interior copper piping in a home, significant EMFs are created.

Another remediation that people undertake to reduce EMF problems in homes is to insert a plastic piece of piping between the water main and the house piping. This stops the flow of current into the home but also eliminates the grounding of the system, so alternative grounding must be installed. (Most newer homes have water mains made of plastic, so electric current cannot flow into the home from the city water system, and alternative grounding is already present.)

SOME RECOMMENDATIONS

- If you live in a house that was constructed before 1978, have the paint in your home and the soil outside tested for lead.

- If you suspect or know that the soil around your home contains lead, do all you can to prevent dirt from coming into the house. Have people take their shoes off at the door, for example.

- Don't sand lead paint.

- Asbestos testing must always be done by licensed professionals. There are kits that home occupants can purchase for asbestos testing, but because of the risk of exposure to the material, we don't recommend the use of such kits.

- Always have lead paint and asbestos removed by licensed professionals.

- Check licensing in your state for paint and asbestos testers and remediation companies.

- If you are considering having SPF (spray polyurethane foam) insulation installed in your home, hire a company that has been doing these installations for at least five years, and do not remain in the property while the product is being installed.

- People with chemical sensitivities should probably be wary of installing SPF in their homes.

23.
TESTING AND REMEDIATION

In this chapter we introduce you to some of the many tests that home occupants as well as indoor air quality (IAQ) professionals can use. We also discuss remediation work that you could consider doing yourself and work that only professionals should tackle.

TESTING: WHAT'S THE GOAL?

The goal of any IAQ testing should be to identify potential sources of indoor contaminants and allergens in order to determine effective remediation steps. Air sampling alone does not reach that goal, though air sampling can certainly be useful in determining what may be in the air that people inhale.

People often ask me what additional services I provide in addition to IAQ consulting work. My answer? None. As far as I'm concerned, investigating building problems should be an IAQ professional's primary business endeavor. Most IAQ professionals are ethical. Still, as a consumer, I would be a little suspicious if an IAQ professional tries to sell me expensive equipment or if the professional owns, works for, or has other business connections with a remediation company. It may be convenient to have a "one-stop shop" when you work with one company, but such business connections could represent a potential conflict of interest.

TESTS THAT HOME OCCUPANTS CAN CONDUCT

There are a number of test kits available. Some are passive devices, meaning that they do not have pumps that move air. Other test kits are direct-read, meaning that the results can be read directly from the device itself, which typically is electrically powered. Depending on the vapor or gas you want to measure, you might find the test you are looking for in a home improvement store or online, or acquire the test kit from a laboratory.

Below are some of the options of tests and equipment you could find in many hardware or building-supply stores or online. Some of these are more expensive than others.

- radon test kit

- thermo-hygrometer to measure relative humidity

- carbon monoxide (CO) detector

Below are some additional test kits and equipment that you could probably find online (keep windows and exterior doors closed while conducting the five tests listed below).

- A kit to test for VOCs (volatile organic compounds). While such a test is running, do not use any fragranced products.

- A formaldehyde test kit. The best conditions for formaldehyde testing are when the relative humidity is above 50 percent and the temperature is above 70°F.

- A TIF8800 combustible gas detector to track odor trails and combustion spillage. I often use the TIF8800 when I go to a site. This instrument produces a ticking rate that depends on the concentration of a gas or vapor. The stronger the vapor or gas concentration, the faster the ticking (like a Geiger counter). If you are wondering where a gas leak might be located, the TIF8800 will find it for you. This instrument is more sensitive than the gas detectors that most gas utility technicians use.

- A moisture meter. This instrument detects dampness in a substrate, but a meter can incorrectly read the moisture content of a substrate if there is metal or salt present or if the temperature of the surface is below 32°F. The resistance to electric current flow that a moisture meter measures depends on wood's moisture content. The wetter the wood, the less the resistance and the greater the electrical conductivity. Salt from urine increases the conductivity of wood and makes dryer wood appear wet to a moisture meter. Frozen moisture in wood does not conduct electricity, so frozen wood appears dry to the meter.

- A "Wizard Stick" to track airflows. This nifty child's toy produces nontoxic smoke, so you can see where air is flowing, which can help you find an odor source. You will be amazed at how much airflow there can be from your basement to the first floor, or from a basement into a crawl space and out of the crawl space into a basement. And when you aren't using this handy device, your children can have fun playing with it.

THE ALUMINUM FOIL/PAPER TOWEL TEST

This test is a great way to see if a surface is off-gassing an odor. Take a white, unscented piece of paper towel, fold it in half twice, and then place it on a surface to be tested (can be a carpet, ceiling, wall, or furniture). Cover the towel with aluminum foil extending at least two inches beyond the towel's edges. Secure the edges of this "package" with removable painter's tape. Leave the package in place for forty-eight hours. When you remove the package, quickly fold the foil in half so that it encloses the paper towel. Take the package outside and open up the foil enough so you can sniff the paper towel. If the surface you tested is off-gassing an odor, the paper towel will have adsorbed the odor. If you have more than one such package positioned here and there, be sure to label each package so you know where it came from when you remove it from a surface (fig. 23.1).

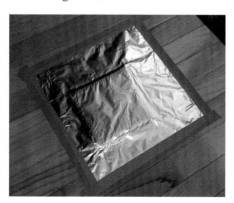

FIGURE 23.1. When there is a pervasive odor indoors, it can sometimes be difficult to find the source. One simple way to test surfaces for odor emissions is to do an aluminum foil/paper towel test, as shown in this photo.

EXHAUST FANS

It can be difficult to identify odor sources because odors can quickly spread throughout the air in a space. An ordinary window exhaust fan can sometimes be a useful tool in discovering the source or sources of a building odor. For example, if there is a dead mouse in one of your wall cavities (and we hope not), air flowing through a nearby electrical outlet can carry the odor of the decaying carcass into the room. If you put a fan on exhaust in a window in that room and close the other windows in the room and the door leading to the room, air will flow out the window, and makeup air will flow into the room from the ceiling, wall, or floor cavities. Then you can sniff outlets and any cracks or gaps to find the general location of the dead mouse.

This isn't exactly the most pleasant testing method, but it's easier, cheaper, and less invasive than removing walls or the ceiling to find an odor source.

PARTICLES: TESTS FOR MOLD

Mold test kits are available in most home- and building-supply stores, and some you can acquire from laboratories or online.

PETRI DISHES (SETTLE PLATES)

I would not attach much importance to the results of settle plate (petri dish) testing that home occupants undertake, because the testing conditions aren't always conducive to accurate results, for several reasons. Many of the most allergenic mold spores in homes, particularly in basements, are dead and therefore will not grow on the agar medium in the plate. But dead mold spores can still be exposure threats and cause allergy symptoms. And many of the mold spores that produce colonies on settle plates are from outdoors, so a plate full of colonies can cause needless concern. (For example, one of our clients placed a petri dish near an open window, so spores from the exterior rather than interior landed in the petri dish.) Lastly, the conditions under which the testing is done may not necessarily be appropriate.

There is one kind of petri dish test that I do encourage you to use, however, that will help you assess whether there is mold growth in exposed fiberglass insulation in a basement or crawl space. (If you have mold allergies, be sure to wear a NIOSH N95 two-strap mask when you do the test.) Gently press a petri dish into the insulation at two or three locations. Then cover the dish and let it sit at room temperature for a few days. If only a few mold colonies appear in the dish, I would not worry, but if dozens of nearly identical-looking colonies appear, then there is mold growth in the insulation. If anyone in your household has mold allergies, the insulation should probably be removed professionally under containment conditions. This is a potentially expensive venture, so you might want to confer with an IAQ professional before taking that step.

QUANTITATIVE TESTING

In order to test the air quantitatively for mold spores, you will need to rent an air pump that is similar to the type that IAQ professionals use. The pump draws air in at a fixed rate through a filter cassette that you buy. Then you return the cassette to a lab for analysis. A quantitative analysis gives you the genus identity of mold spores as well as their concentrations.

ENVIRONMENTAL RELATIVE MOLDINESS INDEX TESTS

Many people call me who have done Environmental Relative Moldiness Index (ERMI) testing in their homes. The test was developed by the US Environmental Protection Agency (EPA) as a means for comparing the moldiness of homes to a number of houses that had been previously tested. In the procedure as originally developed, testers vacuumed up dust in each home from two square meters (about two square yards) of carpet in a bedroom and a living room. They then analyzed the dust for the presence of 36 different molds, which they classified into two different groups. One group of molds consisted of those considered to be present in damp environments; the other group of molds consisted of those considered to be present outdoors as well as primarily in non-moldy homes.

The DNA in the dust was analyzed by PCR (polymerase chain reaction), a complicated methodology to determine the quantitative presence of spore equivalents per gram of dust. A curve was created that consists of a graphical representation of all the homes tested, from non-moldy homes to very moldy homes, based on a scale of minus 10 to plus 20.

To conduct an ERMI test, most homeowners gather dust on a specific type of cloth by wiping many non-floor surfaces. They then send the cloth to a lab for analysis, and they receive specific concentrations (in the spore equivalents per gram of dust) for the 36 molds as well as an ERMI number that places their house on the ERMI curve. In a strict sense this number is questionable for two reasons. First, the dust was probably not collected according to the strict protocol used to create the ERMI curve; second, the dust is almost always collected from surfaces other than the carpet in a bedroom or a living room—spaces in which the carpet must be vacuumed for the ERMI test.

The ERMI test can give you a useful historical view, however, in determining what species of mold may have been present or are still present in the dust in a space. But an ERMI test only identifies the presence of 36 different mold species. There may be other mold species present in any given indoor environment. I've looked at homes that had high ERMI numbers but little in the way of mold problems, and other homes that had low ERMI numbers but contained significant mold growth. This is why I always recommend having an experienced professional investigate an indoor environment to uncover mold problems. The investigation must include a thorough visual inspection of the premises and mechanical equipment. Air and dust samples may have to be taken to determine whether spore exposure risks are present.

TESTING URINE FOR MYCOTOXINS

A number of our clients have had their urine tested for mycotoxins, which are highly toxic chemicals that some molds produce under certain conditions. Ingestion of mold-contaminated foods presents the biggest danger of exposure to mycotoxins. A highly carcinogenic mycotoxin called aflatoxin is produced by the mold species *Aspergillus flavus*, which grows on peanuts, grains, and other foods. Another potent, carcinogenic mycotoxin called ochratoxin A (OTA) is produced primarily by the mold species *Aspergillus ochraceous*, which also grows on grains.

Some research on exposure to mycotoxins by inhalation has been undertaken, but the Centers for Disease Control and Prevention (CDC) is not convinced of the validity of urine testing for mycotoxins. "There is no FDA-approved test for mycotoxins in human urine. . . . Using unvalidated laboratory tests to diagnose work-related illness can lead to misinformation and fear in the workplace; incorrect diagnoses; unnecessary, inappropriate, and potentially harmful medical interventions; and unnecessary or inappropriate environmental and occupational evaluations."[1]

Over the last thirty years, I have worked with hundreds of people who live or work in moldy environments. I am therefore convinced that the inhalation of indoor-generated mold spores can cause health symptoms. Many professionals don't believe in the validity of urine testing for mycotoxins, however, so I worry that

The US Environmental Protection Agency (EPA) agrees with my cautions about using Environmental Relative Moldiness Index (ERMI) test results to determine next steps in cleaning up an indoor environment: "there is a risk that the public may make inappropriate decisions regarding indoor mold on the belief that MSQPCR and ERMI results were based on research tools fully validated and endorsed by the EPA for public use. . . . Informing the public about the ERMI tool and monitoring compliance with license agreements would improve assurance that the public is not misled about the ERMI tool and understands its limitations." (Note that MSQPCR stands for mold-specific quantitative polymerase chain reaction.)

US Environmental Protection Agency, Office of Inspector General, *Policy May Be Making Indoor Mold Cleanup Decisions Based on EPA Tool Developed Only for Research Applications*, Report No. 13-P-0356 (Washington, DC: US Environmental Protection Agency, August 2013).

a dependence on such unvalidated testing techniques can create doubt about the documented connection between mold spore exposures and human health. And as with some other types of sampling, the most widely used technologies for testing urine for mycotoxins cannot determine whether exposure occurred in the past or is current, or where the exposure source is located.

That said, I also think that the question of the threat that inhalation of mycotoxins may pose is serious enough to mandate more research on potential mycotoxin exposures in both workplaces and homes. The determination of mycotoxins in bodily fluids should be undertaken using widely accepted scientific methodology and chemical testing.

Until more research is done, I caution you not to make health or remediation decisions based primarily on urine testing for mycotoxins. The CDC shares my concern: "Persons using direct-to-consumer laboratory tests that have not been approved by FDA for diagnostic purposes and their health care providers need to understand that these tests may not be valid or clinically useful."[2] This is not to say that moldy environments should be discounted as potential health threats. If you are concerned about mold exposures in your indoor environments, consult your physician and have an IAQ professional inspect the space. "To identify possible mold contamination, visual inspection is the first step," states the CDC. "Identification and elimination of sources of moisture and cleaning or replacement of contaminated materials is essential."[3]

TESTS FOR OTHER PARTICLES

You can purchase a particle counter online that will continuously measure particle concentrations. This instrument will not tell you what the particles are, but it can give you an idea of the particle load (PM_{10} and $PM_{2.5}$) in your indoor air. If the load is excessive, you may want to turn to a professional IAQ assessor/inspector for advice and testing.

LEAD

If you want to test for lead, test kits are available in many hardware stores. Be sure to follow the instructions for conducting such a test.

DUST MITES "PLUS"

People who are allergic to dust mites can buy a sampling bag or cassette from a laboratory and send a vacuum sample of the dust from

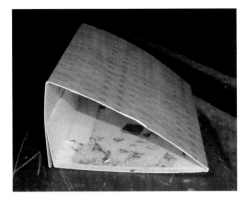

FIGURE 23.2. This sticky trap has a small amount of female sex-attractant pheromone. If there is a wool moth infestation, males fly into the trap. If you see flying moths in a closet but none appear in the trap, the moths are probably not wool moths (unless they are all females).

their mattress, pillows, or carpeting off for testing. This analysis may be more costly than using acaricide powders, but minimum testing may be worth the expense, depending on the size of your home, how many people live there, how much wall-to-wall carpeting you have, and how much of your furniture has fleecy surfaces.

There is also a MARIA (Multiplex Array for Indoor Allergens) allergy test kit, which provides quantitative results for the presence of dust mite, cat, dog, rat, mouse, and cockroach allergens. The dust kit comes with a vacuum collector cassette. You would mail this cassette to a lab for analysis.

OTHER "BUGS"

Most "bugs" use pheromones as a means to communicate. Females emit one type of pheromone (called a female sex attractant) to attract males. Some sex-attractant pheromones for particular species have been installed in sticky traps. The males are attracted to the traps, where they meet their fate but not their mate.

If you want to know whether you have a wool moth infestation, place the appropriate trap in a closet. Similar traps are also available for aphids, pantry (flour) moths, and bedbugs (fig. 23.2).

TESTING DONE BY IAQ PROFESSIONALS

Many IAQ tests are best undertaken by IAQ professionals. Before you make the investment of hiring one, however, you need to be clear about why you want such testing done and what you hope the outcome will be. Let's start with some of the questions that people have asked us when they are considering whether they need professional IAQ testing and our answers to these questions.

QUESTION: *Do I need to test my indoor air quality?*

ANSWER: If you or anyone else living in the house is experiencing allergy or other health symptoms and feels better when away from the building, then you should consider having your home investigated by an IAQ professional. Even if no one is experiencing symptoms but you are concerned about your indoor air quality, conferring with an IAQ professional makes sense.

QUESTION: *What type of samples do you take on an indoor air quality investigation?*

ANSWER: The type of samples I take and the tests I conduct depend on the symptoms occupants are having or the indoor environmental concerns they may have. If people are having headaches or eye or throat irritation, the cause may be volatile organic compounds, whereas if they are having allergy symptoms such as sneezing, coughing, and wheezing, the cause may be airborne particles such as mold spores and pet dander particles. What I want to test for determines the type of testing I do.

QUESTION: *Five different people, including a plumber and a contractor, tried to figure out the source of an awful odor in our entryway. One person said it was a dead animal. Another person couldn't even detect the odor. How can we find the odor source?*

ANSWER: It's not always a simple task to identify potential odor sources because building odors can be intermittent. I've been investigating odor problems in buildings for nearly thirty years. I'm also an organic chemist, so I use my education and professional experience to determine the nature of the odor and its possible source. If you hire someone to identify potential sources of a building odor, the person should be familiar with building science as well as basic scientific principles.

QUALIFICATIONS, EXPERIENCE, AND FEES

Whenever you consider hiring an IAQ professional to investigate your home or another building in which you spend extended time, it's important to do your research. Here are some questions you might ask.

- How long has this person been doing this kind of work?

- What is the person's training and educational background?

- Is the person a member of a professional IAQ organization, such as the Indoor Air Quality Association (IAQA) or the American Industrial Hygiene Association (AIHA)?

- Is the person certified to do this kind of work? If there is licensing in your state for mold or IAQ assessments, does this person have a license? Licenses and certifications are confirmation of a person's training.

- Does the inspector know anything about buildings?

- Does the person also earn fees selling remediation services or mechanical equipment? Such relationships could represent potential conflicts of interest.

- What do the quoted fees include? Some mold inspectors charge extra, for example, for air or dust samples taken over a certain number or for specific tools that are used. Their fees may sound reasonable at the start, but when you add up the costs of the extras, their fees may be more expensive than the fees of some of the other mold inspectors you've spoken to.

- How does the IAQ professional gather samples? If the samples are for spores, does the IAQ professional use swabs? Settle plates? Or does the person use other air-sampling equipment? An IAQ professional should be able to explain the pros and cons as well as the goals of different types of sampling methods.

One client called me because she had received a $10,000 estimate to remediate her basement. The mold inspector was employed by the remediation company. He told her that the mold in the basement was a serious health risk and that she should move out of the house until the remediation work could be completed. The so-called life-threatening mold growth was efflorescence: mineral deposits on foundation walls due to migration of moisture from the exterior through the concrete walls.

TESTING FOR VAPORS AND GASES

Most IAQ professionals own instruments that can test for gases and vapors as well as track airflows. There are also some tests that can be done for VOCs and formaldehyde. Know what vapors and gases for which you'd like your home tested so you won't be paying for unnecessary or irrelevant tests.

Be sure to gather third-party reviews, and not just from the professional's website. Most indoor air quality inspectors are well-meaning and honest professionals, but it's your job to find them. You can start by getting referrals from health professionals, your local health department, or the Indoor Air Quality Association (IAQA).

When hiring someone to do mold testing, make sure that the person tests the clean areas of your home first before testing potentially moldy areas, such as your basement. On more than one occasion, building occupants were upset by the high concentrations of mold spores found in the samples taken. In one situation, it turned out that the mold inspector was in a moldy crawl space before gathering samples in other parts of the home. The high spore concentrations in subsequent samples taken were due to the mold spores on the inspector's clothing—spores that were picked up in the crawl space. In another case the inspector took an air sample in a living room after the heat turned on. The mold spores in the sample came from mold in the duct supplying heat to the room rather than from some source within the room itself.

If you also want testing done for other particles such as pet dander or fiberglass, find out which laboratory the IAQ inspector uses to analyze the samples. Ask what particles the lab will identify in a sample. Some labs only identify mold spores in a sample, while other labs identify a wider range of particles. Asbestos testing should be done by licensed professionals.

LABORATORIES

Though you probably won't have direct contact with the laboratory that analyzes air and dust samples taken in your home, the lab is nonetheless working for you, since you are paying indirectly for lab analyses, and the results can determine "next steps" that you will need to take to cleanse your indoor air. Do your research. Be sure the laboratory that the IAQ professional uses is certified or licensed, according to the requirements in the state where the lab is located.

Tests for the total VOC (TVOC) load are less expensive than VOC tests that identify a few hundred of the particular compounds present. The results of a TVOC test can be useful because you can see how the total load of VOCs in your indoor environment compares to the total VOC load in other environments, but to identify potential chemical sources, you may have to know the particular compounds that are present. In either case, such tests usually add to the fees involved in any IAQ investigation.

I investigated a home in which the occupants were experiencing some symptoms that could be attributed to VOCs. I used the type of testing that identifies many of the compounds in the air. The results were surprising because they listed in relatively high concentrations a number of compounds considered to be fragrances. The wife was sensitive to fragrances and did not use any fragranced products. It turned out that the large plastic vapor barrier in the crawl space was manufactured from recycled shampoo bottles. The company replaced the vapor barrier.

MOLD TEST REPORTS

Laboratories' mold test reports can be confusing; spores can be misidentified, important information can be left out, and the sampling methods can be inconsistent.

MISIDENTIFICATION OF SPORES

Except in the winter, spores outdoors are primarily from a few groups of fungi. Two of the more common groups are basidiospores (from mushrooms) and ascospores (mostly from leaves and parts of plants). Spores from a third group of fungi (from the genus *Cladosporium*, which grows on plant material) often make up as much as 50 percent of outdoor spores. In windy conditions, spores from mushrooms and leaves easily become aerosolized. Soil fungi, which include microfungi such as *Aspergillus*, *Penicillium*, *Chaetomium*, and *Stachybotrys*, grow outdoors, but their spores are not readily aerosolized by the wind because they grow in the soil and are thus much less prevalent in outdoor air.

Most mold samples are identified by microscopy, and *Penicillium* and *Aspergillus* (Pen/Asp or Asp/Pen) spores cannot generally be distinguished from each other, so they are referred to collectively as Pen/Asp or Asp/Pen spores. The Pen/Asp spore concentration outdoors should not typically be more than 5 percent of the total outdoor spore concentration. Unfortunately, many labs misidentify basidiospores, because some small round basidiospores look like Pen/Asp spores. If a mold test report listed elevated concentrations of spores from soil fungi in an air sample taken outdoors, I would question the sampling methods used and even the competence of the lab technician who examined the sample.

MISSING INFORMATION

In some simplified lab reports, only total spore concentrations are given without listing the genera of the spores and their individual concentrations. Depending on the season and weather conditions, the concentration of basidiospores outdoors can be in the hundreds of thousands of spores per cubic meter (meter³) of air. The total concentration of spores indoors can be hundreds of times lower, but if the indoor spores are due to soil fungi, there is still reason for concern owing to potential exposure, particularly since most of us spend more than half of our lives indoors.

If samples are examined by microscopy, find out whether all or only part of a sample is examined. If only part of a sample is examined, important information may be missing from the lab report. With mold spores, some laboratories report only spore concentrations rather than also identify whether the spores are present in chains or clusters, which would indicate the presence of mold growth in the area sampled instead of just settled spores from another source. If a sample contains even one chain or cluster of spores from *Penicillium* or *Aspergillus* mold, the presence of indoor mold is confirmed, no matter what the comparison is to the outdoor spore concentrations of these molds. Does the lab identify the presence of mold conidiophores? A conidiophore is the spore-forming structure of a microfungus, so a conidiophore in a sample also signals indoor mold growth rather than just settled spores.

The results of culture plate (petri dish) samples can be misleading. Dead spores will not grow in the medium, and yet they remain allergenic. If you need to know the species rather than just the genera of molds, find out whether the laboratory can analyze that type of testing.

SAMPLING METHODS

Soil fungi grow indoors in humid indoor environments, and in such environments their spores can become aerosolized, for some genera even with the slightest of air movements or foot traffic. When someone walks across a moldy carpet in a finished basement, microfungal spores will be aerosolized and will be detected in an air sample taken at the same time or within a few minutes. If, however, no one has been in the space for a while and there has been no foot traffic over that carpet, the air sample will probably not include many spores from the growth in the carpet. Then the building occupants may be falsely reassured that the air is spore-free, even though potential mold exposures will occur when someone walks across that moldy carpet. In one crawl space I inspected, I took an air sample without disturbing any dust, and there were no mold spores in the sample. Then I waved my notebook a few times near the floor and the exposed fiberglass insulation at the ceiling and took another sample; it contained 17,000 *Aspergillus* mold spores per cubic meter of air.

People are not generally allergic to basidiospores, but many of our clients appear to be sensitized to *Aspergillus*, *Penicillium*, or other soil fungi. One woman who had mold sensitivities called us because she had done her own agar plate test and was ready to move out of her home because the lab report's summary listed elevated concentrations of basidiospores. The report itself, however, did not identify any Pen/Asp colonies. "Do you have mushrooms growing in your home?" I asked. "No," she replied, meaning that the spores came from the exterior. Perhaps she had the windows open while the agar plate was exposed.

WHAT INFORMATION ARE YOU (OR YOUR PHYSICIAN) LOOKING FOR?

An IAQ inspector should be able to explain the results of IAQ sampling; the results won't be helpful to you otherwise. If you did the testing yourself and don't understand the results, it's worth spending some money on an IAQ consultant who can discuss the implications of the results with you.

REMEDIATION / MITIGATION

GASES AND VAPORS

All surfaces surrounded by air have a thin (motionless) "boundary layer" of air that slows down off-gassing. In order to speed up the off-gassing of solvents in paints and varnishes, you must reduce the thickness of the boundary layer with increased airflow. Isolate the room or area as best you can from adjacent spaces. Put an exhaust fan in one window and a supply fan in another window in that room or area. These fans will provide good air exchange to dilute any contaminants. If you are trying to speed up off-gassing from a floor finish, position one or two box fans on the floor, directing air across the floor. If you are trying to speed up off-gassing from vertical surfaces, use one or two oscillating fans to stir up the air at wall surfaces. The fans blowing air across the floor or wall surfaces will reduce the thickness of the boundary layer of air on those surfaces. The solvents in paint or varnish will therefore off-gas (evaporate) much more quickly, and their fumes will be blown out of the room to the exterior. At the same time, the supply fan will be blowing outdoor air into the room. Isolate the room so that the fumes will vent to the exterior as intended and not flow into adjacent spaces.

You may want to confer with an IAQ professional regarding some odors, such as those that can be emitted from SPF (spray polyurethane foam) insulation, which we discuss in chapter 22.

MOLD

Some very simple remediation work can be done by home occupants. The New York City Department of Health (NYCDOH) states that for areas smaller than 10 square feet, building occupants can undertake remediation.[4] As discussed in chapter 2, molds (microfungi) grow along surfaces, digesting surface nutrients such as dust and spilled foods. You can wipe nonporous surfaces with a dilute bleach solution (one part bleach to sixteen parts water) or with any suitable cleaning agent (see chap. 24 for further discussion of the use of bleach). Still, containment should be set up to minimize the spread of allergenic dust, exhaust fans should be in place to vent dust to the exterior, and surfaces in the room should be HEPA vacuumed when the work is done. Whoever does the work should wear protection such as a NIOSH N95 two-strap mask as well as eye protection and gloves, and should shower and change clothing when the work is done.

If you see a mushroom (a product of a macrofungus, a wood-decaying organism discussed in chap. 2), ask a building or indoor air quality professional to investigate, because there will be hidden decay beneath the surface.

HIRING A PROFESSIONAL: QUALIFICATIONS AND EXPERIENCE

Larger areas with mold growth should be tackled by remediation professionals working under asbestos-level containment. Follow their advice about maintaining that containment for as long as they recommend. Hiring a professional remediation company again requires research.

- Ask what kind of products they use.

- They should be able to describe in detail their containment methods.

- The remediation company should have someone on site to supervise the work.

- Professional remediation work should be done according to some of the published documents, including the American National Standard Institute/Institute of Inspection, Cleaning, and Restoration's *Document S520 Standard and Reference Guide for Professional Mold Remediation*[5] as well as guidelines formulated by the New York City Department of Health, the American Industrial Hygiene Association, and the American Conference of Governmental Industrial Hygienists.

- Ask how they intend to encapsulate any remaining spores that may still be present in rough surfaces after such surfaces have been remediated.

- Be sure that the remediators as well as the testers are certified or hold the required licenses. Legitimate certifying organizations include the American Industrial Hygiene Association, the American Council for Accredited Certification, and the Association of Energy Engineers.

FOGGING

Fogging a moldy space with antimicrobial treatment seems an easy solution, but I have several cautions about this approach. First, in order for the remediation work to be effective, the mold must be removed after it has been fogged, since mold spores remain potentially allergenic even when dead. Second, the substances in the fogging product could be allergenic. I worked with one client who chose to have her moldy home fogged. Unfortunately, she was sensitized to the chemicals (enzymes) in the fogging product, so after her house was treated, she experienced allergic reactions in the home. Some companies claim falsely that fogging can eliminate mold in wall cavities; the only way to eliminate such concealed mold is to open up the wall or ceiling cavity.

PENNY-WISE AND POUND-FOOLISH

One couple hired me because there was a musty smell emanating from their finished basement. Their children had grown up and moved out, so they didn't use the basement much. They weren't controlling the relative humidity down there through dehumidification in humid weather and heat in the heating season. Copious amounts of mold were present on walls, the floor, and on furniture. Unfortunately, the laundry area was in the basement. The woman had mold allergies, so whenever it was her turn to do the laundry, she was exposed to spores from basement mold growth and experienced respiratory symptoms. I recommended that she stay out of the basement until it could be professionally remediated under containment conditions. She honored the "letter of the law" but not the spirit.

As in any basement remediation project, personal goods had to be removed from the basement before the remediation work began. To reduce the cost of the remediation, the couple decided they would empty the basement rather than pay the remediation company to add this work to their list. Their children came home to help. The woman stayed out of the basement, but she and her husband stood in the yard next to the bulkhead. As their children carried goods out of the basement, the couple directed which goods they wanted to keep and clean and which goods they were willing to discard. This project stirred up a lot of dust to which the woman was exposed, even when she was outside, and she touched some of the moldy goods. She wasn't wearing a mask or gloves. In addition, allergenic dust spread up into the house from the basement because the family had not set up containment. The woman became so reactive in the house that she had to move out until the basement was remediated. In the end, the remediation work was even more expensive because surfaces in the entire house had to be cleaned to remove allergenic dust.

In another situation, a woman needed to have her basement remediated, but she chose the least expensive company to do the work. The crew didn't set up sufficient containment, so moldy dust spread throughout the house and even into her duct system. She had to hire another company to finish the job, which now included cleaning the entire house and the mechanical system including the ducts. And she had to move out while the work was being done. She decided to hire a lawyer to sue the company she had originally hired. As of the writing of this book, I don't know the outcome of her suit, but lawyer fees added to the expense she faced as a result of her original choice of remediation companies.

SOME RECOMMENDATIONS

- If you are concerned about chemicals in your indoor environment, avoid using fragranced products and choose paints and sealants that don't contain volatile organic compounds.

- If you have chemical sensitivities and there is an odor in your home that's exacerbating your symptoms, you can wear a charcoal half-face respirator until the source is found and eliminated.

- People with chemical sensitivities should avoid using bleach or products that contain bleach.

- Operate a window fan on exhaust to find an odor source that may be in a wall, ceiling, or floor cavity.

- Identify the problem first before deciding on a solution; otherwise, remediation work could easily be "hit or miss" and more costly than is necessary, either because the work is too broad or the work doesn't solve the problem.

- Air sampling alone does not identify potential sources of contaminants.

- Do your research when hiring a professional IAQ investigator or remediation company.

24.

CLEANING

In many of the homes I have described, the rooms seemed spotless and yet people were experiencing indoor air quality (IAQ) problems. I make my living in part with my microscope, and when I examine dust samples, even from homes that look clean, I often see particles that may be allergenic.

What can you do to keep your indoor environment really clean?

USE THE RIGHT VACUUM CLEANER

One woman had lived in her home comfortably for many years, but two years before she called me she had developed a persistent cough and frequent sinus infections. She thought something in the apartment might be causing her symptoms. She had vacuumed as well as she could, and she had even consulted a psychic (not a step I generally recommend), who suggested cleaning the drains. Nothing seemed to make a difference, so when a similar apartment in the same complex became vacant, she considered moving.

Before she made her final decision, she slept in the empty apartment for several days and was relieved to find that she didn't cough. She committed to the new apartment and had new carpeting and a new refrigerator installed before moving in. Soon after she settled into her new home, her cough returned. She gave up the fight and temporarily moved in with her parents until she could figure out a solution.

Because the woman's allergist found she was allergic to dust mites and other common allergens, she asked me to look for any allergen sources in her new apartment. We decided it would be a good idea to check the level of dust mite allergens in her couch. The woman used her own vacuum cleaner to obtain a dust sample. By the time she had finished collecting the dust (about three minutes), she was coughing so violently that she ran to the bathroom and vomited. I went out on the front stoop and took a Burkard sample of the air at the vacuum exhaust; it was full of mold spores and dust mite fecal pellets. The concentration of dust mite allergens in the couch was almost 25 micrograms (mcg) per gram (g) of dust (above 10 mcg/g is considered a threshold for inducing asthma). Her vacuum cleaner may have been removing surface dirt from the couch, but it was also sucking up mite allergens and spewing them into the air.

We think of a vacuum cleaner as a machine that draws dirt in, but in fact it's pulling in air that contains the dirt. The air flowing into the machine has to flow out, and we hope the dirt and dust particles will remain behind in the vacuum bag. This usually doesn't happen with microscopic particles, however, because most vacuums are leaky. Particles exit around seals and from within the vacuum bag itself. In addition, vacuuming vigorously with any type of equipment disturbs the carpet surface, releasing additional contaminants into the air.

Some vacuum cleaners have special filtration. I prefer a vacuum with a HEPA (high-efficiency particulate arrestance) filter that is supposed to contain all large particles and at least 99.97 percent of the 0.3-micron particles suspended in the air moving through the machine. Connie and I own a Miele vacuum. Whatever kind of HEPA vacuum you choose, be sure to purchase the HEPA filter, even if that involves extra cost. Use a HEPA vacuum for all household cleaning, including in a basement. Never use a shop vacuum indoors unless the vacuum has a HEPA filter. If you hire a cleaning service, insist that the cleaners use your HEPA vacuum. If you have a regular vacuum cleaner and you are allergic to dust, wear a NIOSH N95 two-strap mask and air the house out after vacuuming.

One client spent $800 on a low-quality vacuum that had an "optional HEPA" filter attachment, which she also purchased. The filter holder was secured to the vacuum by two plastic tabs that fit into holes much larger than the tabs. Most of the exhaust air blew unfiltered out of the openings around the tabs, completely defeating the purpose of the HEPA filter. If you do buy a HEPA vacuum, be sure the HEPA filter holder is airtight at the perimeter and that the filter is properly placed in its holder. Follow the manufacturer's recommendations for filter replacement. If you are allergic to dust, wear a NIOSH N95 two-strap fine-particle mask to change the vacuum bag (outside the house), and be sure the inside of the compartment that holds the bag is clean. Avoid using a bagless vacuum; dumping the dust will create potentially allergenic aerosol.

Another costly type of filtering vacuum cleaner uses water to trap the dust. I took an air sample at the exhaust of such a vacuum and found many aerosolized particles. In addition, people don't always follow instructions for the proper use of these vacuums. The water is supposed to be emptied when the vacuuming is completed, but one man left the water with the dust in the vacuum, which he then stored in a closet. You can imagine what grew in this dusty reservoir!

I worked with one family whose cat allergy symptoms were increasing, particularly after their home was cleaned. I took Burkard air samples in the house and concluded there were cat dander particles in the carpets. The couple was astonished because they had never owned a cat and the carpets were relatively new. I asked what type of vacuum they used, and they told me they hired people to clean. The cleaning company first vacuumed the neighbor's house where three cats were happily shedding and then ran the non-HEPA-filtered vacuum in my clients' home, where it spewed out cat dander particles that rained down on all the carpets. If you hire outside cleaners, be sure they use your HEPA vacuum.

Some people prefer to use a central vacuum system rather than using a portable vacuum cleaner. If you have a central vacuum system, be absolutely certain that the exhaust vents to the exterior and not into the garage, basement, or crawl space. (The outside vent should be as close to the motor as possible. If the exhaust path is too long, back-pressure might reduce the airflow.) If dust collects around the unit, your vacuum canister probably has a leak.

How often should you vacuum? I recommend HEPA vacuuming floors and upholstered furniture at least once a week.

KEEP CARPETS AND RUGS CLEAN

WALL-TO-WALL CARPETING

To support claims of benefit, I suppose that if the same amounts of dust were placed in two experimental rooms, one with carpet and one without, and the air was then sampled while a small room fan was operating, you would find less aerosol in the room with the carpet because the fibers trap some of the dust. Such an experiment would not be representative of an actual home where the fibers themselves are regularly disturbed by foot traffic and not just by airflows, however.

Over the last thirty years I've inspected thousands of homes and always find that the air in spaces with wall-to-wall carpeting contains higher concentrations of particles than the air in spaces with hardwood, vinyl, or ceramic flooring. Dust accumulations may be diminished by vacuuming carpets thoroughly once or twice a week with a HEPA vacuum cleaner, but dust (which may contain pet dander particles, mold spores, and dust mite fecal pellets) can never be completely removed by vacuuming.

You may have to replace your carpet if the allergens prove too troublesome. Always replace the pad and HEPA vacuum the floor before installing a new carpet. If there were significant allergens in the old carpet, it's also a good idea to lightly paint the floor if it is unfinished subflooring. This will seal in any residual allergens. If you have lead paint dust or asbestos fibers in a carpet, you will want to have the carpet removed by professionals. Testing for lead and asbestos is relatively inexpensive, so when in doubt, take dust samples.

When carpeting gets dirty enough to wash, be sure to hire a trained professional. When people wash their own carpeting using rented equipment, the machine may either apply too much water or be unable to remove enough water. If carpets stay damp for more than a day, bacteria and fungi will start to grow. Many people have told me that their carpets remained damp for more than a day after being washed and smelled for a while longer. Even though the smell may go away, I believe that such carpets will forever after contain biological organisms, and their by-products will be aerosolized with every footstep.

AREA RUGS

Area rugs should also be HEPA vacuumed once a week, more often if the rugs are located in areas where people eat food. You can send area rugs out to have them washed. Research the methods used, however, and be sure that potentially irritating chemicals won't be used and the rugs will be dried quickly enough to avoid microbial growth.

TREATMENT WITH STEAM VAPOR (OR "DRY" STEAM)

For mitigating allergens, I recommend steam (water vapor) instead of typical carpet cleaning equipment, which uses only hot water. When rugs and carpets are cleaned with hot water (often referred to as "steam cleaning"), the material takes longer to dry out, creating a better opportunity for mold and bacterial growth. In addition, when the hot water hits the room-temperature carpet, the water cools and is thus less effective in destroying organisms. Steam (pure water vapor),

The article "Carpets and Healthy Homes" in the National Center for Healthy Housing's Fact Sheet offers some practical tips about carpeting in homes and discusses the relationship between carpeting and indoor air quality.

D. Jacobs et al., "Carpets and Healthy Homes," National Center for Healthy Housing, Fact Sheet, July 2008, https://nchh.org/resource-library /fact-sheet_carpets-and-healthy -homes.pdf.

however, is an outstanding method for killing dust mites, spiders, carpet beetles, and fleas—anything that may be living in a carpet (or in upholstered furniture or mattresses and pillows, for that matter). A steam vapor treatment can also denature many allergens.

A number of home versions of steam vapor cleaning equipment are on the market. Some machines look like vacuum cleaners and are relatively easy to use. It may be less expensive to treat your carpets with steam vapor than to replace them. One of my clients was having increased difficulty with his allergies when he was at home. He had three floors of wall-to-wall carpeting that I found was full of dust mites. He decided to treat the carpeting with steam vapor, and because this type of cleaning is slow-going, he spent several weekends working at it. It was worth the effort. He told me that after all the carpets had been steamed, his symptoms abated.

Why is steam vapor so much more effective than hot water? This question leads into a brief discussion of the three phases of matter: solid, liquid, and gas (bear with me, reader, please). Water is the liquid form of H_2O; in its solid state, H_2O is ice; in its gaseous state, it is water vapor. When ice becomes liquid water, the H_2O is undergoing a phase change from one state of matter to another. The same is true when H_2O changes from liquid to vapor during evaporation or boiling. (H_2O means that one molecule of water contains two hydrogen atoms and one oxygen atom.)

"Ordered" indicates the way the molecules are arranged. In a solid, the molecules are all spatially arranged in a pattern, often crystalline. In a liquid and a gas, molecules are constantly moving and rotating. In a gas, the molecules are about 10 times as far apart as they are in a liquid or a solid. A solid is in a more ordered state than a liquid is, and a liquid is in a more ordered state than vapor is. Energy is always required to change matter from an ordered to a less ordered phase (ice to water), and energy must be taken away to change matter from a less ordered phase to an ordered phase (water to ice). Heat energy changes ice to liquid water and liquid water to vapor. It takes about five times as much energy to change a cup of water to vapor as to heat the cup of cold water to the boiling point. As the water changes to vapor at the boiling point (212°F or 100°C at sea level), both the liquid and the steam vapor are at the same temperature, but the steam vapor contains far more stored energy (like a stretched spring versus a relaxed spring). Steam vapor thus has much more heat energy to lose than does hot water at the boiling point.

Suppose you treat a sofa with steam vapor. When the steam vapor hits the room-temperature surface, a small amount of it condenses to liquid; the phase change releases the stored energy and heats the couch material to the boiling point of water. In addition, the steam vapor continues to flow, and because it is a gas, it penetrates the cushioning, raising the temperature of the stuffing.

If applied long enough, steam not only kills insects but also denatures many allergens. I tested the effectiveness of steam by applying it for different lengths of time to certain sections of a mattress that contained about 40 mcg/g of dust mite allergens. I divided the mattress surface into quadrants. One part was my control; this section I did not treat with steam vapor. I treated a second part for ten minutes, the third part for twenty minutes, and the last part for thirty minutes. A few hours later, after the mattress dried, I took dust samples from all four sections. I found what I had expected: the longer the steam vapor application, the lower the concentration of allergens. In another experiment, steam vapor reduced the dog allergen concentration in a cushion from more than 30 mcg/g to less than 1 mcg/g.

There are several general cautions to keep in mind when using a steam vapor machine. First, be sure the high temperature will not harm the material you are steaming. If applied too long, steam vapor can damage the finish on a hardwood floor, for example, so area rugs should be treated outside or above the floor. Second, steam vapor may damage carpet and rug fibers or upholstery fabric, so test a small section of the surface first. Third, direct contact with steam vapor can cause burns, so be careful while using a steam machine and follow closely the manufacturer's directions for maintenance and use. And last, don't let moisture build up in an enclosed space, because this can cause paint to peel.

DUSTING AND WIPING SURFACES

Just as walking on a contaminated carpet releases potential allergens into the air, cleaning surfaces with a feather duster only resuspends the settled dust. Dust should be either HEPA vacuumed or wiped away from solid surfaces with a clean, slightly damp cloth.

Studies have demonstrated that regular application of antiseptic sprays drastically reduces the level of viable mold spores and bacteria on surfaces.[1] But in most cases this spraying is unnecessary; in fact, it can introduce irritating fragrances and chemicals from the spray itself into the interior air. Trying to eliminate the background level of microorganisms that can settle on surfaces is futile, because wherever there are people, there is an endless supply of skin scales, and wherever there are skin scales, bacteria and possibly yeast will be present. And this doesn't even take into account the mold spores suspended in the air that infiltrates a home from the outside. To minimize the

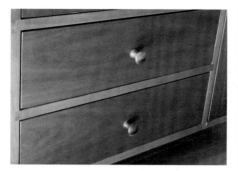

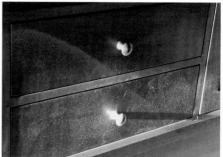

FIGURE 24.1A. Figures 24.1A and 24.1B depict the same dresser. The dresser surface appears clean in diffuse light but looks quite different when the sun is shining on the surface from an oblique angle.

FIGURE 24.1B. The dresser is coated with dust that only becomes visible in bright sunlight. This dust consists of nearly all skin scales (with some lint fibers). Dust collects on all surfaces and can accumulate under and behind furniture in large clumps referred to as "dust bunnies." This dust can serve as food for a host of microarthropods, so the dust over time can become allergenic owing to the presence of microarthropod fecal pellets.

nutrients available for living organisms, just dust surfaces regularly. If an individual is sensitized to particular components in the dust (such as dust mite droppings or mold spores), the source of the allergens should also be eliminated; otherwise, allergens will continue to collect on surfaces. And don't forget to remove dust from the backs, sides, and bottoms of furniture pieces on a regular basis (figs. 24.1A and 24.1B).

Some dust reservoirs present more exposure threats than others do. The "dust bunnies" behind a bed's headboard may not have much impact on your life, but the dust near a hot-air register or in a refrigerator drip tray may find its way to your lungs.

BLEACH

The US Environmental Protection Agency does not recommend the use of bleach for ordinary cleaning tasks.[2] Yet people have been using dilute bleach for laundering and to clean moldy bathroom surfaces for more than 100 years. The regular (not concentrated) bleach sold in supermarkets typically contains about 5 percent sodium hypochlorite (the solid chemical dissolved in water to make bleach) and 95 percent water. If you decide to use bleach, the Centers for Disease Control and Prevention recommends that you mix the bottled bleach with water in a ratio of 1 to 16 (one part bleach to sixteen parts water, or a cup of bleach to a gallon of water),[3] and only use that solution on nonporous surfaces that will not lose their color when wiped.

When bleach reacts with organic materials (such as mold spores, fingerprints, skin, food spills, urine, etc.), toxic fumes are produced, so always use the bleach solution with plenty of fresh-air ventilation. Keep windows open; if you are cleaning a large area, operate a fan on exhaust in a window. Wear eye protection, gloves, and a NIOSH N95 two-strap mask (available at most home improvement stores). Anyone with chemical sensitivities should probably avoid using products or solutions that contain bleach.

Some people argue that the use of bleach encourages mold to grow because commercial bleach is mostly water, and once the chemical (sodium hypochlorite) is inactivated through reactions with organic materials, the moisture left behind fuels fungal growth. On solid, non-porous materials, however, if left in place long enough, the bleach will disinfect the surface before the sodium hypochlorite is inactivated. Then the surface can be rinsed with plain water and dried.

If you are uncomfortable using bleach, you can purchase 27 percent hydrogen peroxide solution (called "pool shock") in pool supply stores and dilute one part of the pool shock with two parts water to make a 9 percent solution for cleaning. (Unfortunately, in the winter, pool supply stores may be closed.) Hydrogen peroxide–containing products like pool shock are unstable and over time decompose to water and oxygen gas. Over time, some peroxide solutions can decompose completely to plain water. Pool-shock bottles therefore always have a small hole at the top to release oxygen-gas pressure. To avoid leakage, bottles of peroxide should always be stored in a vertical position. If you purchase a bottle of pool shock, pour a small amount onto some dirt outdoors; if the solution does not bubble, the bottle should be returned because the peroxide is no longer active. Use great caution when handling pool shock or any hydrogen-containing solution; wear protective gloves and goggles, as the solution can cause burns. Again, be careful not to get the solution into your eyes or onto your skin.

Hydrogen peroxide solutions can also bleach some surfaces; do not use bleach or hydrogen peroxide on porous surfaces. You can always choose to use any suitable cleaning product instead. People with chemical sensitivities should avoid using bleach or bleach-containing products or fragranced cleaning (or body) products.

Store bleach and bleach-containing products as well as pool shock and other dangerous substances in a safe location, where children and pets cannot reach them. Keeping such chemicals locked in a cabinet or in a garage or separate shed is probably best.

DANGEROUS MIXTURES

Ammonia and chlorine bleach should never be mixed together because then they form a poisonous, carcinogenic gas called chloramine. The labels on these products warn against mixing the two, but keep in mind that other cleaning products may also contain ammonia or bleach. For example, some scouring powders contain chlorine bleach, and some dishwashing liquids contain ammonia-like compounds. You may think of cleaning products as benign, but in fact they may be powerful chemicals. Follow label directions, believe the warnings, and use ventilation as needed.

One additional warning: if you have a swimming pool, be extremely careful to keep any bromine- or chlorine-containing biocides out of the house and away from any other chemicals. The fumes alone can be irritating, and the compounds themselves are dangerous. If a chlorine-containing biocide comes in contact with some algaecides (also used in pools) or other household chemicals, the mixture can burst into flames.

MOLDY FURNITURE

Furniture that has been stored in a moldy garage or basement or that has been stored in rooms where the relative humidity (RH) was elevated can contain microfungal growth (see chap. 2). The mold growth is typically present on the backs, bottoms, and legs. Some furniture pieces that contain mold growth or that smell musty can be cleaned. Solid surfaces such as metal or glass can be wiped with any suitable cleaning agent. Finished wood can be cleaned and then polished to adhere residual dust. Unfinished wood can be HEPA vacuumed and then sealed with varnish or clear shellac to encapsulate residual allergens. If you have chemical sensitivities, you can use a glue/water solution (one part polyvinyl acetate glue to one to two parts water). Just don't apply the solution to any surface that may become damp in the future, because the surface will become tacky.

This work is best done outdoors. If the work must be done indoors, the work space should be isolated from adjacent spaces, an exhaust fan should be operating in a window to vent allergenic dust to the exterior, and surfaces in the room should be vacuumed after the work is done. Whether the work is done outside or indoors, whoever does the work should wear a NIOSH N95 two-strap mask and gloves, and change clothes and rinse hair afterward. If you are sensitized to mold, ask someone else to do the work for you.

Furniture with moldy cushions should be re-cushioned and reupholstered or discarded. Musty or moldy mattresses and pillows should be thrown away. We discussed steam vapor treatment for rugs and carpeting earlier in this chapter, but if a rug or carpet contains mold growth, it, too, should be discarded.

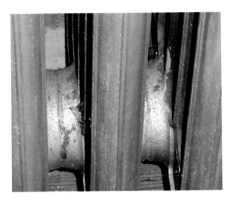

FIGURE 24.2. The dust that accumulates on radiator surfaces consists mostly of skin scales. If there were ever pets or dust mites in a home, their allergens would also be in the dust. If the radiator is below the dew point of the air in the summer, mold may even grow in the dust. In the winter, warmed air rising through the radiator can aerosolize allergens.

HEATING AND COOLING EQUIPMENT

RADIATORS

Radiators can collect allergenic dust, so radiator surfaces as well as radiator covers, if present, should be cleaned before the heat is turned on each year. Remove the cover and HEPA vacuum the radiator; a 36-inch vacuum crevice tool (available on line) will help you access hard-to-reach spots. Don't forget to clean under and behind the radiator, where dust can collect. Damp-wipe the top and bottom surfaces of the radiator cover (if present) before putting the cover back in place (fig. 24.2).

HOT-WATER BASEBOARD HEATING CONVECTORS

Hot-water baseboard heating convectors also collect allergenic dust. When I look at samples of dust taken from hot-water baseboard heating convectors, I often find pet and bird dander particles, skin scales, pollen grains, and mold spores. (These particles and allergens could have collected on the convectors when prior occupants lived in the home.) When the heat is off in the summer, moisture may condense on convectors' cool metal surfaces (especially in basements), and microbial growth can occur in this captured dust. Cleaning hot-water baseboard heating convectors can be important in maintaining healthy indoor air, especially if you have allergies or are moving into a new home with this kind of heating system.

To deep-clean a hot-water baseboard heating convector, remove and clean the cover and place it upside down under the heating fins. Rags or old towels can be placed on top of the covers to catch the grime as the convector's fins are cleaned. HEPA vacuum the fins (taking care not to bend them) and then, using the smallest nozzle, blast the fins with steam vapor from a steam vapor machine. Wipe clean any sheet metal surfaces before reattaching the cover.

One of the best uses for steam vapor is to clean fin tubing in hot-water baseboard heating convectors. Once a baseboard convector has been cleaned in this way, you need only damp-wipe the tops of the covers at the start of every heating season.

ELECTRIC BASEBOARD HEATING CONVECTORS

The top surfaces can be damp-wiped to remove dust, but be sure that the heating convectors have been turned off and have cooled before you do this work.

AIR CONDITIONING UNITS

If your window air conditioner can be removed, take the unit outdoors for cleaning. The cover should be removed and cleaned and the motor and electrical components covered with aluminum foil. Then the interior surfaces should be sprayed lightly with a dilute bleach solution (one part bleach to sixteen parts water) or a 9 percent hydrogen peroxide solution, and washed and rinsed. The filter should also be rinsed and cleaned. The interior of the unit should be dry before the aluminum foil is removed and the cover reattached.

A window or through-wall air conditioner that cannot be removed must be cleaned in place. Unplug the unit and then take off the front plastic grille and clean it in a sink. HEPA vacuum the fins of the cooling coil, being careful not to bend them. Spray the fins with a dilute bleach solution or a 9 percent hydrogen peroxide solution. The coil must then be thoroughly rinsed. Keep in mind that cleaning solution may drip from the exterior of the case to the outside, so make certain that liquid will not drip onto people or anything else that might be affected by the cleaning solution. Put rags or old towels under the unit at the interior in case water drips to the inside. It is also important to keep the coil in a portable air conditioner clean.

If you live in a multi-unit building and are not able to remove your air conditioning unit for cleaning, ask the building's maintenance personnel to do this work for you.

LAUNDROMATS AND DRY CLEANERS

If possible, it's probably a good idea to do your laundry at home if you have serious allergies. If you use a public laundromat, the dryer may contain residues of irritating or allergenic detergent, fragrances, and fabric softener.

I find even walking by a laundromat irritating because the dryer exhaust is always contaminated with laundry chemicals. (I took an air sample at one dryer exhaust and collected numerous respirable detergent particles.) If people who are chemically sensitive live downwind from a laundromat or a dry-cleaning establishment or even live in an apartment near a communal laundry area, the odors and particles could affect them.

Dry cleaning makes use of a solvent, usually tetrachloroethylene (sometimes called perchloroethylene or PCE). When you pick up a suit or a dress at the dry cleaner, the clothing usually retains a chemical smell from the residual PCE. If this odor bothers you, air out the clothing before bringing it into your home, or hang it in a well-ventilated room (remember to remove the plastic bags).

AIR PURIFIERS

People concerned about the conditions in their indoor environments sometimes spend a lot of money on air purifiers in the belief that such machines can clean the air and thus solve indoor air quality problems. If operating a HEPA-filtered air purifier relieves some of your allergy symptoms, then continue to use the machine. But remember that while an air purifier can mitigate the impact of an IAQ problem, it is not the solution for the problem.

AIR PURIFIERS DESIGNED TO REMOVE AIRBORNE PARTICLES

A HEPA-filtered air purifier is designed to remove airborne particles. If you are sitting quietly in a room or sleeping in your bedroom, a HEPA-filtered air purifier will work nicely to clean the air in the space. Imagine, though, that there is a carpet in the room that is contaminated with allergens. Every time you walk across the carpet, you will disturb dust captured in the carpet's fibers, and allergenic particles will be aerosolized. The air purifier will remove the suspended allergens, but every time you walk on the carpet again, more allergens will become airborne. The air purifier may not be able to remove all of these particles before they enter your breathing zone.

Some air purifiers have blowers that exhaust high-velocity air out along the floor. Such machines can actually aerosolize allergenic particles. I've sampled the air in several homes when the air purifiers' blowers were off and on. Initially, I always found higher levels of airborne particles in the air samples when the blowers were on; after the blowers had been operating for a while, of course, the air was cleaner. In a carpeted bedroom of one child with asthma, I started coughing as soon as I entered. An air purifier was operating. I turned it off and left the room. I returned twenty minutes later and had no trouble breathing. I took a sample of the dust in the carpet in the child's bedroom and sent to the sample to a lab for analysis. I wasn't surprised that the sampled dust contained 20 mcg/g of mite allergens.

I also don't recommend any air purifier that produces ozone, a gas that may smell like fresh air but is irritating and is one of the chief components of smog.

Air purifiers with charcoal filters are intended to adsorb formaldehyde, solvents, and other vapors (volatile organic compounds or VOCs) from the air. These types of air purifiers have been used successfully for many years. The hitch, though, is that the filtering ability (adsorption capacity) of the charcoal may only last a few months, so the charcoal medium has to be changed frequently.

There are two recently developed technologies that claim to eliminate VOCs from the air. One professes to use hydroxyl radicals, and the other uses photocatalytic oxidation (PCO). Air purifiers that generate hydroxyl radicals use UV (ultraviolet) lamps. Hydroxyl radical generators are used by the restoration industry to eliminate smoke and other odors. I do not believe that people should be exposed to the air in a room where a hydroxyl radical generator is operating.

The PCO method also uses UV light to irradiate a metal grid with titanium dioxide catalyst. (Ultraviolet lights produce ozone, which is an irritating gas and one of the chief components in smog.) VOCs adsorbed on the grid are supposed to be destroyed. This technology works when there is a large area of catalytic surface and slow airflow over the catalyst. The device is sold to homeowners for installation in air conveyance systems, but it has a relatively small area of catalytic surface, and the duct system airflow over the surfaces is far too rapid to accomplish much (see chap. 18).

In the professional community, the jury still seems to be out as to whether these technologies have more advantages than disadvantages. A position document produced by ASHRAE (American Society of Heating, Refrigerating and Air Conditioning Engineers)[4] summarized existing literature describing various filter and air-cleaning techniques, including photocatalytic technology. While the paper lists some advantages to this technology, the paper also lists some disadvantages, including "the likelihood of ozone generation" and "the potential of an incomplete oxidizing process, which produces by-products of reaction that can be more toxic or harmful than the original constituents."

I would be cautious about telling my clients to install such air purification equipment in their homes until more research has been done on the effects of such technologies on human health. (One of the installed PCO systems I inspected made the entire interior space reek of ozone gas.)

DIRECTED AIRFLOW

A HEPA purifier with a gooseneck or a HEPA purifier that directs the airflow toward a person's breathing zone can be helpful in situations where the person has no control over indoor environmental conditions (such as in a workplace). Air purifiers can be useful in keeping indoor air clean once the sources of contaminants, irritants, and allergens have been removed from an indoor environment. Air purifiers also serve an important function in capturing small (10 microns or less) airborne particles, the inhalation of which can have a deleterious effect on human health (see chap. 2). Gooseneck air purifiers with charcoal filters can also filter out gases and vapors from someone's breathing zone.

CLEANING OURSELVES

Some of my clients with serious allergies report having symptoms when they are near certain people with an allergic dust aura. People who have pets carry pet dander particles on their clothing and in their hair. People who sleep on pillows contaminated with dust mite allergens can carry dust mite fecal pellets in their hair. In chapter 2 we wrote about yeast that causes eczema and dandruff as well as asthma symptoms. Good old-fashioned soap has biocidal properties; the longer you keep soap on your body, the more effective it will be in killing bacteria and yeast. If you soap yourself thoroughly in the shower, turn the water off, and wait a minute before turning the water back on to rinse, the soap will have a chance to do its work. (Just keep soap off the bottom of your feet so you don't slip.)

While we're on the subject, hair collects allergens and can be an allergen source long after the initial exposure. For example, on most typical non-winter days, mold spores and pollen grains are in the air. If you go outside, your hair will accumulate these particles, and when you disturb your hair, allergens can become airborne. If you are particularly sensitive, your allergy symptoms may increase. When you put your head on a pillow, your hair is around your face. If you have allergies, it's a good idea to shampoo your hair after you've spent time outside in the pollen or mold season (fallen leaves can be moldy) or after you've been in moldy spaces or spent time with pets. Don't go to bed with wet hair, because mold may grow in a damp pillow. If you don't like washing your hair so often, wear a hat when you're in an environment that may contain allergens.

WAGING THE WAR

Having to fight microscopic life forms can turn people into fanatics. For example, to deal with dust mites, people sometimes do the equivalent of bombing an entire village to capture one soldier. They eliminate their curtains, shades, carpets, bedding, and stuffed furniture. They buy new mattresses and pillows. They apply acaricide powders (which kill mites) to all fleecy surfaces. Such steps are indiscriminate. If a mattress and pillows are the sources of dust mite allergens, the allergens will also be in the dust in the curtains. Encasing the mattress and pillows in dust mite covers will eliminate the source, and then the curtains can be washed and rehung. The curtains should never again be a problem.

Identifying the source or sources of allergens is vital in a successful cleaning campaign.

SOME RECOMMENDATIONS

AIR PURIFIERS

- Find and eradicate the sources of indoor allergens and contaminants before primarily depending on an air purifier to achieve healthier indoor air.

CLEANING

- Avoid using fragranced cleaning products.

- See chapter 10 for recommendations regarding laundry products.

- Dilute 1 cup of bottled bleach with 16 cups of water to make a cleaning solution.

- If you have chemical sensitivities, it's best not to use bleach or products containing bleach.

- You can purchase 27 percent hydrogen peroxide (called "pool shock") in pool supply stores and dilute it with two parts water to make a 9 percent solution for cleaning.

- Never mix bleach or hydrogen peroxide with ammonia, and don't store products containing bleach or ammonia near each other.

- Store pool chemicals, bleach, bleach-containing products, and other potentially hazardous products in a safe place that children and pets cannot access, preferably not in the house.

- It's a good idea to HEPA vacuum floors, carpets, and rugs, and to dust surfaces once a week.

- Use a HEPA vacuum with a bag. Change the bag outdoors, and be sure that the inner compartment is clean. Change the HEPA filter on the recommended schedule.

- If you hire people to vacuum your home, insist that they use your HEPA vacuum.

- If you have a central vacuuming system, be sure it vents to the exterior.

- HEPA vacuum the backs and bottoms of furniture on at least an annual basis.

- If necessary, wear a NIOSH N95 two-strap fine-particle mask when vacuuming or dusting.

- Refer to part III of our book *The Mold Survival Guide: For Your Home and for Your Health*, which discusses mold removal including from personal goods.

DRY CLEANING

- If you are chemically sensitive, don't live downwind from a commercial laundry or dry-cleaning establishment.

- Hang up recently dry-cleaned items of clothing to air them out.

STEAM VAPOR

- Use steam vapor to reduce allergens and pests in furniture and carpeting as well as to clean radiator and hot-water baseboard heating convectors.

- Don't use a steam vapor machine to clean area rugs on hardwood floors. Hang rugs up off the floor or treat them outside.

- Spot-test fabrics and carpeting first to be sure they will not be damaged by steam vapor.

CLOSING REMARKS

Take Charge

We'll be pleased if you purchased a HEPA vacuum after reading this book. We'll be upset, however, if you threw out your mattress or couch before having it tested to see if it contained allergens. We wrote the book not to cause hysteria but to help people gain greater control over the quality of indoor air.

Your home won't contain all the problems identified in this second edition. Your story won't be the same as the stories we've included in the book. But we hope that our advice will help you identify and eradicate some of the sources of indoor air quality problems. The following steps should help guide you in your crusade.

BELIEVE YOUR BODY

If you have headaches or rashes, if you sneeze or cough, or if you have trouble breathing in a certain indoor space, believe what your body is telling you. Even if someone standing next to you has none of these symptoms and thinks that you may be imagining things, trust your nose and believe your lungs. The first step toward taking charge is accepting that we are all different and that we respond to our environments in individual ways. (And, please, if you are living or working with someone who experiences symptoms that you do not share, believe and support the person.)

STUDY YOUR BODY'S REACTIONS

Be a scientist and objectively observe how your body responds to its environment. Might there be any connections between the symptoms you experience in a particular space and the activities occurring around you? Do you have particular difficulty at certain times of the day, in certain seasons of the year (including when the heat or air conditioning is running), or under certain weather conditions (such as a windy day)? Do you cough more frequently when one of your friends is near you? Don't be discouraged if it's hard to make connections between what you are feeling and what may be happening around you; some people only have allergic reactions hours after being in contact with allergens. Keep a journal to identify when and where you experience some physical reactions that may be caused by indoor environmental conditions.

IDENTIFY AND REMOVE PROBABLE SOURCES OF IRRITANTS AND ALLERGENS

Use this book as a guide to help you identify and remove some of the sources of irritants and allergens.

TURN TO A PROFESSIONAL WHEN NECESSARY

You may need a professional to help you identify or solve an IAQ problem. Be sure, though, to depend on someone who knows what he or she is doing.

One man with asthma called us after he had employed two environmental testing companies to determine whether his home had air quality problems. Technicians from these companies tested for benzene, ammonia, formaldehyde, and carbon monoxide, and they measured relative humidity and temperature (in one case, a technician even measured oxygen!). The two technicians never inspected the property for allergens or irritants that might have caused asthma symptoms. I found mold and mites in the carpet in the finished basement.

In another property, an indoor air quality inspector took air samples in an unfinished basement under quiescent conditions (he did not create airflows). The samples he took did not contain allergens. I took a sample in the same basement, but only after creating some airflow by walking around and gently waving a notebook (anyone entering the basement would have likewise stirred up air). My sample contained hundreds of *Penicillium* and/or *Aspergillus* mold spores, which easily become airborne with even slight airflows. I also took dust samples from the joists and exposed fiberglass insulation. Both samples contained copious amounts of mold spores.

I've been an IAQ professional for more than thirty years. In that time, I've examined by microscopy more than 40,000 air and dust samples and offered advice to hundreds of people. I've received numerous messages from those who have followed my advice—much of which I include in my books on indoor air quality. One client wrote, "My daughter's asthma has dramatically subsided to the point where she has not had an attack in a very, very long time." Another sent this encouraging news: "My nose and lungs are happier now and my repeated sinus infections are gone." And here's a message from a woman whose symptoms were debilitating. She cleaned up her environment and experienced great relief. "I am now walking four miles a day," she wrote. "Feeling good. Sleeping well and happy!"

Let me share two more stories: one involving a simple solution to an indoor air quality problem and the other a story with a less promising result.

I'll start with the first scenario. The owner of a large suburban house called us because her toddler was experiencing repeated bouts of respiratory symptoms and had been diagnosed with asthma. Part of the house dated back to the early 1800s but had been extensively renovated; the rest of the house was a recent addition. The property was impressive and very, very clean. I expected to find a problem with the HVAC (heating, ventilation, and air conditioning) system, but the real culprit ended up being a small, expensive antique rug that the child played on nearly every afternoon. The rug was full of mold and mites, and every time the little boy thumped the rug, mold spores and mite fecal pellets were aerosolized. The boy's parents had the rug cleaned and then put it into storage, and the little boy's symptoms almost disappeared.

The other story is more complicated. A middle-aged social worker was perfectly healthy until she moved into a condominium in a new building. She had exercised regularly, but after living in her new home for a few years, she found it increasingly difficult to exercise. She began to have trouble concentrating at work. By the end of her seventh year in the condominium, she had to take a leave from her job and was barely able to lift herself from her couch. She had also acquired a chronic cough and asthma.

I found many sources of contaminants in her home, and her physician confirmed that she was allergic to mold. She cleaned up her home environment, and most of her symptoms disappeared. Yet when she returned to work, she became ill again and was forced to remain on leave. She insisted there was mold in her basement office, but few believed her until the soggy, moldy ceiling tiles above her desk collapsed under their own weight. Now that her condo is cleaned up and she remains away from the office, her health has continued to improve.

Unfortunately, however, an entire world beyond her condominium contains contaminants, irritants, and allergens, as well as unsympathetic listeners and poorly qualified technicians. The woman has therefore become a more active advocate for her own well-being and has a sharper sense of when her symptoms reappear. If she walks into a store or another indoor space and experiences symptoms, she leaves. And I don't think she'll ever agree to work in a basement office again. I hesitated to use this story as the last one in the book because it's a story of a person's continuing struggles. But her story also illustrates the progress she made in protecting her own health.

Even in my own home, the struggle is ongoing. I have many allergies, including to mold and pets. I have had to abandon rugs that contained mold growth, and after some visitors leave, I have to open up several doors and windows to air the house out because the visitors had pet dander particles or mold spores on their clothing. Sometimes I even have to clean surfaces to remove allergenic dust.

At least I know I'm not crazy, because I can see with my microscope the allergenic particles that haunt me. For many of you, this will not be true. The irritants, contaminants, and allergens that cause health symptoms may appear to be phantoms but are real, and you must believe you can eliminate many of them if you try.

WHAT ABOUT COVID-19?

The droplets that people infected with COVID-19 emit when they speak, cough, and sneeze contain virus particles. Larger droplets settle out of the air within a few seconds; smaller droplets can dry out, leaving virus particles suspended in air. Though it has not yet been documented with certainty, some infective particles may be picked up and distributed by HVAC systems. Installing MERV-11 filtration in an HVAC system can capture many of these particles. (And a well-fitting face mask acts as a particle filter over your mouth and nose, protecting you and others.) What about germicidal UV-C lamps? In residential HVAC systems, installation of these costly lamps does not disinfect the air stream.

We completed this second edition before COVID-19 changed our lives, but our advice throughout the book has hopefully helped you create a healthier indoor environment, one in which exposures to contaminants and allergens are greatly reduced.

TAKE CHARGE

This book may not provide you a miracle cure, but we hope that it will give you the confidence that you can better control conditions in your indoor environment. Don't be like that woman who said on our voicemail, "My house is killing me." Trust and believe in yourself. Make the effort and begin to take charge.

NOTES

APPRECIATION

1. T. Godish, *Indoor Air Pollution Control* (Chelsea, MI: Lewis, 1989).

CHAPTER 1. SEEING THE INVISIBLE

1. "Allergy Statistics," American Academy of Allergy, Asthma & Immunology, accessed January 6, 2020, https://www.aaaai.org /about-aaaai/newsroom/allergy-statistics.
2. "Most Recent Asthma Data," Centers for Disease Control and Prevention, last updated March 2019, https://www.cdc.gov /asthma/most_recent_national_asthma_data.htm.
3. A. Steinemann, "National Prevalence and Effects of Multiple Chemical Sensitivities," *Journal of Occupational and Environmental Medicine* 603, no. 3 (March 2018): e152–e156.

CHAPTER 2. CAST OF SMALL CHARACTERS

1. "Health and Environmental Effects of Particulate Matter (PM)—Health Effects," US Environmental Protection Agency, accessed January 6, 2020, https://www.epa.gov/pm-pollution /health-and-environmental-effects-particulate-matter-pm.
2. J. Anderson et al., "Clearing the Air: A Review of the Effects of Particulate Matter Air Pollution on Human Health," *Journal of Medical Toxicology* 8, no. 2 (June 2012): 166–175.
3. R. Rylander, "Symptoms and Mechanisms—Inflammation of the Lung," *American Journal of Industrial Medicine* 25 (January 1994): 19–23.
4. T. Leino et al., "Occupational Skin and Respiratory Diseases among Hairdressers," *Scandinavian Journal of Work, Environment and Health* 24, no. 5 (October 1998): 396–406.

CHAPTER 3. "TROJAN HORSE" ALLERGENS

1. D. Ownby, "A History of Latex Allergy," *Journal of Allergy and Clinical Immunology* 110, no. 2 (August 2002): S27–S32.

2. H. Ormstad, "Suspended Particulate Matter in Indoor Air: Adjuvants and Allergen Carriers," *Toxicology* 152, nos. 1–3 (November 2000): 53–68.

3. J. Woodfolk et al., "The Effect of Vacuum Cleaners on the Concentration and Particle Size Distribution of Airborne Cat Allergen," *Journal of Allergy and Clinical Immunology* 91, no. 4 (April 1993): 829–837.

4. M. Hew et al., "The Melbourne Thunderstorm Asthma Event: Can We Avert Another Strike?," *Journal of Internal Medicine* 47, no. 5 (May 2017): 485–487.

CHAPTER 4. CREEPY CRAWLERS

1. J. Cuesta et al., "Asthma Caused by Dermestidae (Black Carpet Beetle): A New Allergen in House Dust," *Journal of Allergy and Clinical Immunology* 99 (1997): 147–149.

2. E. Ebeling, *Urban Entomology* (Davis: Division of Agricultural Sciences, University of California, 1978).

3. Y. Fukutomi et al., "Allergenicity and Cross-Reactivity of Booklice (Liposcelis bostrichophila): A Common Household Insect Pest in Japan," *International Archives of Allergy and Immunology* 157, no. 4 (November 2011): 339–348.

4. D. Do et al., "Cockroach Allergen Exposure and Risk of Asthma," *Allergy* 71, no. 4 (April 2016): 463–474.

5. M. Clark, "Cross-Reactivity between Cockroach and Ladybug Using the Radioallergosorbent Test," *Annals of Allergy, Asthma and Immunology* 103, no. 5 (November 2009): 432–435.

CHAPTER 5. THE THREE Ps

1. P. Salo et al., "Indoor Allergens in Schools and Daycare Environments," *Journal of Allergy and Clinical Immunology* 124, no. 2 (August 2009): 185–194.

2. K. Cummings et al., "The Changing Public Image of Smoking in the United States: 1964–2014," *Cancer Epidemiology, Biomarkers and Prevention* 23, no. 1 (January 2014): 32–36.

3. "What Are the Effects of Secondhand Exposure to Marijuana Smoke?," National Institute on Drug Abuse, last updated December 2019, https://www.drugabuse.gov/publications /research-reports/marijuana/what-are-effects-secondhand -exposure-to-marijuana-smoke.

4. K. Nguyen et al., "Perceptions of Harm to Children Exposed to Secondhand Aerosol from Electronic Vapor Products, Styles Survey, 2015," *Preventing Chronic Disease* 14 (2017): 160567.

5. K. Nguyen, "Two Common Flavoring Chemicals in E-Cigarettes Can Damage Lung Cells," *Chemical and Engineering News,*

February 4, 2019, https://cen.acs.org/biological-chemistry
/genomics/Two-common-flavoring-chemicals-e/97/web/2019/02.

6. D. Lockwood, "Controversy Clouds E-Cigarettes," *Chemical and Engineering News*, March 10, 2014, 32–33.

7. "Surgeon General's Advisory on E-cigarette Use among Youth," accessed January 6, 2020, https://e-cigarettes.surgeongeneral .gov/documents/surgeon-generals-advisory-on-e-cigarette-use -among-youth-2018.pdf.

8. "Outbreak of Lung Injury Associated with E-Cigarette Use, or Vaping," updated February 11, 2020, Centers for Disease Control and Prevention, https://www.cdc.gov/tobacco/basic _information/e-cigarettes/severe-lung-disease.html.

CHAPTER 6. THE SET

1. J. Hirzy et al., "Carpet/4-Phenylcyclohexene Toxicity: The EPA Headquarters Case," in *The Analysis, Communication, and Perception of Risk*, vol. 9 of *Advances in Risk Analysis*, edited by B. J. Garrick et al., 51–61 (New York: Springer Science+Business Media, 1991).

2. D. Karimian-Teherani et al., "Allergy to Ficus Benjamina," *Bulletin of Social Scientific Medicine* 2 (2002): 107–113.

CHAPTER 10. ROOMS WITH WATER—THE LAUNDRY

1. B. Hileman, "What's Hiding in Transgenic Foods?," *Chemical and Engineering News* 80, no. 1 (January 2002): 20–23.

2. K. Sarlo et al., "Proteolytic Detergent Enzymes Enhance the Allergic Antibody Responses of Guinea Pigs to Nonproteolytic Detergent Enzymes in a Mixture: Implications for Occupational Exposure," *Journal of Allergy and Clinical Immunology* 100, no. 4 (October 1997): 480–487.

3. D. Basketter et al., "The Toxicology and Immunology of Detergent Enzymes," *Journal of Immunotoxicology* 9, no. 3 (2012): 320–326.

4. Private communication with researcher, 2014.

5. A. Steinemann, "Fragranced Consumer Products: Exposures and Effects from Emissions," *Air Quality, Atmosphere and Health* 9, no. 8 (October 2016): 861–866, https://link.springer.com /article/10.1007/s11869-016-0442-z.

6. E. Heuberger, "Effects of Chiral Fragrances on Human Autonomic Nervous System Parameters and Self-Evaluation," *Chemical Senses* 26, no. 3 (March 2001): 281–292.

CHAPTER 11. BEDROOMS

1. A. Falleroni et al., "Bean Bag Allergy Revisited: A Case of Allergy to Inhaled Soybean Dust," *Annals of Allergy, Asthma and Immunology* 77, no. 4 (October 1996): 298–302.

CHAPTER 16. FINISHED BASEMENTS

1. E. Kern et al., "Diagnosis and Treatment of Chronic Rhinosinusitis: Focus on Intranasal Amphotericin B," *Therapeutics and Clinical Risk Management* 3, no. 2 (June 2007): 319–215.

CHAPTER 17. ATTICS

1. "Histoplasmosis," Mayo Clinic, January 27, 2018, https://www.mayoclinic.org/diseases-conditions/histoplasmosis/symptoms-causes/syc-20373495.
2. M. Horwath et al., "Histoplasma Capsulatum, Lung Infection and Immunity," *Future Microbiology* 10 (June 2015): 967–975.

CHAPTER 18. HEATING AND COOLING WITH DUCTS

1. J. Richard et al., "The Occurrence of Ochratoxin A in Dust Collected from a Problem Household," *Mycopathologia* 146 (1999): 99–103.
2. "Should You Have the Air Ducts in Your Home Cleaned?," US Environmental Protection Agency, accessed January 6, 2020, https://www.epa.gov/indoor-air-quality-iaq/should-you-have-air-ducts-your-home-cleaned.
3. J. Davis et al., *Furnace Mount Humidifier Testing: July 1990 through April 1991* (Arlington, VA: Humidification Section of the Air Conditioning and Refrigeration Institute, June 1991).
4. J. Burkhart et al., "Microorganism Contamination of HVAC Humidification Systems: Case Study," *Applied Science and Environmental Hygiene* 8, no. 12 (1998): 1010–1014.
5. J. Lee et al., "Outbreak of Bioaerosols with Continued Use of Humidifier in Apartment Room," *Toxicological Research* 28, no. 2 (June 2012): 103–106.
6. C. Yang et al., "Fungal Levels on Interior Surfaces of Ventilation Ductwork: Closed Cell Foam Insulation versus Fibrous Glass Insulation and Galvanized Metal," presented at the American Society of Heating, Refrigerating and Air Conditioning Engineers Conference, San Francisco, California, November 4–7, 2001.

CHAPTER 21. RENOVATION AND NEW CONSTRUCTION

1. "Deaths Linked to a Common Paint Stripper Chemical Go Back Decades, So Why Isn't It Banned?," *CBS News*, April 2, 2018, https://www.wivb.com/news/local-news/deaths-linked-to-a-common-paint-stripper-chemical-go-back-decades-so-why-isnt-it-banned/1094520001.

CHAPTER 22. MORE ENVIRONMENTAL HAZARDS

1. P. Gajsek et al., "Review of Studies Concerning Electromagnetic Field (EMF) Exposure Assessment in Europe: Low Frequency Fields (50 Hz-100kHz)," *International Journal of Research and Public Health* 13, no. 9 (September 1, 2016): E875.

2. "Electromagnetic Fields (EMF)," World Health Organization, accessed January 6, 2019, https://www.who.int/peh-emf/en/.

CHAPTER 23. TESTING AND REMEDIATION

1. M. Kawamoto et al., "Notes from the Field: Use of Unvalidated Urine Mycotoxin Tests for the Clinical Diagnosis of Illness," *Morbidity and Mortality Weekly Report* 64, no. 6 (February 20, 2015): 157–158.
2. Kawamoto et al., "Notes from the Field."
3. Kawamoto et al., "Notes from the Field."
4. New York City Department of Health and Mental Hygiene, *Guidelines on Assessment and Remediation of Fungi in Indoor Environments* (New York: New York City Department of Health and Mental Hygiene, November 2008), https://www1.nyc.gov/assets/doh/downloads/pdf/epi/epi-mold-guidelines.pdf.
5. American National Standard Institute/Institute of Inspection, Cleaning, and Restoration (ANSI/IICRC), *Standard and Reference Guide for Professional Mold Remediation*, IICRC S520 (Las Vegas, NV: ANSI/IICRC, 2008), https://www.claimsparency.com/learning/wp-content/uploads/2013/05/IICRC-S520-standard-and-Reference-Guide-for-Professional-Mold-Remediation.pdf.

CHAPTER 24. CLEANING

1. G. McDonnell and A. Russell, "Antiseptics and Disinfectants: Activity, Action, and Resistance," *Clinical Microbiology Reviews* 12, no. 1 (January 1999): 147–179.
2. US Environmental Protection Agency, "Should I Use Bleach to Clean Up Mold?," last updated August 20, 2019, https://www.epa.gov/indoor-air-quality-iaq/should-i-use-bleach-clean-mold-0.
3. Centers for Disease Control and Prevention, "If You Have Mold in Your Home," last reviewed August 29, 2017, https://www.cdc.gov/mold/control_mold.htm.
4. American Society of Heating, Refrigerating and Air-Conditioning Engineers (ASHRAE), *Position Document on Filtration and Air Cleaning* (Atlanta, GA: ASHRAE, January 13, 2018).

GLOSSARY

ACARICIDE: A chemical (usually benzyl benzoate or a borate) used to control mites.

ACM: Asbestos-containing material.

ACTINOMYCETE: An organism that produces small spores and grows like mold but is actually a filamentous bacterium.

ADSORB: To collect onto a solid surface, usually from a vapor state. Adsorbed water is invisible and is always present so long as there is water vapor in the air.

AEROSOL: Any suspended airborne particulate.

AFLATOXINS: A series of toxic chemicals (mycotoxins) produced by molds. Produced by *Aspergillus flavus*, aflatoxin B1 is a potent carcinogen and may be responsible for liver cancer in regions where contaminated grains are abundant.

AIR-HANDLING UNIT (AHU): A device that circulates air as part of a ducted system.

AIR PRESSURE: The force that air exerts upon a surface.

ALLERGEN: Anything that causes an allergic reaction. Many allergens are proteins. Cat and dog dander, mold spores, pollen, and dust mite fecal pellets all contain protein allergens.

ALLERGENCO AIR SAMPLER: A device that separates particulates such as pollen and mold spores from the air in which they are suspended. The particulates are trapped on a greased microscope slide. Sample times and intervals can be programmed, and multiple samples can be taken on the same slide.

ALTERNARIA: A genus of fungi with large spores that generally contain allergens. Spores from one allergenic species, *Alternaria alternata*, are occasionally found in house dust, but the spore sources are typically outdoors.

AMERICAN SOCIETY OF HOME INSPECTORS (ASHI): A professional national association of home inspectors.

AMINE: A nitrogen-containing class of organic chemicals related to ammonia. Amines are added to boiler water to minimize rust accumulation. Many amines are irritating or have a "fishy" smell. Cadaverine and putrescine are two malodorous amines produced by bacterial decomposition of muscle and other protein.

ANAPHYLAXIS: A life-threatening allergic response.

ANDERSEN SAMPLER: An air-sampling instrument that uses petri dishes for determining the concentration of "live" (viable) mold spores in the air.

ARTHROPODS: An invertebrate animal of the large phylum Arthropoda. Arthropods are animals with exoskeletons, segmented bodies, and jointed appendages.

ASBESTOS: A naturally occurring carcinogenic mineral that exists in several forms, including amosite, chrysotile, and crocidolite. Chrysotile, believed to be the least carcinogenic form of asbestos, was used in thousands of products, including insulation and construction composites.

ASPERGILLUS: A genus of allergenic fungi. The spores grow in chains that are usually attached to a globular structure. *Aspergillus* is frequently found in homes with damp basements. One species, *Aspergillus fumigatus*, is associated with a lung disease called aspergillosis.

BACHARACH MONOXOR II: An instrument containing an air pump that is used to measure the concentration of carbon monoxide in combustion gases and the air.

BACTERIA: Usually single-celled microscopic organisms that reproduce by division. Some bacteria are round; others are rod shaped or spiral. Bacteria cause syphilis, pneumonia, tuberculosis, infections of the skin, and many other diseases.

BIOAEROSOL: Any suspended particulate in the air that comes from a living organism. Bioaerosol can consist of pollen, mold spores, human and animal dander, insect body parts, and fecal material.

BIOEFFLUENTS: The chemicals produced by natural processes on and in the human body that can pollute the air in an indoor space.

BOOKLOUSE: A small, nonbiting insect in the biological family Psocidae (psocids) that subsists on house dust.

BORESCOPE: An optical instrument consisting of a long tube and a light, used for seeing into cavities.

BUDDING: The process by which yeast reproduces asexually. A small part of the parent cell forms a "bud" that enlarges and then separates and forms a new individual cell.

BUILDING-RELATED ILLNESS (BRI): A specific disease or illness (such as Legionnaire's disease or hypersensitivity pneumonitis) caused by exposures to chemical or biological agents, the sources of which are the building or its components. *See also* Sick building syndrome (SBS).

BURKARD AIR SAMPLER: A device that separates particulates such as pollen and mold spores from the air in which they are suspended. The particulates are trapped on a greased microscope slide.

BUTYRIC ACID: An unpleasant-smelling acid with the odor of stomach contents, produced by digestion of fats. Butyric acid is found in rancid butter and in perspiration, where it is produced by bacteria. Ceiling tiles made from cellulose (paper) contaminated with butyric acid have caused sick building symptoms and building odor problems.

CARBON DIOXIDE (CO_2): A colorless gas produced by combustion and animal respiration. High levels of carbon dioxide indoors are often an indication of inadequate building ventilation.

CARBON MONOXIDE (CO): A colorless, odorless combustion gas that in low concentrations causes headaches and nausea and in high concentrations can cause coma and death.

CHASE: A vertical or horizontal space created to house pipes or ducts. A chase can be open from the basement all the way up to the attic.

CHEMICAL CHANGE: A change in matter that produces one or more new substances. Thermal decomposition, digestion, and chemical reactions between substances are all chemical changes. Grinding, melting, and boiling are physical, not chemical, changes.

CHEMICAL SENSITIVITY (CS), also referred to as multiple chemical sensitivities (MCS): An increased sensitivity to chemicals and other irritants found in the environment. Symptoms may include respiratory distress, muscle pain, headache, fatigue, neurological problems, and cognitive difficulties.

CHLORAMINE: A toxic chemical produced when ammonia and chlorine bleach are mixed.

CHLORDANE: A persistent chlorinated hydrocarbon pesticide, often noticeable because of its odor. Now banned, chlordane was once used as a treatment for termites.

CHLORINATED HYDROCARBON: Generally, a compound containing the elements carbon, hydrogen, and chlorine, typically used as a solvent or pesticide.

CHRONIC FATIGUE SYNDROME (CFS): A syndrome characterized by extreme and constant fatigue, thought to be caused by an immune system disorder. CFS is possibly linked to environmental triggers, such as viral infections and mold. Symptoms include impairment of short-term memory, sore throat, and joint pains.

CLADOSPORIUM: The most common genus of outdoor fungi. Spores of some species are allergenic, and others contain a mycotoxin, epicladosporic acid. Two species, *Cladosporium cladosporioides* and *C. herbarum*, grow well at low temperatures and can be found living in the dust in air conditioning systems.

CLOSED-CELL FOAM: A foam in which each "bubble space" is separate from every other one. Gas cannot be squeezed out of closed-cell foams, and they don't absorb water the way open-cell foams do. *See also* Open-cell foam.

COMBUSTION CHAMBER LINER: A refractory (high-temperature melting) material, usually ceramic, placed in the combustion chamber of an oil-fired furnace or boiler. The liner shields the metal from the intense heat of the flame.

COMPOSITE: A mixture of two or more materials whose properties are different from those of the separate ingredients.

COMPOUND: A chemical combination of elements in a fixed atomic ratio. For example, carbon dioxide is a compound of carbon and oxygen atoms in a 1:2 atomic ratio, written CO_2. Carbon monoxide is a compound of carbon and oxygen atoms in a 1:1 atomic ratio, written CO.

CONDENSATE PUMP: A small pump and reservoir containing a float switch. The pump is used with air conditioning equipment to collect and eliminate water condensed from the air during cooling. Condensate pumps may also be used to eliminate water from high-efficiency gas furnaces and dehumidifiers.

CONDENSATE TRAY: A shallow metal tray tipped to a drain opening beneath an air conditioning coil to collect condensed water.

CONDENSATION: A change of state from gas (vapor) to liquid; condensation is the opposite of evaporation. Clouds and fog form from condensation of water vapor to liquid water droplets in air. In a bathroom after someone has showered, the haze on a mirror is formed by condensation of water vapor onto a surface.

CONDITIONED AIR: Air that has been heated or cooled to the comfort range.

CONDUCTION: Energy transferred by collisions, usually between "atomic" particles (electrons, atoms, molecules). Conduction occurs in all three phases of matter and is the principal method of heat energy transfer through solids (for example, a metal pot on a stove transfers heat from the burner to the food inside the pot).

CONIDIOPHORE: The microscopic spore-forming structure of a micro-fungus (mold). Technically speaking, the "spores" from microfungi are called conidia.

CONTAINMENT: A means by which dust is contained during the mitigation of a contaminated area, usually involving (among other steps) isolation of the space with plastic sheeting, cleaning with HEPA vacuums, and depressurization of the space with HEPA-filtered exhausts.

CONVECTION: Heat transfer associated with bulk movements of matter owing to differences in density. Convection takes place only in gases and liquids, not in solids.

COPPER ARSENATE: A compound of copper, arsenic, and oxygen in pressure-treated wood that is toxic to plants and animals as well as to fungi and bacteria.

CREOSOTE: An oily liquid with a powerful odor produced when wood is burned or heated and used with solvent to preserve telephone poles and railroad ties.

DAMPER: A movable obstruction built into a pipe or duct to vary the flow of air or gases.

DEHUMIDISTAT: A variable control that senses relative humidity and regulates the operation of a dehumidifier.

DENSITY: The amount of mass per unit volume. Oil floats on water because the two don't mix and because oil is less dense than water.

DERMATOPHYTES: Fungi that cause skin conditions such as dermatitis and dandruff. Species include *Pityrosporum ovale* and *P. orbiculare*.

DEW POINT: The temperature at which water vapor in the air condenses to liquid water on a surface that is cooler than the air.

DIFFUSER: A round metal louver, usually in the ceiling, that spreads out the flow of air from a duct in an air conditioning or hot-air heating system.

DOWNDRAFTING: Airflow down instead of up a chimney flue.

"DRY" STEAM (STEAM VAPOR): At one atmosphere of pressure, pure water vapor at or above 212°F, containing no liquid water.

DUST MITE: *See* Mites.

ELECTRONIC FILTER: A highly efficient filter that works on the principle of attracting charged particles using opposite-charged electrodes. Electronic filters cease to function when dirty.

EMULSION: A stable mixture of two or more immiscible liquids. Cream, for example, is primarily an emulsion of microscopic butterfat droplets in water.

ENVIRONMENTAL PROTECTION AGENCY (EPA): A division of the US government concerned with air quality, among other issues.

ENZYMES: Chemicals, usually protein, synthesized by an organism to facilitate chemical reactions. Enzymes help organisms synthesize and digest protein, carbohydrate, and fat. Some enzymes are used within cells, and others are secreted to be used outside the cells.

EPICOCCUM: A genus of allergenic molds with large brown spores. Chronic inhalation of Epicoccum spores is associated with increased respiratory problems.

EPINEPHRINE: A hormone produced by the adrenal glands and used in emergency treatment of severe allergic reactions (anaphylaxis) to insect bites or foods.

ETHYLENE GLYCOL: A toxic, barely volatile, and sweet-tasting chemical used in automobile antifreeze to lower the freezing point of water.

EVAPORATION: A change of state from liquid to gas; evaporation is the opposite of condensation.

EXFILTRATION: Pressure-driven flow of air out of a building or other defined space; exfiltration is the opposite of infiltration.

EXTERIOR WALLS: Walls that face the exterior.

FAN COIL: A device that provides heated or cooled air or both. A fan coil consists of one or more heat exchange coils, a blower, and typically a filter.

FASCIA BOARD: A vertical trim board parallel to the edge of a roof but perpendicular to the soffit board.

FIBERGLASS: A nonwoven mixture of threadlike fibers made from molten glass and often held together by microscopic droplets of glue.

FIN TUBE: A copper pipe with numerous parallel aluminum plates (fins) attached. In a forced hot-water heating system, hot water is pumped through the copper pipe. Heat from the water is transferred by conduction to the copper and from there to the fins. Air between the fins is heated and rises by convection.

FLAME ROLL-OUT: A flame that appears on the outside of a combustion chamber when a gas appliance such as a boiler or water heater is lit. Many conditions can cause flame roll-out, including inadequate draft and delayed ignition of the gas.

FLASHING: Metal or other material used in construction to make watertight a joint or intersection that is exposed to rain.

FORMALDEHYDE: An extremely irritating gas that is soluble in water. Formaldehyde off-gasses from adhesives found in some wood composites, such as fiberboard.

FRASS: "Bug" droppings or powdery refuse from wood-boring insects.

FUNGUS (PL. FUNGI): A plantlike life form that lacks chlorophyll and thus depends on other living or dead organisms for its nourishment. Fungi include mushrooms and microscopic molds.

GAS: One of the three states of matter (gas, liquid, and solid). Most (but not all) gases are colorless and can't be seen. Some gases, like helium, are less dense than air, and other gases, like propane and chlorine, are denser than air.

GENUS: A category of biological classification comprising various species.

GLOW PLUG: An electric heating element that ignites the burner in an oven without a pilot light.

GLUCAN (BETA-GLUCAN): A component of the cell wall of all molds. Respirable bits of mold cell walls cause inflammation in the lung when inhaled.

GRAM, MILLIGRAM, AND MICROGRAM: Measures of mass. There are 1,000 micrograms in a milligram and 1,000 milligrams in a gram. A US copper penny has a mass of about three grams.

GRILLE: An opening in the floor, ceiling, or wall at the end of a return duct in a hot-air heating system. Unlike a register, a grille does not usually have a damper and cannot be closed.

GUANINE: A water-insoluble substance that is the major component in the excretions of some animals, including birds (*guano* means bird droppings) and insects.

HEAT EXCHANGER: A device that either adds or takes away heat from a fluid that flows through it. The radiator on a car is a heat exchanger that transfers excess engine heat to the outside air. An air conditioning coil is a heat exchanger that cools the circulated air by removing heat from it.

HEPA VACUUM: A vacuum cleaner with a high-efficiency particulate arrestance (HEPA) filter. A HEPA filter is supposed to remove

99.97 percent of 0.3-micron particulates from the air flowing through it and 100 percent of the particulates larger than 1 micron.

HISTOPLASMOSIS: A lung disease caused by a fungus, *Histoplasma capsulatum*, spores of which are found in bird droppings.

HUMIDISTAT: A variable control that senses relative humidity and regulates the operation of a humidifier.

HVAC: Heating, ventilation, and air conditioning.

HYDROCARBON: A compound of carbon and hydrogen. Hydrocarbons can be gases, liquids, or solids. Propane (a gas), octane (a liquid), and wax (a solid) all consist of hydrocarbons.

HYDROGEN PEROXIDE: A compound made up of molecules, each molecule having two hydrogen atoms and two oxygen atoms (H_2O_2). A 3 percent hydrogen peroxide solution is available in many drug stores for use as a disinfectant. A 27 percent hydrogen peroxide solution is used to disinfect pool water.

HYPERSENSITIVITY PNEUMONITIS (HP): A pulmonary disease characterized by inflammation and fibrosis, often caused by an allergic response to inhaling bioaerosols.

HYPHAE (SING. HYPHA): The rootlike threads of fungi.

IAQ: Indoor air quality.

IMMISCIBLE: Not mixable. Two liquids (such as oil and water) that separate into layers are immiscible.

IMMUNOGLOBULIN: A protein having antibody activity, found in the blood or other body fluids.

INCOMPLETE COMBUSTION: Combustion that results in the formation of soot, carbon monoxide, or both. In contrast, when combustion is complete, all carbon is combined with oxygen to form carbon dioxide.

INFILTRATION: Pressure-driven flow of air into a building or some other defined space; infiltration is the opposite of exfiltration.

INFRARED ENERGY: A form of light energy associated with radiant heat transfer through a vacuum or a gas. Infrared energy can be felt as heat on the skin and can be reflected by a mirror and focused like light, but it cannot be seen except with the aid of a "night scope."

LARVA (PL. LARVAE): The juvenile form of some insects and animals. The larvae of many insects are wingless and look like small worms. A maggot is a fly larva.

LINSEED OIL: A nonedible vegetable oil obtained from flaxseed and used as a binder in oil-based paint.

MACROFUNGI: Fungi that produce fruiting (spore-producing) bodies that we call mushrooms or toadstools. Unlike almost all microfungi, macrofungi degrade wood.

MEDIA FILTER: A pleated filter made from fiberglass that looks like a thick piece of folded paper.

MEDIUM-DENSITY FIBERBOARD (MDF): A composite of wood and formaldehyde-containing glue.

MERV: Minimum-efficiency reporting value. MERV is a numerical scale in a range of about 1 to 16 that is used to rate filter efficiency.

MESOTHELIOMA: A type of chest cancer caused by inhalation of asbestos fibers.

METER: A unit of measurement equal to about 39 inches.

METHYLENE CHLORIDE: A very volatile chlorinated hydrocarbon solvent that was a component of many paint strippers.

MICROARTHROPODS: Small (usually smaller than two millimeters) members of the phylum Arthropoda. A microarthropod is an invertebrate animal with a segmented body, jointed appendages, and usually a chitinous exoskeleton molted at intervals.

MICROBIAL GROWTH: Growth of microbes such as mold, yeast, and bacteria.

MICROFUNGI: Fungi (typically referred to as mold or mildew) that produce fruiting bodies (conidiophores) all along the surface of the organism. Conidiophores release conidia (spores). For the most part, microfungi subsist on surface nutrients and do not degrade wood.

MICROGRAM: *See* Gram.

MICROGRAPH: A photograph taken with a microscope. A light microscope uses a beam of light to form the images, and a scanning electron microscope uses a beam of electrons to form the images. *See* Scanning electron microscope.

MICRON: A measure of length equal to one-millionth of a meter, about 0.00004 inch.

MILDEW: Technically, mildew fungi only grow on living organisms. In common usage, "mildew" and "mold" are used interchangeably. *See* Microfungi.

MILLIGRAM: *See* Gram.

MITES: Tiny members of the arachnid family. Most species live in the soil, but others are associated with animals and insects. Dust mites, found in pillows, mattresses, and carpets, subsist on skin scales and cause asthma symptoms.

MIXTURE: A combination of materials that can be separated by physical means (such as a strainer or filter).

MOISTURE METER: A device used to determine the moisture content of wood or other materials.

MOLD: Microfungi, which require oxygen, moisture, and a source of nutrients such as bread or plant materials to flourish.

MOLD SPORE: *See* Spores.

MUD TUBE: Hollow tubes constructed of sand and termite secretions; also rcfcrrcd to as a shcltcr tubc.

MULTIPLE CHEMICAL SENSITIVITY (MCS), also referred to as multiple chemical sensitivities. *See* Chemical sensitivity.

MYCELIUM: A fungal network of fine white filaments (hyphae) that grow around a food source.

MYCOTOXIN: A toxin produced by a fungus. Some mycotoxins are carcinogens, others are immunosuppressants, and some are both carcinogens and immunosuppressants.

OCHRATOXIN A: A mycotoxin made by species of *Aspergillus* and *Penicillium*.

OFF-GASSING: Emission of a solvent or other chemical from the surface of a solid into the air; also referred to as out-gassing.

OIL SAFETY VALVE (OSV): A control placed on an oil tank or line that prevents oil from leaking through a punctured oil line when the burner pump is not operating.

OPEN-CELL FOAM: In an open-cell foam such as a sponge, all the bubble spaces are connected. When the foam is compressed, the gas is forced out. *See also* Closed-cell foam.

OUT-GASSING: *See* Off-gassing.

OZONE (O₃): An unstable form of oxygen (O₂) formed by electric sparks or ultraviolet light in air.

PANNED BAY: A return duct that is formed by installing sheet metal between two or more joists.

PARTICULATE MATTER (PM): Suspended particles classified by size. PM_{10} refers to particles less than 10 microns in size. $PM_{2.5}$ refers to particles less than 2.5 microns in size.

PENICILLIUM: A genus of fungi. Some *Penicillium* species produce the antibiotic penicillin; one species, *P. camemberti*, is used to make Camembert cheese.

PHASE CHANGE: The changing of a substance from one state of matter to another. Phase changes include freezing and melting, condensation, and boiling and evaporation. During a phase change, a substance is not chemically altered, but its physical properties (or characteristics such as color, density, or conductivity) change.

PHASES OF MATTER: States of matter. The three states or phases of matter are solid, liquid, and gas.

PHEROMONE: A chemical substance released into the environment by an animal or plant that affects the behavior of others of its species.

PIGMENT: In paint, pigment is a powder used to hide or to introduce color. Originally, most pigments were ground-up minerals, but now many pigments are made from synthetic chemicals.

PLENUM: Part of the air-conveyance system in which the pressure of the air is greater (as in supply ducts) or less (as in return ducts) than that of the outside atmosphere. In office buildings the space between the suspended ceiling and the floor above serves as a return plenum.

POLYETHYLENE: A solid combustible hydrocarbon "polymer" (a long chain of molecules or atoms) of ethylene that burns with the odor of wax. Most garbage bags are made of polyethylene.

PRESSURE-TREATED WOOD: Wood containing a preservative that permeates much of the wood structure rather than simply coating the surface. Copper arsenate was typically used as the preservative.

RADIANT HEAT: Heat energy that is infrared. All objects, unless at a temperature of absolute zero, radiate heat, which is a form of energy. The hotter something is, the more heat it radiates. If the temperature of an object is high enough (above 1,000°F), light is radiated as well as heat.

RADIATION: The emission of energy. There is an entire spectrum (from low to high energy) that includes radio waves, microwaves, infrared, visible light, ultraviolet light, X-rays, and gamma rays. Note that nuclear radiation may refer to subatomic particles as well as energy.

RADON: A radioactive cancer-causing gas released from soils containing uranium.

REGISTER: A rectangular device with louvers (slats) at the end of a duct in an air conditioning or a hot-air heating system that spreads out the airflow. A register usually has a damper to control the intensity of the flow.

RELATIVE HUMIDITY (RH): A measure of how saturated with moisture the air is at any given temperature or how close the air temperature is to the dew point.

RESPIRABLE PARTICLE: A suspended particle under about 3 microns (0.00012 inch) in size and therefore small enough to enter deeply into the lungs.

RIDGE VENT: A simple device installed at the ridge of a roof to cover an opening along the ridge and designed to let air flow out of the attic as well as to prevent rain from wetting the structure. Ridge vents are usually installed in conjunction with soffit vents.

SCANNING ELECTRON MICROGRAPH (SEM): A micrograph taken with a scanning electron microscope, which uses a beam of electrons rather than a beam of light to form the image. *See* Micrograph.

SICK BUILDING SYNDROME (SBS): Symptoms (such as headache, nausea, and eye and throat irritation) experienced by building occupants for no apparent reason. Symptoms seem to lessen when people are away from the building. *See also* Building-related illness (BRI).

SILL (OF A HOUSE): A horizontal piece of framing wood, usually resting on the foundation or other masonry, at the bottom of an exterior wall. The sill is the first piece of wood the wall framing is attached to.

SLAB-ON-GRADE BUILDING: A building that is constructed on a concrete slab at grade (at ground level) with no basement or crawl space present.

SLEEPERS: Strips of wood installed on a concrete floor to support a subfloor (typically plywood or oriented strand board).

SMOKE: Suspended particulates in air that may be either a liquid or solid.

SOFFIT: The lower enclosed portion of a roof overhang. The soffit consists of a lower horizontal piece (the soffit board) and a long perpendicular attached vertical board (the fascia) that together create the enclosure. The fascia board is nailed to the rafter ends, and a gutter is usually nailed to the fascia.

SOFFIT VENTS: Openings in the soffit board that allow air to flow into the soffit to ventilate an attic.

SPORE: A reproductive cell released into the air by macrofungi. The reproductive cells released by microfungi are conidia but in common usage are also referred to as spores.

SPORULATION: The production of spores as a fungus or mold colony matures.

STACHYBOTRYS: A dark brown or black genus of mold that may be associated with sudden infant death syndrome (SIDS). The species *Stachybotrys chartarum* (also known as *S. atra*) produces trichothecene mycotoxins and is referred to as "toxic black mold."

STACK PIPE: A vertical pipe three or four inches in diameter that goes from the basement through the roof (where is it called the plumbing vent). All wastewater flows through drainpipes into the stack and from there into the sewer or septic system.

STYRENE: An irritating and possibly carcinogenic volatile hydrocarbon used to manufacture the polystyrene plastic found in many products, including computer and television cases and insulating foams.

SUMP PUMP: Typically, a pump that sits in the sump (a hole in the basement floor) to remove water from beneath the floor.

SURROGATE ALLERGEN: A particle (such as cornstarch, rust, plaster, or drywall dust) coated with allergen from another source (such as latex, pollen, or microbial growth) that was in contact with the particle.

SWALE: A depression excavated at the base of a contoured mound of earth, often used to channel water away from a house.

SWAMP COOLER: A device that uses the evaporation of water to cool air. Swamp coolers are found mainly in the Southwest and function the way evaporative-pad humidifiers function.

THERMAL DECOMPOSITION: A chemical change caused by the addition of heat energy. When food is thermally decomposed, charcoal is produced.

THERMO-HYGROMETER: An instrument that measures relative humidity.

THOROSEAL: A Portland cement product that is mixed with water and used to seal foundations at the inside.

TREATED WOOD: Wood to which chemicals such as creosote, copper arsenate, and disodium octaborate have been added. These chemicals make the wood resistant to decay caused by fungi and insects. *See also* Pressure-treated wood.

TRICHOTHECENES: A series of toxic chemicals (mycotoxins) produced by fungi such as *Stachybotrys chartarum* (common on chronically wet drywall) and *Fusarium graminearum* (common on damp stored corn). The latter fungus produces vomitoxin, a powerful emetic (causing vomiting) for pigs that eat the contaminated corn.

ULTRAVIOLET (UV) LIGHT: UV light is invisible and is part of the continuous electromagnetic energy spectrum that extends from radio waves and infrared (heat) to visible light, UV light, X-rays, and gamma rays.

UREA FORMALDEHYDE FOAM INSULATION (UFFI): A friable (easily reduced to dust), low-density open-cell foam. UFFI was banned by the US Consumer Product Safety Commission (CPSC) because it off-gassed formaldehyde, a toxic gas that causes illness.

VADOSE ZONE: The zone of soil above the water table where pores in the soil are filled with air and water vapor, not liquid water.

VAPOR: The gaseous state of a liquid. Pure steam in a pipe is water vapor, a colorless gas.

VENTILATION RATE: The amount of fresh air supplied to a space. The ventilation rate is commonly expressed as cubic feet of air per minute (cfm) or air changes per hour (ACH).

VIABLE: Having the capacity to germinate and grow. Viable spores, under appropriate conditions, lead to fungal growth. Nonviable spores are dead and usually outnumber viable spores in indoor air by a factor of between 3:1 and 10:1.

VISCOSITY: The resistance to flow ("thickness") of a liquid or gas. Water has a low viscosity compared with honey and ketchup.

WATER TABLE: The level in the soil below the vadose zone in which all pores in the soil are filled with liquid water rather than air and water vapor.

WATER VAPOR: Water in its gaseous state.

YEAST: Single-celled microscopic organisms, many of which reproduce by budding.

RESOURCE GUIDE

ORGANIZATIONS AND WEBSITES

    Milwaukee, WI | 414-272-6071 | www.aaaai.org
Provides information on allergies as well as pollen and mold-spore levels.

AMERICAN INDUSTRIAL HYGIENE ASSOCIATION (AIHA)
    Falls Church, VA | 703-849-8888 | www.aiha.org
*Anticipates health and safety concerns in work environments and
offers education and other services and products to its members.*

AMERICAN LUNG ASSOCIATION (ALA)
    Chicago, IL | 800-586-4872 | www.lungusa.org
Fights lung diseases and promotes tobacco control.

AMERICAN SOCIETY OF HEATING, REFRIGERATING AND
AIR CONDITIONING ENGINEERS (ASHRAE)
    Atlanta, GA | 800-527-4723 | www.ashrae.org
*Focuses on building systems, energy efficiency, indoor air quality,
refrigeration, and sustainability within the industry.*

AMERICAN SOCIETY OF HOME INSPECTORS (ASHI)
    Des Plaines, IL | 847-759-2820 | www.homeinspector.org
*Has chapters nationwide and provides the names of member
home inspectors.*

BUILDING SCIENCE CORPORATION

Westford, MA | 978-589-5100 | www.buildingscience.com

A consulting and architecture firm specializing in building technology. The company's website contains a wealth of information, including specifications for many construction projects, such as finishing a basement.

CHEMICAL SENSITIVITY FOUNDATION (CSF)

Topsham, ME | www.chemicalsensitivityfoundation.org

Runs a website that offers information and resources for those with multiple chemical sensitivity (MCS).

CHILDREN'S ENVIRONMENTAL HEALTH NETWORK (CEHN)

Washington, DC | 202-543-4033 | www.cehn.org

Works to protect children and the unborn from environmental health hazards.

HEALTHY SCHOOL NETWORK, INC.

Albany, NY | 518-462-0632 | www.healthyschools.org

Promotes the development of policies, regulations, and funding for healthy school facilities.

INDOOR AIR QUALITY ASSOCIATION

Mt. Laurel, NJ | 844-802-4103 | www.iaqa.org

Maintains a list of indoor air quality professionals in or near your area.

INSTITUTE OF INSPECTION, CLEANING AND RESTORATION CERTIFICATION (IICRC)

Las Vegas, NV | 844-464-4272 | www.iicrc.org

Certifies cleaning technicians and publishes industry standards for cleaning and restoration.

MAINE INDOOR AIR QUALITY COUNCIL (MIAQC)

Augusta, ME | 207-626-8115 | www.maineindoorair.org

Is committed to creating healthy and environmentally sustainable indoor spaces and offers a resource list as well as an annual conference.

MASSACHUSETTS ASSOCIATION FOR THE CHEMICALLY INJURED (MACI)

Andover, MA | 978-681-5117 | www.maci-mcs.org

Offers support, education, and referrals for people who are sensitive to chemicals in the environment, as well as for those who care about the prevention of chemical injuries.

EQUIPMENT

Airflow tracking
A Wizard Stick that produces nontoxic "smoke,"
available from Zero Toys in Concord, CA
978-371-3378 | www.zerotoys.com

Carbon dioxide (CO_2) monitor
Extech CO200, available from W. W. Grainger, Inc.,
at many locations across the United States
800-472-4643 | www.grainger.com

Combustible gas detector
TIF8800, available from W. W. Grainger, Inc.
800-472-4643 | www.grainger.com

Particle counter to detect and measure airborne particles
Available from Dylos Corporation in Riverside, CA
877-351-2730 | www.dylosproducts.com

PRODUCTS

Air purifiers
Including Atem models for smaller spaces as well as HealthPro
and HealthPro Plus for larger spaces, available from
IQAir in La Mirada, CA
562-903-7600 | www.iqair.com

Austin Air in Buffalo, NY, sells other models of air purifiers
800-724-8403 | https://austinair.com

Allergy products
Allergy Buyers Club in Bristol, CT
888-236-7231 | www.allergybuyersclub.com

Allergy test kits
For a variety of indoor air quality issues
Indoor Air Test in Clearwater, FL
727-572-4550 | https://indoorairtest.com

Carpet protector
A plastic carpet covering that is self-adhesive
Pro Tect Associates in Northbrook, IL
800-545-0826 | www.pro-tect.com

Dehumidifiers
Therma-Stor Products in Madison, WI
800-533-7533 | www.thermastor.com

Filters for air-conveyance heating and cooling systems
Trion Air Bear five-inch pleated media filter (requires an Air Bear filter holder), manufactured by Trane and available from many distributors. Call 844-365-8054 to find a distributor near you, or check online.

Portable heaters
Lasko manufactures a 200-watt portable heater that is small enough to insert into a washing machine and that is available from many distributors. Call 800-233-0268 to find a distributor near you, or check online. Follow the recommendations at the end of chapter 10 for safe use of such a heater.

Pleated media filter
Fits standard one-inch filter slots.
AllergyZone: 888-704-2112 | www.allergyzone.com

PUBLICATIONS

Feiza, Tom. *How to Operate Your Home.* Mr. Fix-It Press, 2013
262-303-4884 | www.misterfix-it.com
Everyone should have a copy of this book!

Johnson, Alison. *Amputated Lives: Coping with Chemical Sensitivity*
Brunswick, ME: Cumberland Press, 2008
www.alisonjohnsonmcs.com

———. *Gulf War Syndrome: Legacy of a Perfect War.*
Brunswick, ME: Cumberland Press, 2001
www.alisonjohnsonmcs.com

May, Jeffrey C. *My Office Is Killing Me! The Sick Building Survival Guide*
Baltimore: Johns Hopkins University Press, 2006
www.myhouseiskillingme.com

May, Jeffrey C. and Connie L. *Jeff May's Healthy Home Tips: A Workbook for Detecting, Diagnosing, and Eliminating Pesky Pests, Stinky Stenches, Musty Mold, and Other Aggravating Home Problems*
Baltimore: Johns Hopkins University Press, 2008
www.myhouseiskillingme.com

———. *The Mold Survival Guide: For Your Home and for Your Health*
Baltimore: Johns Hopkins University Press, 2004
www.myhouseiskillingme.com

INDEX

191–92, 216; and boilers, 266–72; cleaning of equipment for, 347–48; cooling connected to, 274–75; cooling not connected to, 276–77, 279; and dryers, 130–31; electric convectors for, 264–65; gas-fired, 266, 282; history of central systems, 240–42; hot-air systems for, 10, 11, 148, 188, 208, 249, 251, 296, 303, 311; hot-water systems for, 173, 265, 303, 347–48; in kitchens, 118–19; in multi-unit buildings, 173–75; portable electric heaters, 280; radiant floor heat, 266; and radiators, 265–66; recommendations for, 278–79; and steam distribution, 272–74; wood stoves for, 281. *See also* central heating and air conditioning; ducts; hot water heaters

heating, ventilation, and air conditioning (HVAC) systems, 254, 257, 275, 280, 358

heat loss, 150, 195, 212, 243; in attics, 161, 233, 234; from basements, 168, 278

heat pumps, 239, 242, 261; about, 258–59; mini-splits, 275, 279; water heated by, 278

HEPA (high-efficiency particulate arrestance) air purifiers, 14–15, 28, 349, 351

HEPA (high-efficiency particulate arrestance) vacuums, 62, 91, 191, 196, 201, 207, 219, 235, 248–49, 302, 309, 334, 347, 348, 352, 353; about, 339–40; for carpeting and rugs, 231, 340–41; and renovation work, 298, 306

Histoplasma capsulatum, 223, 235

histoplasmosis, 223

home offices, 301, 305

hot tubs, 89–90, 92

hot water heaters, 94, 118; about, 281–83; connected to boiler, 277–78; and dryers, 130–31, 132; flooding from broken, 208, 247; and heat pumps, 278; leakage from, 282; not connected to boiler, 278; recommendations for, 291; and toilets, 93; warranties for, 282

house and building exterior, 153–71; chemicals and particles from neighbors, 158–59; and do-it-yourself disasters, 157–58; and gutters,

164–69; mold growth on, 163–64; recommendations for, 169–71; and rodents, 63, 153–57; vegetation around, 159; water threats to, 159–63

HRVs (heat recovery ventilators), 260–61, 263

humidifiers: central, 251–54, 262; evaporative-pad, 138–39; furnace, 230, 235, 251, 262; mold growth in, 251–53; portable, 137, 140, 143, 253; recommendations on, 143, 262–63; steam, 138, 139–40; ultrasonic, 138; warm mist, 139–40

humidistat, 140

humidity. *See* moisture; relative humidity

hydro-air systems, 274–75

hydrogen peroxide, 187, 193, 345, 348, 352

hypersensitivity pneumonitis (HP), 23, 29–30, 189, 205

hyphae, 21–22, 24, 114, 141, 188, 198

ice damming, 229–30, 234, 276

incomplete combustion, 84, 92, 266, 268

indirect-fired system, 277–78

indoor air quality (IAQ) professionals: hiring of, 1, 209, 311, 326, 334–35, 356–58; qualifications, experience, and fees of, 328–29; samplers used by, 15; scientific method used by, 11

Indoor Air Quality Association, 380

indoor air quality (IAQ) testing: done by home occupants, 321–27; done by professionals, 327–30; goal of, 320; test kit for, 158; for vapors and gases, 321–23

indoor pools. *See* swimming pools

insulation, 233, 249, 254–55, 256, 301; and asbestos, 233; in basements, 211–12; fiberglass, 10, 54, 56, 144, 150, 152, 187–89, 208, 214, 216, 220, 254, 255, 262; and foundation walls, 189, 195, 211–12, 313; and new construction, 302; open-cell foam, 313, 314; pests in, 47, 56, 144, 150, 187, 214, 219, 220; sheet foam, 195, 211–12, 302; spray foam, 313–17, 319; urea formaldehyde foam, 316–17; XPS, 301–2

Related Titles

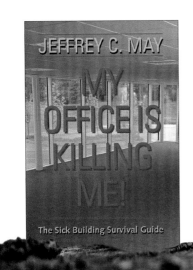

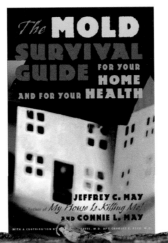

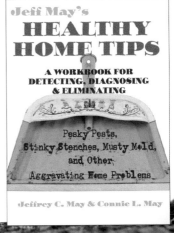

MY OFFICE IS KILLING ME!

The Sick Building Survival Guide

Jeffrey C. May

THE MOLD SURVIVAL GUIDE

For Your Home and for Your Health

Jeffrey C. May and Connie L. May

with a contribution by John J. Ouellette, M.D., and Charles E. Reed, M.D.

JEFF MAY'S HEALTHY HOME TIPS

A Workbook for Detecting, Diagnosing, and Eliminating Pesky Pests, Stinky Stenches, Musty Mold, and Other Aggravating Home Problems

Jeffrey C. May and Connie L. May

 @JHUPress

 @JohnsHopkins UniversityPress

 @JHUPress

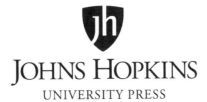

JOHNS HOPKINS
UNIVERSITY PRESS

For more health and wellness books, visit **jhupbooks.press.jhu.edu**

Contents

Part I   Building a Foundation   1

Part II   Gaining Information